Nursing the elderly

A care plan approach

J. B. Lippincott Company   Philadelphia
London   Mexico City   New York   St. Louis   São Paulo   Sydney

Acquisition/Sponsoring Editor: Patricia Cleary
Coordinating Editorial Assistant: Diana Merritt

Manuscript Editor: Lorraine D. Smith

Indexer: Nancy Weaver
Design Coordinator: Anita Curry
Designer: Anne O'Donnell
Cover Designer: Anne O'Donnell

Production Manager: Kathleen P. Dunn
Production Coordinator: Charlene C. Squibb

Compositor: Bi-Comp
Printer/Binder: R. R. Donnelley & Sons Company

6 5 4 3 2 1

Library of Congress Cataloging-in-Publication Data

Nursing the elderly.

  Includes index.
  1. Geriatric nursing.   I. Burggraf, Virginia.
II. Stanley, Mickey.   [DNLM: 1. Geriatric Nursing.
2. Nursing Assessment.   WY 152 N9748]
RC954.N894 1989   610.73'65   87-37937
ISBN 0-397-54670-X

Any procedure or practice described in this book should be applied
by the health-care practitioner under appropriate supervision in
accordance with professional standards of care used with regard to
the unique circumstances that apply in each practice situation. Care
has been taken to confirm the accuracy of information presented
and to describe generally accepted practices. However, the authors,
editors, and publisher cannot accept any responsibility for errors or
omissions or for consequences from application of the information
in this book and make no warranty, express or implied, with respect
to the contents of the book.

Every effort has been made to ensure drug selections and dosages
are in accordance with current recommendations and practice.
Because of ongoing research, changes in government regulations,
and the constant flow of information on drug therapy, reactions, and
interactions, the reader is cautioned to check the package insert for
each drug for indications, dosages, warnings, and precautions,
particularly if the drug is new or infrequently used.

SB 43203 12.95 7-89

I dedicate this book to my husband, Otis,
my daughter, Kristi, and my parents, Dorsey and June Smith,
whose unending love and support
have taught me the true meaning of caring.

Mickey Stanley

Dedicated to Thomas Burggraf, Sr., my husband,
who supported me in all my endeavors
and never had a chance to grow old.

Virginia Burggraf

The little boy and the old man

Said the little boy, "Sometimes I drop my spoon."
Said the little old man, "I do that too."
The little boy whispered, "I wet my pants."
"I do that too," laughed the little old man.
Said the little boy, "I often cry."
The old man nodded, "So do I."
"But worst of all," said the boy, "it seems
Grown-ups don't pay attention to me."
And he felt the warmth of a wrinkled old hand.
"I know what you mean," said the little old man.

Shel Silverstein
A Light in the Attic

Contributors

Sister Rose Therese Bahr, *PhD, RN, FAAN*
Professor of Nursing
Catholic University of America
Washington, DC

Chapter 8: Musculoskeletal System

Jéanne Bauvette-Risey, *RN, BNS*
Neuroscience Nurse Clinician
Ochsner Foundation Hospital
New Orleans, Louisiana

Chapter 13: Nervous System

Virginia Burggraf, *RN, C, MSN*
Nursing Instructor
Veterans Administration Medical Center
New Orleans, Louisiana

Chapter 5: Sensory System
Chapter 9: Hematology and the Immune System

Barbara Donlon, *RN, MPH*
Director of Faculty Practice and
    Development
Louisiana State University Medical Center
School of Nursing
New Orleans, Louisiana

Chapter 1: Health History

Shirley Graffam, *RN, EdD*
Associate Professor
University of Texas Health Science Center
San Antonio, School of Nursing
San Antonio, Texas

Chapter 14: Pain in Elderly Patients

Joyce T. Harden, *RN, MSN*
Assistant Professor
University of Texas Health Science Center
San Antonio, School of Nursing
San Antonio, Texas

Chapter 15: Psychosocial Care

Mildred Hogstel, *RN, C, PhD*
Professor of Nursing
Harris College of Nursing
Texas Christian University
Fort Worth, Texas

Chapter 4: Integumentary System

Mary Jackle, *RN, MS*
Director of Continuing Education
University of Texas Health Science Center
San Antonio, School of Nursing
San Antonio, Texas

Chapter 12: Genitourinary System

Katherine K. Kim, *RN, PhD*
Associate Professor
Kirkhof School of Nursing
Grand Valley State College
Allendale, Michigan

Chapter 3: Patient Education

Adrianne Linton, *RN, MSN*
Assistant Professor
University of Texas Health Science Center
San Antonio, School of Nursing
San Antonio, Texas

Chapter 10: Gastrointestinal System

Elizabeth Miller, *RN, MPH*
Assistant Professor of Nursing
Louisiana State University Medical Center
School of Nursing
New Orleans, Louisiana

*Chapter 16: Caring for the Dying Elderly
and Their Families*

Grace Olmsted, *RN, MEd, MS*
Assistant Professor of Nursing
Louisiana State University Medical Center
School of Nursing
New Orleans, Louisiana

*Chapter 9: Hematology and the Immune
System*

Barbara K. Penn, *RN, MS*
Lieutenant Colonel, U.S. Army Nurse Corps
Director, Practical Nurse Course
Brooke Army Medical Center
Ft. Sam Houston, Texas

Chapter 11: Diabetes Mellitus

Elizabeth Reed, *RN, MN, CCRN*
Assistant Professor of Nursing
Loyola University City College
New Orleans, Louisiana

Chapter 7: Respiratory System

Mickey Stanley, *RN, PhD, CCRN*
Assistant Professor
University of Texas Health Science Center
San Antonio, School of Nursing
San Antonio, Texas

Chapter 6: Cardiovascular System
Chapter 7: Respiratory System

Bernita Steffl, *RN, MPH*
Professor of Community Health Nursing
  and Gerontology
Arizona State University College of Nursing
Tempe, Arizona

*Chapter 2: Discharge Planning and the
Elderly*

Preface

This book, *Nursing the Elderly: A Care Plan Approach,* originated from the class-room experience of teaching a gerontological nursing elective to undergraduate students. In each class session the nursing process was applied to the topic under consideration and, as we attempted to review the literature on the nursing process specific to the elderly, we found a sparsity of information. The creative effort of developing nursing care plans for our classes sparked the idea for this text.

Because the nursing process is undergoing a major metamorphosis, we struggled with the question of how to present the nursing process and have selected the approach that was presented by Carpenito (1st edition). Therefore, we are defining those content areas that need intervention from both nursing and medicine as *clinical nursing problems.* A problem that requires independent nursing actions is defined as the *nursing diagnosis.* Some readers may take exception to the use of the medical diagnosis to structure our nursing content. In our view, health care of the elderly requires an interdisciplinary focus, with nursing assuming the primary responsibility for coordination and continuity of care; therefore, we are comfortable with this approach. However, we understand the views of our colleagues who have challenged us on this issue.

Nursing the Elderly: A Care Plan Approach is organized according to the body systems and subject areas in which today's gerontologic nurses are required to be knowledgeable. We have provided a consistent approach by presenting the normal age-related changes and assessment variables, as well as drug information and care plans in most chapters. The selection of care plans included in the following chapters is not intended to be exhaustive. We have chosen not to reiterate problems and care plans for which there are no unique nursing approaches or distinct nursing knowledge that applies to the elderly. The nursing diagnosis and clinical nursing problems chosen for inclusion in these chapters represent those most frequently experienced by elderly patients and those requiring a specialized knowledge of gerontological nursing.

Read and use this text in the manner in which we originally intended: to not only understand the elderly physiologically and emotionally, but also to develop appropriate plans to manage their nursing care. The book is designed for those who work with the elderly, and it can also be a valuable addition to any nursing curriculum in which students are learning to understand and care for the elderly in the United States. In this way, the quality of care we all desire for our elderly patients will be achieved.

As complete as one attempts to be in writing a book, there will always be gaps in material, areas that could benefit from expansion, and new knowledge to be incorporated in future editions. We invite you to address us through our publisher, and look forward to opening a dialogue that will ultimately benefit elderly patients.

This text is only a beginning into a process that is now the "language of nursing." Take this language and speak it clearly as advocates for the elderly.

Virginia Burggraf, RN, C, MSN
Mickey Stanley, RN, PhD, CCRN

Development of a nursing care plan

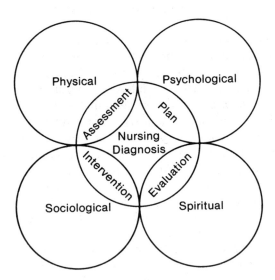

Every elderly person has an individual orientation towards life, which has been developed as a result of years of physical, psychological, sociological, and spiritual experiences. During illness, this orientation presents a challenge to the elderly patient and to care-takers. It must become a useful element of the effort to help the patient stay healthy in the face of chronicity and loss.

The four large dependent circles represent the physical, psychological, sociological and spiritual components of the elderly patient that must be considered when developing a nursing care plan.

The interdependent circle intersects these components to represent the nursing process with its integral four components of assessment, planning, intervention, and evaluation. The nursing diagnosis forms the central core pulling the entire process together.

Acknowledgments

Many persons deserve an accolade for their patience and understanding throughout this endeavor. Our families, for giving us up for long periods of writing, deserve the first thank you. Paul Hill, our original nursing editor at Lippincott, and Patricia Cleary provided periodic encouragement and truly made this endeavor pleasant. To all the contributors, a resounding thank you for your perseverance in meeting our deadlines.

Mildred Hogstel, an invaluable, creative and efficient consultant, provided additional input to all the content presented. We are indebted to her for all her hours of reading and timely suggestions. Carlos Tam and Nancy Meadow, our pharmacy consultant and medical illustrator from the VA Medical Center in New Orleans, were always amenable to all our requests and worked diligently.

The final thank you goes to the Louisiana State University Medical Center Editorial Office, especially Chuck Chapman, Virginia Howard, and Susan Rogers, for their every effort in reviewing copy and revising revisions for over a year.

Many thanks to all of you; we could not have done it alone.

Virginia Burggraf

Mickey Stanley

Contents

Nursing the elderly
A care plan approach

Barbara Donlon

Health history

The health history or data base obtained through patient interview provides the basis for the nursing diagnosis, nursing care plan, and discharge plan. For the elderly patient, this history is vital to comprehensive care, appropriate follow-up, and quality of life. Several aspects of the geriatric health history differ from those of other age groups. This health history is a story of many years, and will require the nurse's time, patience, and vigilance to gather the important details that will begin and ultimately complete the nursing process.

The environment

The nurse has the responsibility of controlling factors that have the potential to influence the quality of the interview and the data collected. These factors include both the physical setting and the psychological tone of the interview.

Physical setting

Patients need to be comfortable during the interview so that they can react to questions naturally, with both verbal responses and body language. Chairs should be easy to get into and out of, provide armrests, and be roomy enough for the patient to shift positions. The area designed for interviewing should be conducive to the confidential nature of the task. Doors that can be closed or partitions that allow private conversations are important elements in the history-taking process. The placement of the furniture and equipment in the interviewing area should compensate for the common sensory restrictions that accompany aging, such as presbyopia and presbycusis. Proper lighting, elimination of extraneous noises, and facilitation of good eye contact with the patient are important. Patients who tire easily should be scheduled early in the day. It may be necessary to take only a partial history, and follow up at a later date to complete the process. A problem that often occurs when time is a factor is the intermingling of the history-taking and the actual physical examination. When the data collection is complete, the patient should be allowed the time and privacy to undress before preceding. Although a family member may be present to assist with disrobing, the nurse should nevertheless offer assistance.

Psychological tone

One of the most significant aspects of a person's sense of self is his or her name. Often, for an older person, the use of full name and title connotes respect. Pronouncing and spelling a person's name correctly is an important part of building rapport. Determine what the patient would like to be called; most people do not appreciate overfamiliarity from nurses or other health-care providers. Nurses should address the patient by the full name, preceded by a proper title—*Mr., Mrs., Ms.,* or *Miss.* Nicknames or first names should be used only if it is suggested by the patient. Nurses who work with elderly patients should wear a name tag with large, easy-to-read letters that will reinforce the pronunciation and spelling.

An explanation of what is about to happen and the reason for the interview should precede any personal questions. The patient who is being interviewed will generally be more cooperative and participate more if he or she understands the reason for the interview. The natural resistance that patients often feel when they have been asked the same questions by different interviewers, (*e.g.,* admitting nurse, physician, resident, clinical specialist, nursing student, medical student) can be avoided if the nurse reads all available data before the interview. Old charts can be particularly helpful.

The nurse must be acutely alert to facial expressions, posture, tone, mood, and affect; body language should validate what is being verbalized. Also, remember that patients will pick up body language that suggests the nurse is hurried, uninterested, or distracted. If the nurse has negative attitudes or stereotypes about the elderly, they will be recognized by the patient and will affect the interviewing process. The nurse should give the patient complete attention, interrupting only for clarification or to redirect the interview if the patient seems distracted.

Communication techniques

Direct, close-ended interviewing is of limited use in the geriatric setting, and should be used sparingly. The preferred manner of questioning should be one that encourages patient responses that are reflective and thorough. Questions should be stated in such a way as to gather facts, feelings, inferences, and to allow assessment of the patient's level of cognitive functioning.

If the patient presents with a specific complaint, it is usually best to use the initial stage of the interview to explore the significance of the presenting symptom. People usually contact health-care providers because an episodic event has occurred, and they are most comfortable when they see a clear relationship between the questions being asked and the reason they sought help.

It is important not to group questions together and hope to get a single response. Each question should be asked separately, and the patient should be allowed sufficient time to think and respond before proceeding to the next question. For example, it is not always possible to answer the question, "Do you ever have nausea or vomiting after meals?" with a "yes" or "no." Perhaps the patient has one but not the other.

The nurse should strive to use only terminology that the patient understands, and that understanding should be verified frequently, especially if the answers given do not seem to fit the questions. People are often reluctant to admit that they do not understand what is being said; the nurse should be particularly alert to this possibility. The feelings and cultural background of the patient will often dictate the use of words and phrases. For example, terminology surrounding elimination has long been the subject of humor, misunderstanding, and embarrassment. The nurse must recognize and accommodate these cultural differences while at the same time obtaining the necessary data.

Controlling the interview is a challenge for the nurse. The patient may not understand the value of a complete health history and may become distracted (*e.g.,* begin to reminisce about important past events). When such a situation occurs, the interview must be redirected; this can usually be done with a gentle touch to the arm or shoulder to slow the patient down, followed by a restatement of the question.

The interview is a fact-gathering process, but facts are most useful when they can be associated with the resulting feelings. The nurse's ability to plan and care for Mrs. Jones will be influenced by knowing that her husband died six months ago, and that Mrs. Jones wishes she had died, too. The feelings that accompany life events will not always be manifested overtly, but should be identified by the nurse during the interview.

Occasionally interview questions will uncover memories and feelings that have been forgotten or purposefully avoided, and silence is a common response. Silence is not necessarily an obstacle to be overcome or ignored. The best approach often will be to wait and see how the patient deals with the question and the accompanying silence. Nurses must learn to become comfortable with silence; it can be a valuable tool.

Feelings of understanding and empathy during an interview can best be conveyed through body language, such as leaning toward the patient, holding the patient's hand or patting his or her shoulder, making direct eye contact, and synchronizing breathing. These feelings can also be transmitted through verbal responses that encourage the patient to continue. Comments such as "Yes?," "Go on," or "And what happened then?" can be used. Reflective statements that address the patient's mood or reaction can also be used to validate what is being said. If the nurse suggests to Mrs. Jones that she must be very lonely since the death of her husband and Mrs. Jones replies "Yes, I am, but having the grandchildren near has helped some," the patient has indicated to the nurse the existence of a support system that can assist in coping with change and loss.

Components of the health history

Interview data fall into pertinent general categories that are incorporated into most standardized care plans. These components constitute the historical data needed to develop nursing diagnosis or clinical nursing problems for the care plan. Forms are helpful in recordkeeping and promote easy access to information by other care-givers, but should not be relied on exclusively.

Standardized formats for data collection often miss the unique patient characteristics that are vital to individualized care planning. For example, a form will provide space to indicate that the patient uses a laxative periodically, but generally will not include space to describe the time of the day or the special routine that is preferred by the patient (*e.g.,* four prunes soaked in mineral oil after breakfast on Monday, Wednesday, and Friday). These general categories of interview data are discussed in detail below.

Biographical information

Patient-identifying data generally include, at the minimum, address, telephone number, age, race, place of birth, marital status, occupation, and religion. More detailed information can be included—next of kin, social security number, or source of referral, and so forth. The date of the interview should be recorded.

Reason for visit

This component is a clear statement by the patient about the problem that prompted the visit. It should be concise and in the patient's own words. If the patient says he or she "has a hell of a belly-ache," use that statement as the reason for seeking health care.

Present illness or problem

The goal of this part of the interview is to describe clearly the problem or complaint that has prompted the patient's visit. This detailed narrative should be recorded chronologically, either by beginning at the point when the patient last remembers not being troubled with the problem and moving to the present, or by tracing events backward from the day of the visit to when the problem first appeared.

Most complaints that cause elderly patients to seek help involve pain, sensory changes, structural inability, or perceptual difficulties. The presenting complaint must be thoroughly explored early in the interview. Patients should be asked to identify the following:

1. The onset of the problem—where and when it first started
2. What type of treatment has already been tried
3. The effectiveness of any treatment that has been tried
4. The impact the problem has had on the patient's pattern of living

If the patient has been self-treating at home with a medication, ask if the drug is something that was previously prescribed, or if it was borrowed from a friend or family member.

When pain is involved, the problem should be further described to obtain the clearest possible picture of what has prompted the patient to seek help. By framing directed, close-ended questions in an analytical way, the nurse will obtain the data necessary for patient-centered care planning (see the boxed material below).

Often, the patient has some idea about what is causing the problem. By asking the client about his or her ideas on the source of the problem, the nurse

---

Exploring pain symptoms

Onset
　　When did the pain first start?
　　Was the onset sudden or gradual?

Frequency
　　Is the pain present now?
　　Is it constant, or does it come and go?
　　If it is not constant, how often does it occur?
　　　　Once a week?
　　　　Monthly?

Location
　Localized
　　　Can you point to where the pain is?
　Generalized
　　　Soreness that is diffuse and widespread?
　　　Pain that radiates from one area to another?

Character
　Description of the pain
　　　Sharp, dull, deep, hot, shooting, throbbing
　　　Twinge, tingling
　　How much does the pain interfere with activities of daily living?
　　Have you experienced pain like this before?

Setting
　　What were you doing when the pain first started?
　　Do you always get the pain when involved in this activity?

Associated symptoms
　　Do you get sick to your stomach (shortness of breath, dizziness, etc.) when pain is present?
　　Have you noticed anything else that seems to be related to the pain episode?

Aggravating/Alleviating factors
　　What seems to make the pain worse?
　　What seems to help relieve the pain?
　　Does the pain seem to change during some times in the day?
　　Does aspirin help?
　　Does eating make it worse?

may discover opportunities for patient education that might otherwise go unnoticed, providing an opportunity to give new information or to correct faulty information.

All aspects of the present illness should be explored analytically to determine the impact the problem has on the patient's ability to function and cope. Often, elderly people manage fairly well despite apparently severe disability. Identifying clearly why the current problem has changed the coping pattern is a necessary part of planning care.

Past health history

This portion of the history is often the most difficult to obtain from elderly clients. Keeping events in chronological order, with clear recall about names and places, can be difficult for the patient, if not impossible. In addition, most people of this age group have not been as involved in their health care as younger people are today, and they may not be sure what procedures they have undergone or why the procedures were performed. This information is often understood by the patient in basic lay terms (*e.g.*, "female surgery"). The presence of a friend or relative of the patient can be helpful as a source of information. However, if the companion is a child or younger sibling of the older person, the additional data that is provided may be useful only when exploring the recent past.

General state of health

How does the patient view his or her present health status compared with a year ago? This is the opportunity to ascertain how the person views himself or herself in relation to the environmental constraints of day-to-day living. The question is general rather than specific. If the patient is being seen on a frequent basis, make comparisons based on a briefer time frame (*e.g.*, six months ago, last month, or even last week). The terms "good health" or "bad health" have different meanings to different people. Elderly patients will usually measure health changes by the degree to which they are able to function as independently as in the past. When their ability to accomplish the tasks of personal care or social interaction has been compromised, they will often report poor health.

Childhood disease and immunizations

Many older people cannot recall when or if they had specific infectious diseases commonly associated with infancy and early childhood. Significant data regarding susceptibility can be obtained from an immunization record, if one exists. Persons who served in the armed forces will have been desensitized to the usual communicable diseases. Recent immunizations against the flu and pneumonia should be noted.

Adult illness, injuries, and hospitalizations

Elderly patients have had a 50- to 100-year history, some of which may be difficult to recall or describe accurately. The important data will focus on conditions that, contracted and treated as an adult, may have resulted in complications or disability. Serious or chronic illnesses often compromise the patient's functional patterns or ability to cope. A history of the condition, the treatment, and approximate dates and places of past hospitalization will often be available from previous health records. The nurse will want to use the existing information sources when they are available.

Medications

Elderly people generally take more prescribed medications and over-the-counter drugs than do younger people. An accurate medication history is extremely important in monitoring and preventing health problems. The nurse should recommend that the patient bring all medications on the first visit, and review the medication regime on subsequent visits. Patients should be encouraged to carry a list of all current drugs: the name of each drug, the dose, and the frequency of administration in case of an emergency. The medication history should include both prescription and over-the-counter drugs. Patients often overlook those preparations that are self-prescribed—a practice that can be dangerous. Eliciting an accurate medication history may be difficult because patients may not know which medication is being taken for which condition, and they frequently refer to drugs by color and shape as a means of recognition (many drug names are difficult for lay persons to pronounce and spell). The boxed material on page 8 lists useful questions for taking an accurate geriatric drug history.

Allergies

An allergy history should be obtained, including medications, foods, and environmental elements. A description of how the hypersensitivity is manifest (*e.g.*, rash, respiratory complications, or central nervous system indicators) is a part of the history. As the immune system becomes less efficient with age, the number of allergies tends to increase.

Family history

Examining the health problems of other family members can be helpful in identifying familial health/illness patterns and risk potential. However, this component of the health history is more crucial with children and young adults.

It is often difficult to get more than the most superficial historical data because the elderly population today lived most of their years in an era when medicine was less exact and medical information was not always given to the patient

---

Open-ended questions for use in a geriatric drug history

- When you have a drug reaction, what happens to you? Do you have trouble breathing? Do you get a rash? Do you get an upset stomach?
- Have you noticed any changes in yourself since you began taking this medicine?
- What would you say is your greatest problem in taking your medicine?
- What do you usually swallow your medicine with and what seems to be the best time for you to remember to take your medicine?
- Do you use any medicine that is brewed from roots, teas, alcohol, or any household combinations or vitamins? How many of these do you take and how do they work for you?
- When you have a pain, what is the first medicine that you think about taking?
- Who is most helpful in assisting you with buying and taking your medicine? What kind of advice do they give you?
- Are most of your medicines prescriptions or from the drug counters in the store?
- How do you manage your mid-morning dose while out of the house?
- How often would you estimate you miss a dose?

(Burggraf V, Pedego N: Pharmacotherapeutics in the elderly: Aging and drug action. Pharmacology for Nurses by Home Study 3:1–13. Kansas City, MO, PRN Learning System, 1982)

---

or family. Medical records are frequently no longer available, and sometimes memories have dimmed. The cause of death of family members will often be identified only as "old age" or other nebulous diagnoses.

Family history, when collected, should cover the immediate family, generally considered to be parents, siblings, spouse, children, and grandparents. Because some illnesses can be traced to a genetic origin or a family tendency (*e.g.,* adult-onset diabetics), it is often helpful to draw a family tree. The information being sought about family members include state of health, or cause of death if deceased. The focus of these questions is the occurrence of major diseases such as those listed below.

Diabetes	Cancer
Tuberculosis	Arthritis
Coronary heart disease	Anemia
High blood pressure	Seizure disorders
Stroke	Alcoholism
Renal problems	Depression/suicide

As a starting point, inquire about the people who presently live with the patient. If there are persons who live in the same home but are not related, either through blood or by marriage, do not consider them part of the family, but do inquire about their state of health because contagion and susceptibility are important elements in the overall history.

Review of functional health patterns

Carnevali and Patrick (1986) suggest that by the conclusion of the interviewing process, which may take more than one contact, the nurse should have both subjective and objective data that describe how the patient sees his or her present state of health, usual or preferred lifestyle, the activities and demands of daily living, functional ability, and the support systems that exist. The framework that addresses the patient's strengths or deficits in these five areas constitutes the "Functional Health Framework" identified by Gordon (1982). Each of the 11 functional areas (see the boxed material below) will direct the nurse to information about the patient that is significant to the care planning process. The use of the functional health patterns as a tool for assessment is essential to the development of a nursing diagnosis or a clinical problem list.

Health perception and health management patterns

Data regarding the patient's perceived state of health will be verified with objective data obtained from the physical examination, laboratory results, and other

---

Gordon's functional health patterns

Health perception—Health management

Nutrition—Metabolic

Elimination

Activity—Exercise

Sleep—Rest

Cognitive—Perception

Self-perception

Role—Relationship

Sexuality—Reproductive

Coping—Stress tolerance

Value—Belief

(Adapted from Gordon M: Nursing Diagnosis: Process and Application. New York, McGraw-Hill, 1982)

diagnostic tests. The nurse can inquire further about any health maintenance practices that are important to the patient. Are there any activities or remedies that the elderly patient believes are important to his or her health status, or that predispose him or her to pain, disability, or illness? The taking of yeast tablets, "little liver pills," or a "morning constitutional" can be viewed as having a major influence on the health of some elderly people. Folk remedies or even "old wives' tales" can play a large role in a person's perception of health and illness, especially when they have been a part of early childhood experience.

When the elderly person is on long-term therapy or medication for any illness or disability, it is important to determine if he or she is complying with the treatment. Does the patient take the medication as prescribed; does he or she adhere to the treatments or activities that have been ordered? The nurse should ask the patient questions about the treatment regime that are designed to ascertain if he or she understands the goals of the therapy and is able to comply.

The potential for injury is a major concern when planning for care of the elderly patient. Identify potential safety hazards that are present in the patient's environment such as: area rugs; items that are frequently used, but stored out of reach; sensory deficits such as low visibility or decreased ability to hear; and lifestyle concerns such as need for transportation, social activities, and appropriate clothing.

Nutritional and metabolic patterns

A 24-hour dietary recall, if taken for a typical day, will be helpful in determining the eating patterns and preferences the elderly person has chosen. These patterns frequently reflect lifelong practices that may be difficult to change. Because fluid is sometimes overlooked when discussing dietary intake, the nurse should ask about the amount, type, and time that both food and drink are consumed. Identify any alterations in eating patterns that have occurred in the recent past and determine if the patient is concerned about these changes. Elderly people who are having trouble with denture fit will sometimes change their eating patterns because of the discomfort, or neglect to wear dentures altogether, limiting their selection of food to that which can be managed without vigorous chewing.

The following areas that address eating practices should be included: the usual number of meals consumed in the day, a typical menu, food preferences, who does the shopping or cooking, and who shares the meal time. Many life events revolve around food and its preparation, giving the subject psychosocial implications.

During the physical examination there will be an opportunity to assess the oral structures and observe for adequate mastication; however, good history-taking includes information about the last dental visit and past or present problems with dentures.

Both coffee and alcohol are known to have central nervous system effects and many vague complaints can be traced to frequent or excessive use of these substances. Attempt to get a past history of consumption and verify it with family members if possible. Determine if the pattern of use has changed recently. Coffee, tea, and alcohol are addictive substances and a change in the intake pattern can cause symptoms that are related to other body systems (*e.g.,* gastrointestinal, musculoskeletal, integument, and sensory problems) to name a few of the more obvious possibilities.

Some clinicians think that patients of all ages routinely under-report their use of alcohol; therefore this area may require further investigation.

Elimination patterns

Nutritional patterns will influence proper elimination. In the absence of structural problems or bowel disease, elderly people should maintain lifelong, established patterns of regularity. The assessment data that are gathered should address the frequency of laxative use or enema administration, the bulk content of the diet consumed, the amount and source of fluid intake, and any routines that are a part of usual bowel habits. The nurse should keep in mind that change in long-established bowel patterns, either toward constipation or diarrhea, needs medical investigation.

Changes in the pattern of urinary elimination, however, occur as a result of the aging process. There may be a tendency toward involuntary leaking (especially in women), which requires additional protection. The nurse should ask the elderly woman if she experiences incontinence, pain, urgency, or retention with overflow. Elderly men will find that they are awakened one or more times during the night to go to the bathroom. This pattern can prove to be a major obstacle to achieving uninterrupted sleep. Complaints that can indicate the need for medical intervention include frequency, nocturia, reduced size and force of stream, hesitancy and interruption of voiding, dribbling, or hematuria.

Activity and exercise

Assessment criteria for this functional pattern encompass those areas that, when working efficiently, require an expenditure of energy (*i.e.,* cardiovascular and respiratory activities). Ask the patient about the activities that he or she participates in during the course of the day. What kinds of things does the patient do in an average day? How much can the patient do without becoming excessively tired, being out of breath, or feeling pain? If the patient indicates that he or she gets chest or calf pain when climbing stairs, ask how many stairs can be managed before the pain starts, or how many blocks he or she can walk without a rest period. Inquire about activities that have previously been easy and enjoyable but can no longer be managed. What are the activities that the patient is able to do without being taxed? Ask if he or she ever experiences a reluctance to move about because of a lack of energy or of a feeling of weakness or dizziness. Is the patient able to manage the usual self-care activities of feeding, bathing/hygiene, dressing/grooming, and toileting independently, or with partial assistance; or must he or she be cared for by others? Are family members or others available to assist with the management of household activities, yardwork, transportation, and social commitments? To what degree are these activities being met by the patient? Are there activities that the patient would like to participate in but is not, either because he or she is physically unable or because the assistance necessary to do so is unavailable?

Sedentary interests such as knitting, checkers, and whittling do not reveal a great deal about exercise endurance; however, they can be good indicators of outside interest and the ability to concentrate and focus.

Smoking is becoming less socially acceptable, and can be another area in which the patient may under-report present or past use. Determine at what age he or she started smoking, and how many packs per day for how many years of use (*e.g.,* 2 packs per day for 40 years). If there has been a change in the pattern of use, indicate the significance of the change (*e.g.,* 2 pk/day × 40 years; only 1 pk/week × past 5 years). If the patient had a long history of smoking but has since stopped, record that information. If the question is asked, "Do you smoke?" and the answer is, "No," be sure to follow up by asking, "Have you ever been a smoker?" Someone may have smoked for 50 years, but quit last year. It is also useful to know what type of cigarette is preferred—filter, nonfilter, kingsize, and so forth. Chewing tobacco or "dipping snuff" are no less harmful or addictive activities than cigar or pipe smoking.

Sleep and rest

Sleep patterns change significantly with advancing age. The most notable difference is experienced in the Stage 4 deep sleep state, which virtually disappears in the older person. When elderly patients and family do not understand this normal aging phenomenon, they often worry that poor sleep will result in serious illness (Clapin-French 1986). Interview questions should assess the sleep pattern that presently exists, identify what changes have occurred in the recent past, and determine how the patient perceives these changes. Nighttime sleep patterns can be influenced by daytime activities. What is the usual waking and retiring time? Is there an established pre-sleep routine that has been interrupted? Does the patient take naps during the day? Other factors that can influence the quantity and quality of sleep include the noise level in the sleeping area, temperature, pain, anxiety, and dependency on hypnotics. Sleep that exceeds what has previously been an established pattern may suggest depression, withdrawal, inappropriate medication levels, or other medical problems.

Cognitive and perceptual changes

Since many of the most obvious changes that accompany the aging process involve diminished sensory function, questions focus on visual and auditory acuity, and the elderly patient's ability to taste, smell, and touch. Explore each area separately, inquiring about changes of which the patient is aware. Because these changes have often occurred slowly over time, the patient may be unaware that significant alterations in the ability to see, or hear, or taste are a problem. In others, however, these changes are apparent and frustrating. For example, the 88-year-old man who has always enjoyed "a good cup of coffee" will try numerous brands in an effort to find one that tastes right, and yearn for the days when it did.

For most people, visual changes have been fairly steady over the years, and the need for prescription glasses is almost universal. How has this restriction affected the patient in day-to-day activities? Is the patient able to read with the use of a magnifying tool? Does he or she still drive? Are there safety concerns because of diminished visual ability? When was the last eye exam? Many age-related changes are fairly common, such as recession of the eyeball into the orbit because of decreased orbital fat, and the formation of "bags" under the eyes and "crow's feet," resulting from muscle and skin changes over time. These changes, like others mentioned above, have usually been so gradual that the patient sometimes does not even notice them. Ask if the patient has ever had cataracts, glaucoma, or injury to the eye. Note excessive tearing, a common condition in older people.

Auditory acuity, like visual acuity, decreases gradually over a long period, and the degree of change is sometimes not apparent to the patient. The nurse might find that the family is more aware and concerned about how "hard of hearing" the elderly person has become. Before assuming that hearing loss is age-related, other potential causes should be explored. For example, toxic doses of some medications can cause hearing changes, including hearing loss, ringing, popping, and other unusual sounds. The accumulation of cerumen can also interfere with sound transmission. With advancing age, certain pitches and tones become difficult to discriminate. This can be frustrating for the patient because often he or she will be able to hear only part of what is being said.

Other sensory changes that are part of the aging process include diminished olfactory acuity and tactile sensations that involve pain, pressure, and temperature. Recognizing that these sensory deficits exist has significant implications in terms of patient safety. Elderly patients may not be as quick to detect the smell of smoke, or pain after a fall from bed, or excessive heat in a hot water bottle. Care must be taken to identify these perceptual changes and plan nursing care that will protect the patient from injury. Ask patients if they have noticed any changes in their ability to recognize temperature changes or identify odors. Whenever possible, verify this information with a family member.

Self-perception

As persons age, many things happen that cause them to question the images that they have of themselves. These life events include a growing dependence on others, a devaluation of their contribution to society, and loss of their loved ones or treasured possessions. This creates anxiety, fear, powerlessness, and an overall diminished quality of life. Inquire specifically how the patient feels about the events that are happening. Ask about the important past experiences that have been meaningful and what plans are being made for the future. Determine how and how much control the patient maintains over the activities in his life. Does the patient participate in any work or task activity that helps make a valid contribution to his or her environment?

Roles and relationships

This functional pattern investigates the usual living arrangements in which the patient is involved and attempts to identify how these can be strengthened. Where, and with whom, does the patient live? Is the arrangement satisfactory? How long has the present living arrangement been in place? If the elderly person's spouse or other loved one has died recently, altering past living arrangements, the resulting grief will often cause some changes in communication, social interactions, or sociability. Who does the patient call for emergencies? Who is called for transportation or recreation?

Inquire about all forms of support systems that may exist, not only the one that is identified as primary. Friends and other relatives can contribute to the overall care planning process, as well as enhance the well-being of the patient. Pets often play a significant role in the life of an elderly person, and will sometimes assume equal importance with immediate family. A patient will often commit a great deal of energy and resources to the care and nurturing of a pet, a fact that requires consideration when long-term care or relocation is necessary.

Sexuality and reproductive patterns

Historical data about sexual activity are often neglected during the course of the assessment, a fact that some authors attribute to discomfort on the part of the practitioner rather than the patient (Mezey et al 1980). Although the nurse will occasionally encounter persons who do not want to discuss the physical aspect of intimacy, each patient should have the opportunity to discuss his or her level of satisfaction or dissatisfaction, pain, discomfort, or recent changes in sexual encounters. Most elderly persons will report a diminished response to intercourse and an altered capacity to perform, but they continue to experience sexual encounters with enthusiasm.

Coping and stress tolerance abilities

Illness, or the fear of illness, can be stress-producing, and a primary goal of the history-taking process is to determine how the elderly person is coping with the situation that has precipitated this visit. Some key indicators of how the stress is being handled will be apparent in the communication patterns, body language, and the answers to direct questioning during the course of the interview. It is a good practice to periodically ask the patient about his or her feelings as they relate to significant events.

People often develop specific patterns in response to distressing situations and continue to use these coping mechanisms into their later years. The nurse can attempt to determine how the patient has reacted and dealt with stress in the past, and sometimes gain valuable insight that can be applied to successful care planning for the present problem.

It is also important to determine how effectively the family has managed the stress of illness or disability in the past. Many elderly persons depend to a large degree on assistance from their family members. Physical or psychological demands placed on family as a result of changes in health can affect everyone involved.

Values and beliefs

Carpenito (1983) defined a value or belief system as that source of strength and hope that is part of a person's life state. Any experience that calls that system into question causes the patient to be at risk for spiritual distress. Nurses often feel unprepared to address the spiritual needs of patients, but nevertheless are frequently the first ones to identify the need for intervention. Indications that the elderly person may be having a conflict with this functional health pattern are usually expressed by feelings of doubt, fear, hopelessness, or even anger. It is important to determine if these feelings are a temporary attempt to cope with an overwhelming situation (loss, disease, trauma, confinement), or are in fact a true disturbance in the value belief system.

Elderly people who have been active and involved in church devotions and rituals often view hospitalization or institutionalization as barriers to meeting their spiritual needs, placing them at risk for conflict.

Careful interviewing centered around the patient's view of his or her present situation, sense of power and spiritual guidance, and the extent to which his or her past life has been spiritually directed, will provide data to help the nurse plan for overcoming ambivalent feelings about this important aspect of care.

Summary

The patient interview is a vital component of nursing care planning. The data base derived from an examination of the 11 functional health patterns will provide information that is specific to the individual patient with direction for nursing interventions. It is important for the assessment process to go beyond history-taking and the physical examination, and to address the ways in which the patient is actually able to function in the environment when away from the hospital or institution. It is the best mechanism nurses have for understanding the uniqueness of each person.

The elderly person seeking assistance with health problems brings with him or her a rich past. To appreciate this gift, the nurse must invest time and energy to develop a relationship that encourages openness while promising compassion.

References

Burggraf V, Pedego N: Pharmacotherapeutics in the elderly: Aging and drug action. Pharmacology for Nurses by Home Study 3:1–13. Kansas City, MO, PRN Learning System, 1982

Carnevali D, Patrick M: Nursing Management for the Elderly, 2nd ed, p 28. Philadelphia, JB Lippincott, 1986

Carpenito L: Nursing Diagnosis: Application to Clinical Practice, p 451. Philadelphia, JB Lippincott, 1983

Clapin-French E: Sleep patterns of aged persons in long-term care facilities. J Adv Nurs 11:57–66, 1986

Gordon M: Nursing Diagnosis: Process and Application. New York, McGraw-Hill, 1982

Mezey M, Rouchhart L, Stokes S: Health Assessment of the Older Individual, p 93. New York, Springer Publishing, 1980

Bernita Steffl

Discharge planning and the elderly

2

What is discharge planning?

The American Nurses' Association (ANA) describes discharge planning as

> *The part of the continuity of care process which is designed to prepare the patient or client for the next phase of care, and to assist in making any necessary arrangements for that phase of care, whether it be self care, care by family members, or care by an organized health care provider (ANA 1975).*

The basic purpose of discharge planning is to provide continuity of care for patients of all ages and in all settings.* For decades, public health nurses and Visiting Nurse Association (VNA) nurses have pleaded for discharge planning for continuity of care, but they did not receive much support until the 1970s. The implementation of Diagnostic Related Groups (DRGs) in the early 1980s has focused more attention on discharge planning because many elderly patients are leaving the hospitals after shorter stays and are still in need of a considerable amount of nursing care. This older group of patients is the most vulnerable and in greatest need of comprehensive discharge planning for continuity of care. They suffer the most physically, psychosocially, and economically in the absence of discharge planning.

The first books on the topic were published in the 1970s (Bristow and Stickney 1974; Steffl and Eide 1978; McKeehan 1980). In 1985, the National League for Nursing (NLN) published a revised, compact, comprehensive new edition of *Discharge Planning for Continuity of Care* (Hartigan and Brown 1985), summarizing a

---

* There is a Hospital Discharge Planner Association. Information is available from: Hospital Discharge Planner Association, 1600 East Pacific Highway, Suite 169, Long Beach, CA 90806; Telephone: (213) 491-9050.

number of publications on the topic. It serves as an excellent quick reference and resource for guidelines.

Comprehensive, coordinated continuity of care

The concept of comprehensive, coordinated continuity of care is the basis for discharge planning (Fig. 2-1). The continuum in this figure involves the delivery of services within the community and between all health-care service agencies and institutions.

The ultimate goal of discharge planning is to restore the patient to a maximum state of wellness and to restore his or her ability to function independently in the community or institutional setting. Discharge to the patient's home should always be the first goal; and alternatives to home, especially longterm-care institutional placement, should be a last resort. Of course, in some situations discharge to a nursing home is the best decision (*e.g.,* an 85-year-old man who has had a cerebrovascular accident and requires total personal care, but his only family is an 80-year-old wife who has both heart disease and arthritis).

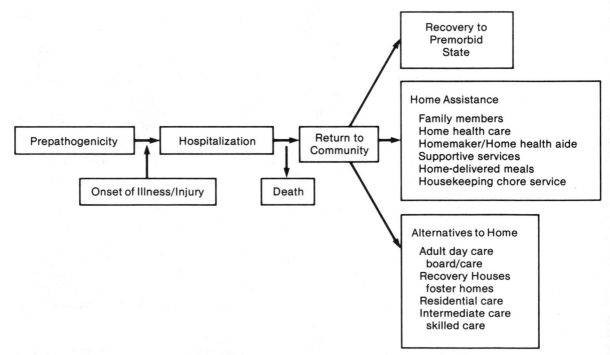

Figure 2-1. Illness–Wellness continuum through discharge planning. (Steffl B, Eide B: Discharge Planning Handbook, p 20. CB Slack, Thorofare, New Jersey, 1978)

The right to continuity of care

Citizens of the United States regard good health and quality health care to be the right of every person. The following statement is included in the "Patient's Bill of Rights" adopted by the American Hospital Association (AHA) in 1972.

> *The patient has the right to expect reasonable continuity of care. He has the right to know in advance what appointment times and physicians are available and where. The patient has the right to expect that the hospital will provide a mechanism whereby he is informed by his physician or a delegate of the physician of the patient's continuing health care requirements following discharge (Hartigan and Brown 1985).*

Organized continuity of care is crucial to the elderly, particularly the frail elderly. It becomes literally a matter of life and death in some situations. For example, pneumonia and dehydration develop rapidly without prevention follow-up care when a frail, confused elderly patient is discharged from an acute-care setting. Unintentional accidents and or problems such as pressure ulcers frequently result from events that occur because of a lack of the kind of discharge planning needed for this group of elderly. This planning should include (1) professional assessment of individual and age-related needs, (2) health education, (3) personal preventive services, (4) diagnostic and therapeutic services, and (5) rehabilitation and restorative services.

Patients at risk

Age itself is a high-risk factor in regard to potential need for discharge planning. Being old, female, and a member of a minority triples the jeopardy. Income, housing, transportation, and nutrition have all been documented as critical variables in health maintenance for the elderly. Linking up with resources in their areas may be difficult for some persons, so families need to be involved.

Case study

Jose Garcia, age 71, had surgery for carcinoma of the colon and was discharged with a colostomy to his home (50 miles from the hospital). Colostomy care had been taught and the patient was supposedly "adapting well." The third day after discharge from the hospital, the agency's home-care office received a frantic call from one of Mr. Garcia's friends, saying that Mr. Garcia was in distress and frightened. The friend could not explain what was wrong. When it was suggested that Mr. Garcia should come in to the clinic, it was learned that he would have to come by bus and there was only one bus daily coming and going. He would have to stay overnight. Sending a nurse 50 miles was also expensive and a risk because he might need to be brought in anyway. The nurse went, however, and discovered the problem was simply a colostomy bag that had not been changed for two days. The patient had not completely understood the procedure for colostomy

---

Conditions almost always requiring discharge planning

High-risk medical conditions	*High-risk social factors*
Amputations	Unstable living arrangements
Colostomy, mastectomy, radical surgery	Living alone
Disabling chronic disease	No family support system
Diabetes	Relocation
Cancer	
Stroke	Substance abuse
Chronic renal problems	Poverty
Dialysis	Abuse or neglect
Complicated medical regimen	Lack of transportation
Medical and medication	
Noncompliance	Minority status
Mental illness	Ethnic and cultural patterns of behavior
Depression	Language barriers
Confusion	
Home oxygen therapy	Rural versus urban locations
Intravenous therapy	Lack of availability of existing support systems
Incontinence	

---

care. The discharge planners had failed in their teaching and recognition of the language barriers. Even though Mr. Garcia had appeared to understand their instructions, the staff had overlooked the impact of his transportation situation and his residence in a rural area. See the boxed material above for a list of high-risk medical conditions and high-risk social situations of the elderly that require discharge planning.

Settings for discharge planning

Discharge planning is not limited to hospital settings. It should be part of patient-centered planning in all longterm-care institutional settings, including nursing homes, ambulatory care settings, and emergency departments.

Discharge planning is of special importance to the elderly patient presenting at the emergency department. Individualized discharge planning from an emergency department and referral to other agencies for continuity of care and prevention or recurrence are cost-effective to the patient, the hospital, the emergency department, and the physician. Only about 19% of patients seen in the emergency department are admitted to the hospital (Genie 1986). More concern should extend to those not admitted. Even in excellent facilities, a patient may receive medication and leave the department without knowledge of his or her medical condition or what to expect from the medication. Without referral for further care, the patient may leave the hospital with a broken leg in a cast without plans for getting to or managing in his or her second-floor, walk-up apartment. Figures about the number of emergency departments with specific discharge planning programs are unavailable, but most emergency departments have social services that provide discharge planning. The number seems to have increased since the implementation of Medicare prospective payments. Some hospitals or emergency departments offer a plan of service that allows the patient to stay for 24 hours at a reduced rate, thus providing more time for discharge planning.

Rationale for more discharge planning in the emergency department include reduction of

Complications for elderly patients

Abuse of emergency facilities. They are often used because they are open 24 hours a day. If the patient has been linked to the proper resources and supports, he or she may be able to take care of potential emergencies.

Hospital admissions

Medical-care cost to the patient

Professional liability—because emergency department physicians and personnel are vulnerable to malpractice actions

Discharge planning in longterm care appears to be limited. Two reasons are that the very old are often not expected to get well enough to go home, and that the possibilities of home care are underestimated. This attitude has been changing since the implementation of prospective payments. Because of DRGs, Medicare patients are leaving the hospital sooner and are more apt to be discharged to a longterm-care facility. Health professionals need to be especially careful to consider this procedure only as a step toward the patient's returning to his or her home or regaining as much independence as possible. Nurses and social workers should begin discharge planning for these patients on admission. Medicare has required discharge planning in longterm-care facilities for some time but most patients in longterm care are not eligible for Medicare because it pays only for skilled nursing-home care for a limited time. Therefore many longterm-care facilities have given up their Medicare certification and may not be as committed to discharge planning. Data about discharge planning and discharge to home or home care from longterm-care and ambulatory-care settings are lacking.

An increase in discharge management has been predicted for all of these settings, with ensuing new definitions and roles for nurses in the future (Berke 1984). Gerontological nurses should assume more leadership, and demonstrate their professional knowledge and skills in case management for continuity of care (see section below on team planning).

The impact of diagnostic related groups

Until the advent of DRGs institutional and medical concern for discharge planning had been equivocal (Rehr 1986). The most influential factor for the development of the DRGs was cost containment. Their implementation has had a profound impact on discharge planning, particularly in hospitals. Elderly patients are leaving the hospital "sicker and quicker" and the number of newly developed home-care agencies is skyrocketing (Table 2-1). Critics charge that the program is leading to serious abuses such as premature discharge, but the Government Office of Beneficiary Services for Medicare and Medicaid claims otherwise (Carlson and Oriel 1985–1986; Health Care Financing Administration 1985).

How do DRGs work?

On April 20, 1983, President Ronald Reagan signed House Bill 1900, which became Public Law 98-21, an Amendment to the Social Security Act. Title IV of the law stipulates that Medicare payments for hospital inpatient service will now be determined under a prospective payment system, replacing the old retrospective per diem cost system. Under the DRG system, the government stipulates in advance how much it will pay toward hospital bills for Medicare patients. The amount is determined primarily by the patient's principal diagnosis; however, age, surgery, and complications are also considered. The government has established 23 major diagnostic categories (Caterinicchio 1984).

Each category consists of a number of diagnoses that are given code numbers. There are a total of 470 code numbers, and the government has determined

Table 2-1. **Number of medicare-certified home health care agencies**

Sponsor	7/1/83	1/3/86	6/1/86
VNA	519	518	514
Public	1216	1217	1200
VNA/Public	58	57	62
Rehabilitation	19	20	19
Hospital	541	1260	1333
Skilled nursing facility (SNF)	112	129	116
Proprietary	871	1927	1922
Private nonprofit	671	831	835
Other	40	5	4
Total	4047	5964	6005

(National Association for Home Care: Report #168. Washington DC, 1986)

how long a patient should be hospitalized for each. Hospitals are reimbursed accordingly. The amount of money the hospital receives is based on this calculated length of stay (Smith 1985; Carlson and Oriel 1985–86). Hospitals may keep whatever portion of the reimbursement that has not been spent when they treat and discharge patients in fewer days than the DRG allowance. Consequently, more patients leave hospitals in need of more care. How well these patients fare depends a great deal on *discharge planning* and home-care services. If the patient's length of stay and costs exceed the DRG allowance, the hospital must absorb the cost. Ultimately, the DRG system is expected to save the government about 13 billion dollars per year (Smith 1985).

The new system is accused of skimping on quality care. For example, Senator John Henry, Chairman of the Senate Special Committee on Aging, stirred controversy in March 1985 when he declared that a peer-review group had reported to the Health Care Financing Administration (HCFA) as many as 3700 inappropriate patient discharges or transfers, including several that resulted in deaths (Carlson and Oriel 1985–86).

Trends

Another movement receiving some scrutiny is the development of skilled (nursing home) facilities within or attached to the hospitals so that elderly patients may be discharged within the DRG guidelines, but actually remain in the same system. On the surface, this approach appears to be the continuity of care being advocated, but it also harbors some potential problems of abuse of the system. For example, what happens to the patient when all the benefits are used up? Where does he or she go? A point is reached where discharge planning, which supposedly begins in the hospital, may be lost.

There is a move toward the development of "one-stop shop systems" linked to hospitals, which provide a variety of services including durable medical equipment (DME). For example, large hospitals are developing extended-care and home-care departments (or agencies) that keep the elderly patient, particularly the Medicare patient, within one system until the patient is independent or until funding is exhausted. The patient may receive home nursing care, special therapies, DME, medications, and various supported services. Because of need for more social services, there is a movement toward the development of agencies referred to as Senior Health Maintenance Organizations (SHMOs), as an alternative to the regular Health Maintenance Organizations (HMOs). SHMOs are structured to anticipate seniors needs. They feature comprehensive social and home care, choose physicians knowledgeable in geriatrics, and stress active involvement of the patient in self-care. Presently, there are only four demonstration SHMOs nationwide (Nassif 1986):

- Elderplan, Inc. (Metropolitan Jewish Geriatric Center), Brooklyn, New York
- Kaiser—Permanent Medical Care Program, Portland, Oregon

- Medicare Partners (Ebenezer Society/Group Health, Inc.), Minneapolis, Minnesota
- SCAN Health Plan (Senior Care Action Network), Long Beach, California

Governmental agencies deny that Medicare is ordering patients out of hospitals and that quality of care to Medicare patients is declining. However, the HCFA has recognized this as a possibility and is taking steps to prevent abuses. Because the system is just reaching full operation, it is too early to draw unbiased conclusions. The DRGs do affect nursing responsibilities in care of the elderly in a number of ways. Nurses need to keep costs in mind when giving care; coordinate more preadmissions; and, after discharge testing and treatment, carefully document uses of supplies and time; and begin discharge planning, including patient teaching, from the time the patient is admitted. See the boxed material below for a list of the ten most frequent reasons that DRGs are used by the elderly.

Other regulatory influences on discharge planning

A number of social policies and governmental regulations control the delivery of health services to the elderly and indirectly affect nursing practice. Nurses tend to

---

The ten most frequent reasons that DRGs are used by the elderly

What patients are you most likely to see under the new DRG system? According to the U.S. Department of Health and Human Services, the DRG uses most frequently reported are

1. Heart failure/shock
2. Lens implant
3. Esophagitis, gastrointestinal/miscellaneous digestive disease in patients over 69
4. Specific cerebrovascular disorders, except transient ischemic attack
5. Simple pneumonia and pleurisy in patients over 69
6. Angina pectoris
7. Chronic obstructive pulmonary disease (COPD)
8. Cardiac arrhythmia and conductive disorders in patients over 69
9. Back problems
10. Bronchitis or asthma in patients over 69

(Smith CE: DRG: Making them work for you. Nursing 85:34, 1985)

consider this content rather mundane and in general remain quite uninformed about policies and regulations pertaining to health care of the elderly. The following is a brief description of regulations other than the law concerning DRGs, which has already been discussed in this chapter.

The most influential incentive for discharge planning has been the need for cost controls, which have led to reimbursement regulations. Some of these mandatory controls are professional standard reviews, utilization reviews, quality assurance, and nursing audits. *The development and implementation of all quality assurance and cost-containment programs have demonstrated the need to strengthen discharge planning and to educate both the consumer and professionals for such planning.*

The Joint Commission on Accreditation of Hospitals (JCAH) has had specific requirements for discharge planning for more than a decade. For example, their Nursing Services Standard IV reads

> *The nursing care plan shall include nursing measures that will facilitate the medical care prescribed that will restore, maintain, or promote the patient's well being. As appropriate, such measures should include physiological, psychological and environment factors; patient/family education, and patient involvement in discharge planning (JCAH 1984; Hartigan and Brown 1985).*

The rules and regulation for Medicare and Medicaid have conditions of participation for hospitals, skilled nursing facilities, and home-health-care agencies that include requirements for discharge planning. These conditions have been a major factor in the development of discharge planning. In other words, for agencies competing for Medicare and Medicaid dollars, discharge planning has become mandatory. Because these laws and rules and regulations are widely published and are readily available in the Federal Register, they have not been reproduced here.

The discharge planning team

Implementation of discharge planning requires a multidisciplinary team with ongoing interdisciplinary networking. Essential team members and their overall responsibilities are summarized in the boxed material on page 26.

Currently, 80% of the collaborative aspects of discharge planning for the elderly is done by social workers (O'Sullivan 1986). It is unclear why nurses have not taken more leadership in the activity. Nurses need to be more involved in discharge planning, and they are perhaps the professionals who are best prepared for the coordinator role. The nursing profession has an opportunity to strengthen its position in this area because industry, commercial insurers, and consumers are depending more on nurses not only for preventive services, assessment skills, utilization review, but also for case management, which includes discharge planning (Peck 1986). The computerization of planning and recordkeeping in health-care delivery is also creating new roles and career opportunities for nurses in the realm of HMOs and insurance companies (Berke 1984).

Eval

Professional roles in discharge planning

Coordinator

The coordinator is a program planner, implementor, facilitator, and evaluator of discharge planning. The coordinator also needs to be an advocate, crusader, mediator, and counselor. Currently socialworkers and nurses most often hold this position.

Physician

The physician is a key person, the director/leader. His or her orders and medical directions are the most essential ingredients in discharge planning. The physician's role is twofold: informing the patient of the diagnosis and possible risks in treatment, and predicting outcomes and expected changes in lifestyle.

Hospital nurse

Nurses who serve a role in discharge planning are usually head nurses or team leaders on the unit. Because nurses have more direct contact with the patients than do other team members, they are in a key position for getting input from the patient and staff for the discharge planning conference.

Social worker

The social worker assists with the social, emotional, and economic problems related to illness or injury, concentrates on the whole person, and is a facilitator and counselor in using community resources. Illness or injury, that often persists indefinitely for the elderly, disrupts family functioning; preventive and therapeutic assistance from a social worker may prevent family breakdown.

Dietician or nutritionist

They are assessors, teachers, counselors, and interpreters. They are often researchers and are always important team members. Nutritional counseling is a priority for elderly clients in any setting.

Physical, occupational, and respiratory therapists

The therapists will collect and disseminate information to and from the physician and other members of the discharge planning team, pertinent to a realistic program and plan of discharge for the patient and for posthospital rehabilitative follow-up care.

Community health nurse

The community health-care nurse acts as the patient advocate and liaison to provide continuity of care in the patient's home. He or she is also a planner, facilitator, implementor, evaluator, and personal counselor for the patient and a support person for the family. The community health nurse may come to the hospital for discharge planning conferences before the patient's discharge, make home assessments, and serve as hospital (medical) link to the family. He or she may work directly with the hospital nurse or discharge planning coordinator.

Nursing roles in discharge planning for the elderly

The gerontological nurse must be an advocate, astute assessor, and assertive intervenor. These roles are critical for effective discharge planning for elderly patients, especially the frail elderly.

The nurse advocate role

There are many advocacy roles for nurses in the care of the elderly. Acting as an advocate is a relatively new role for nurses. Until recently they perceived themselves more as followers of doctors' orders, but nursing leaders say this attitude is changing.

> *Nurses have always been in the forefront of patient care. They are the providers who are with patients for 24 hours a day in acute-care and long-term care facilities, the providers who make home visits, and the providers committed to patient education. They are patients' advocates, and, now more than ever before, patients need providers who will look out for their interests (Ostrander 1986).*

The nurse discharge planner, especially when working with the elderly, must be ready to question hospital administrators and home-health agencies regarding their mission, purpose, and responsibilities (Runner-Heidt 1984).

Nurses must voice their opinions when they observe care that does not meet standards of practice or when situations arise that might influence the quality of life of an elderly patient.

Case study

Mr. James Henry Patterson was 84 years old, black, had no family, and lived alone. He had multiple health problems and was frequently seen in the emergency department of the large city/county hospital. The discharge-planning team had strongly recommended a longterm-care facility where food and housing needs would require less effort for him. In spite of extreme shortness of breath and painful ambulation, Mr. Patterson always refused to consider the team's suggestion and returned to his home. A sensitive nurse discovered this dignified old gentleman was refusing to move and accept a more comfortable situation because he could not take his dog (who was his "most significant other") with him. On Mr. Patterson's last trip to the hospital, he collapsed when he reached the emergency room, yet he had managed to carry his dog to the vet before he came. Unfortunately, Mr. Patterson died before he could move to the home the nurse had found for both him and his dog.

The nurse assessor role

The assessment of elderly patients gives the nurse a unique role in discharge planning. The assessment stage is where the identification of targeted outcomes begins. Much of what the nurse does in discharge planning dovetails with the assessment and intervention of other professionals; however, nurses' skills are unique in the day-to-day assessment of physical status. Most patients are not all sick or all well at one time, and it takes astute evaluation to determine needs in situations such as a diabetic who looks and sounds well, but has an elevated blood sugar level. See Table 2-2 for a list of vital nurse assessments in regard to discharge planning for elderly patients.

Nurses also need to be able to effectively communicate and document what they assess. Ability in these skills is related directly to obtaining funding, assessing the cost of nursing care, and measuring quality care. Since health care has become a highly competitive big business—540 billion dollars in 1986—nurses must have the skills to document and project needs to compete in the marketplace. That is, they must be able to document, and justify their expenditure and direct hospital efforts toward the financial incentives in the marketplace that benefit both the patient and the care-giver. An example is Senate Bill 2920, The Advanced Nursing Service in Nursing Home Act, which was introduced at the 99th Congressional Sessions and passed in December of 1987. This legislation, drafted by ANA and Sen. Daniel Inouye (Democrat, Hawaii), allows a nurse practitioner (NP) or clinical nurse specialist (CNS), working in collaboration with a physician, to certify and recertify the need for patient care in nursing homes, as well as perform the mandatory patient visits under both Medicare and Medicaid (Bonaparte 1986; ANA 1986).

The nurse intervenor role

The nursing intervention role in discharge planning includes intervening with the family as well as with the patient. It means fostering team collaboration and being an instigator and facilitator for the benefit of the patient (or the family). Intervention roles for discharge planning generally fall into the following categories:

- Giving holistic nursing care, which includes "the person" as well as the diseased part
- Modifying what is needed for the patient such as preventive skin care, exercises, sensory stimulation, and rehabilitation activities
- Modifying environmental forces that threaten the older person's well-being such as physical hazards to safety and preventing social isolation
- Facilitating medical management such as implementing the medical treatment plan and monitoring the health–illness status
- Doing health teaching and health promotion
- Articulating community resources (finding the best support services and assuming the role of coordinator or care manager)

• Reporting potential elder abuse. Clues for identifying abusive situations are frequently observed at time of discharge. The five main categories of elder abuse are physical, psychological, material, violation of rights, and denial of basic needs (neglect). Neglect is the most common form.

Table 2-2. **What the discharge planning nurse assesses in the elderly client**

Physical and biological status	Psychological status	Socioeconomic status

Day-to-day physical changes
  Vital signs
  Integument
  Hydration
  Nutritional status
  Bowel and bladder continence
  Elimination patterns
	Sensory alterations and deficits:
	  Vision and hearing
	  Self-image
	  Coping patterns
	  Losses
		General financial status
		  Eligibilities

Nutrition–diet	Cognitive functioning:
	  Orientation
	  Mental status
	  Communication abilities
	  Aphasia/confusion
		Relationships
		  Significant others
		  Family
		  Widow–widower

Dental status		Cultural differences
		  Language limitations
		  Food preferences

Mobility
  Level of mastery of self-care
	Coping capacities and strategies, past and present	Support systems
		  Available
		  Accessible

Activities of daily living
  Supplies for treatment and care
  Adaptive equipment needed
  Durable medical equipment needed
	Health teaching needs
	  Knowledge and understanding of condition
		Home assessment
		  Environmental/safety
		  Atmosphere

	Family coping patterns Family needs and problems	Transportation needs
Pain Tolerance and control	Counseling needs	

Medication regimen
  Compliance
  Therapeutic response
  Contraindications
  Adverse reactions		

Rest and sleep patterns
  In hospital
  At home		

←———— Present and future resources and referrals needed ————→

Note: Some of the above are unique to nursing, but most will dovetail with assessments of other professional team members.
(Adapted from Steffl BM, Eide B: Nurses' role in discharge planning. Discharge Planning Update 1:4, 1981)

What do elderly patients expect from a nurse? I have found that first, patients want someone who is kind and willing to listen to them as they try to describe and understand their physical condition; and second, they expect a nurse to care about their feelings. In some situations, such as the patient on a cardiac monitor, the technical skills of the nurse are of life-and-death concern to the patient, but the issue that is of prevailing importance is that of understanding the feelings and behaviors of elderly people in all interventions, including discharge planning (Steffl 1984).

The nurse evaluator role

The following key words for evaluation of the discharge plan and recommendations remain timely even though proposed more than a decade ago (Bristow and Stickney 1974). Is the discharge plan

Realistic—obtainable—economical?

Functional—efficient—organized?

Flexible—effective—productive?

Nursing diagnosis and discharge planning

The nursing process, including the use of nursing diagnoses, is an essential component of discharge planning. Most patients who require discharge planning will require a nursing care plan. Therefore, even though discharge planning is a multidisciplinary and interdisciplinary affair, the nursing diagnosis, the ensuing nursing care plan, and actual nursing care become most critical variables in the elderly patient's recovery and maintenance of health after discharge.

Nursing diagnoses are directed toward identification of specific imbalances between demands of daily living and coping resources in health and illness. Nursing management of the elderly patient involves mobilizing him or her and outside resources to replace or supplement inadequate coping abilities, support systems, and resources (Carnevali and Patrick 1986). The nursing diagnosis directs the provision of nursing care and assistance and suggests a broad spectrum of ancillary services. Vaughn-Wrobel and Perkins (1986) describe nursing diagnosis as a "pivotal point" in the nursing process.

A study by Hallal (1985) identified the following as the six most frequently occurring nursing diagnoses in a sample of elderly (average age, 76.6 years) medical/surgical patients. These factors have relevance for discharge planning and home-health-care needs:

Impaired physical mobility

Alteration in comfort: pain

Alteration in nutrition: less than body requirements

Fear

Alteration in bowel elimination

Alteration in pattern of urinary elimination

Nursing priorities in discharge planning for older persons

Medications

A safe and viable plan for acquisition, administration, and monitoring of medications is a crucial and high-priority part of discharge planning for elderly patients.

Elderly persons consume 25% of all drugs purchased in the United States today. Eighty-five percent of all noninstitutionalized persons over age 65 use prescription drugs. Elderly persons are taking an average of two to three prescription drugs in addition to a variety of over-the-counter drugs. Shimp and coworkers (1984) interviewed 53 such users. The subjects had an average of five chronic illnesses and used an average of 11 drugs each. They had an average of over ten medication-related problems, which could be grouped into three broad categories: drug toxicity; physician prescribing; and patient behaviors with medication, such as compliance and self-prescribing. The study pointed out a need for health professionals to take a more specific role in helping patients plan a daily medication regimen, and a need for more specific information for patients, including clear, readable information provided on labels. These plans and regimes should be included in the discharge plan.

Patient education regarding medications should have been a part of the daily nursing care plan and the discharge plan; however, the patient frequently reaches the time of discharge and goes home without a clear understanding, ability, or willingness (*e.g.,* giving own insulin) to comply with physicians' orders. This situation requires skilled nursing assessments, evaluation, and communication with other members of the health team, and must include the patient and his or her family or significant others.

Nutrition and hydration

This area of continuity of care requires interdisciplinary collaboration and knowledge of community resources such as how to obtain Meals-on-Wheels and the location of senior centers and daycare centers that provide meals for the elderly.

Most of the elderly population is at nutritional risk. A majority of elderly persons have one or more chronic diseases that may alter nutritional needs and behavior that impacts on nutrition.

Other obstacles to adequate nutrition and hydration that the discharge planning nurse needs to recognize are as follows

- Limited income
- Inadequate dentition
- Immobility
- Reduced activity—loss of appetite
- Sensory alterations in taste and smell
- Drugs (medications) and alcohol use
- Fluid intake and elimination
- Loneliness, anxiety, and fear (Cadigan 1984)

Nutrition is one of the basic elements of health, health maintenance, and health care for older persons in all settings. It is a strong contributor to mental and emotional health. Counseling the elderly regarding this subject is a challenge. Professionals often fail to recognize that elderly persons become more individualistic with age and that what they eat and what they believe about food is strongly instilled and may be difficult to change. Myths and magic about food have existed throughout history and are still common in every ethnic group today (Evenesko 1984; Carnevali and Patrick 1986).

Unintentional injury

Unintentional injury includes injuries ranging from falls to the development of pressure ulcers. These are extremely costly monetarily and even more detrimental to the physical and psychosocial comfort of the elderly person. Because prevention is the only real intervention and many of these unintentional injuries result from accidents in the home, it becomes increasingly important to include assessment of mobility needs and environmental hazards in discharge planning for the frail elderly. Falls that result in bone fractures are most frequent on the list of accidents in the elderly population and are often the turning point for total disruption of lifestyle. The health teaching for the prevention of falls should include information designed to prevent the physiological situations that cause falls such as postural hypotension and hyperextension of the neck, as well as removal of environmental hazards such as scatter rugs and electric and telephone cords on the floor. Even the very old can be taught to take safety measures such as rising slowly from a bed or chair to prevent postural hypotension and dizziness, which may cause them to fall.

Mobility and transportation

Maintaining independence is a major goal for elderly persons and losing it is their greatest fear. Mobility and transportation are two of the greatest contributing factors to independence and therefore need to be considered in all discharge planning. Assessment of mobility and transportation again requires knowledge of community resources and home health equipment. A most valuable resource regarding equipment to facilitate mobility for the discharge planning team is the *Sears Home Health Catalog*. The discharge planner must also search for community resources that provide transportation for the elderly with special needs. Because federal funding is available for such services, most communities have at least limited service such as Dial-a-Ride.

Supportive services in the home

Well-organized home health care has assisted many elderly people in independent living. Home health care in itself, however, is not all that is needed. Many of those with multiple chronic impairments need more than health care, they need support services to remain in their home environment. Funding for these support services has been more difficult to obtain than for medical care, although they are less expensive. The discharge-planning nurse needs to know how to locate these services. If they are unavailable, the discharge planner may be instrumental in facilitating their initiation. Services that assist elderly persons in remaining in their home include, but are not limited to, the following

- Supervised home health nursing and aides
- Homemaker grocery shopping
- Home-delivered meals
- Chore services—minor repairs
- Cleaning and laundry services
- Transportation

Case study

Willie Mae Jenkins is in her late 70s, an insulin-dependent, obese diabetic with severe stasis leg ulcers that limit her mobility. She is unable to fill her insulin syringes because of poor vision and cannot change the dressing on her leg. With a support system arranged through discharge planning, she has been able to function independently at home for over two years. A public health nurse fills a supply of syringes for her weekly. The home health aide changes her dressing and assists her with bathing, shopping, and chores once or twice a week, as needed. Ms. Jenkins is happy and busy. She manages most of her own housework, cooks her own meals, and nurtures plants. She is still able to do for others, which is important to her. For example, she presented a pie to her aide as a gift.

Summary

Discharge planning is an essential part of gerontological nursing. Almost every encounter of an elderly person with health-care agencies calls for some discharge planning for optimum continuity of care. This chapter has provided rationales for discharge planning and described the nurse's role in discharge planning. Because of the rapidly increasing number of frail elderly, and the current content of federal legislation and social policies, discharge planning is now in the spotlight as the major vehicle for moving patients through the acute phase or stage of institutionalization to more economical and sometimes more appropriate modes of care such as home care.

Large hospitals are becoming more mobile and decentralized. The key to survival for institutions is to offer many services from a centralized location, which are deliverable to many settings. Nurses and consumers will need to be educated to this shifting scene of health-care delivery. Nurses will need to demand (as consumers) and provide (as professionals) discharge planning for the comprehensive, coordinated continuity of care for the elderly. Basic preparation in professional nursing lends itself to discharge planning, perhaps more than that of any other helping profession, yet professional nurses have been comparatively slow to see themselves in leadership roles in discharge planning. This attitude is changing. Nursing leadership in discharge planning is growing (Berke 1984).

References

American Nurses' Association: Continuity of Care and Discharge Planning Programs, 3. New York, ANA 1975

American Nurses' Association: Capital Update 5(24):2. Washington DC, ANA, 1987

Berke J: The spread of discharge management: New definitions, new careers, new power. The Coordinator 3:16, 1984

Bonaparte BH: Preparing nurses to win in a competitive system. Nursing and Health Care 7:471, 1986

Bristow O, Stickney C: Discharge Planning for Continuity of Care, pp 51–71. Richmond, Virginia Regional Medical Program, 1974

Cadigan M: Nutrition and the elderly. In Steffl BM (ed): Handbook of Gerontological Nursing. New York, Van Nostrand Reinhold, 1984

Carlson E, Oriel E: DRGs: Surviving Medicare's new obstacle course. Modern Maturity 28:25, Dec 1985–Jan 1986 edition

Carnevali DL, Patrick M: Nursing Management for the Elderly. Philadelphia, JB Lippincott, 1986

Caterinicchio RP: DRGs: What They Are and How to Survive Them. Thorofare, New Jersey, Charles B Slack, 1984

Eveneshko V: Ethnic and cultural considerations. In Steffl BM (ed): Handbook of Gerontological Nursing, pp 425–449. New York, Van Nostrand Reinhold, 1984

Genie E (Director of Home Health Services, Admission records statistics, Maricopa County Hospital, Phoenix, Maricopa County Health Services): personal interview, 1986

Hallal JC: Nursing diagnosis: An essential step to quality care. J Gerontol Nurs 11:35, 1985

Hartigan EG, Brown DJ: Discharge Planning for Continuity of Care. Columbus Circle, New York, National League for Nursing Publication No. 20-1977, 10, 1985

Health Care Financing Administration: Medicare/Medicaid Notes. DHHS Publication, Washington DC, 1985

Joint Commission for Accreditation of Hospitals (JCAH): Accreditation Manual for Hospitals. Chicago, American Hospital Association, 1984

McKeehan KM (ed): Continuing Care: A Multidisciplinary Approach to Discharge Planning. St. Louis, CV Mosby, 1980

Nassif JZ: Social health maintenance organization. Caring 5:34, 1986

National Association for Home Care: Report #168. Washington DC, 1986

Ostrander VR: Consumers look to nurses for affordable quality care. Nursing and Health Care 7:369, 1986

O'Sullivan J: Planning the discharge with the elderly. Quality Review—Bulletin, Journal of Quality Assurance 12:68, 1986

Peck SB: Nursing: On the cutting edge of opportunity. Nursing and Health Care 7:365, 1986

Rehr H: Commentary. Quarterly Review Bulletin: Journal of Quality Assurance 10:546, 1986

Runner-Heidt CM: Where does the hospital discharge planner go from here? Home Health Care Nurse 2:34, 1984

Shimp L, Ascione F, Glazer H, Atwood B: Potential medication: Related problems. Drug Intelligence and Clinical Pharmacy 19:5, 1984

Smith CE: DRGs: Making them work for you. Nursing 85:34, 1985

Steffl BM: Handbook on Gerontological Nursing. New York, Van Nostrand Reinhold, 1984

Steffl BM, Eide B: Discharge Planning Handbook. Thorofare, New Jersey, Charles B Slack, 1978

Steffl BM, Eide B: Nurses' role in discharge planning. Discharge Planning Update 1:4, 1981

Vaughn-Wrobel BC, Perkins SB: Nursing diagnosis: The pivotal point of the nursing process in cardiovascular nursing. Cardiovas Nurs 22:25, 1986

Katherine K. Kim

Patient education

3

Because elderly people are the most likely to suffer from chronic diseases and because their self-care management tends to be complex, teaching health care to the elderly is a special challenge to nurses. The challenge is to both minimize potential problems in the learning–teaching process by understanding elderly patients' needs, and simultaneously to maximize their strengths and talents.

Recent research on learning in old age has suggested that many factors influence learning by elderly persons. Age-related changes in sensory processes, memory, and health status affect learning; and other factors also have impact, such as intellectual ability, meaningfulness and difficulty of tasks, cautiousness, the speed of information presentation, and response time allowed during the learning presentation.

Several points should be kept in mind when teaching the elderly. First, the factors that influence learning are usually interrelated (however, for the purpose of this discussion each factor will be explored separately). Second, nurses, because they usually work with elderly people who are sick, may hold erroneous beliefs about the aged. Aging is not necessarily a process of decline; thus, it is important not to stereotype the elderly person. Because the experiences and capabilities of the elderly vary significantly, some patients may not have any learning difficulties, and others may have disabilities. In many learning situations, some elderly perform as well as or even better than younger adults. Therefore, the learning experience must be shaped to meet the abilities of each patient. Third, the inferior learning performance found in some studies on elderly populations may not be the result of diminished learning ability, but may be caused by other factors such as basic educational differences. Decreased learning performance may also be caused by unfamiliarity with test-taking, a decline in visual or auditory perception, or an altered physical state. By knowing how these factors affect health-care learning by elderly patients, nurses can choose appropriate teaching strategies.

Age-related changes

Sensory processes

Sense perception declines with age. Although perception diminishes in all senses, it is the visual and auditory changes that most effect an elderly person's learning abilities.

Visual perception

Visual acuity remains relatively unchanged up to ages 40 through 50, but after this time there is a sharp decline. This deterioration of visual acuity is most probably the result of changes in the crystalline lens and vitreous humor (Corso 1975). A marked loss of the eye's adjustment capacity for seeing objects at various distances (*accommodation*) occurs up to the age of 30. The rate of accommodation loss slows between 30 and 40 years, but increases sharply between the ages of 40 and 50 (Corso 1975; Fozard et al 1977). Because the eye's lens yellows with age, causing a filter effect for the shorter light wavelengths, color discrimination declines. Consequently, many elderly persons are unable to discriminate among blue, green, or violet, but less deficiency is demonstrated in red, orange, and yellow discrimination (Corso 1975). The ability to adjust to glare also decreases with age, and thus a lighting situation with glare may make it difficult for some elderly persons to perform visual tasks (Fozard et al 1977). Therefore, loss of clear vision can result from too much illumination, as well as from too little. In addition, the incidence of vision-impairing diseases such as cataracts and diabetic retinopathy increases with age.

If an elderly patient wears glasses, it is important to make sure the glasses are clean and properly fitted. Visual materials that are used to teach elderly patients should consist of large-scale elements. Unfortunately, most health-teaching materials, because they often involve small print, are unsuitable, and it may be necessary to develop materials. It is important that lighting be adequate and glare-free.

Color discrimination is another area of visual ability that requires consideration. Elderly diabetic patients who have poor color discrimination may encounter special problems in using the urine test for sugar and acetone. The chart for checking urine color includes blue, green, and violet, which are particularly difficult shades for some elderly to discriminate. Consequently, diabetic patients should be examined for defects in color vision before they are instructed about their self-care. In addition, teaching materials that use color are more interesting and effective. But patients who have poor color discrimination, or who are presented with materials in poorly discriminated shades might find them to have decreased effectiveness as teaching materials. Color also can be used as a learning aid, for example, a color-coding system helps elderly patients with self-admin-istration of their medications (Freeman 1974; Gimble 1967). In uses such as this, it is clear that the patient's ability to discriminate color must be assessed. Poor color perception might also cause communication problems between the elderly patient and the nurse. For example, a patient might refer to, "My gray pill," when the drug is actually a pale green. Unless the patient's problem with color discrimi-nation is known, the nurse might think that the patient is referring to a different drug. On the other hand, the nurse might say, "Mr. X, take your sedative, the blue pill, at bedtime." The patient with poor color discrimination could find such in-struction confusing.

Auditory perception

Research reports a wide variation of hearing loss in the elderly. A significant num-ber of elderly persons have serious hearing impairment and need rehabilitation (Maurer and Rupp 1979). In old age, high-pitched tones are progressively less audible for the elderly, whereas low-pitched tones are heard better (Corso 1971). Thus, speech discrimination among the aged is poorest for those consonants that have high-frequency components in their acoustic patterns (*e.g., s, z, t, f,* and *g*), as well as consonants that do not carry much acoustic power (*e.g., thin, sing*). Together, these factors produce a situation in which some elderly persons are unable to discriminate among phonetically similar words and, consequently, have difficulty in following normal conversation (Corso 1971). Comprehension of speech is also influenced by the rate of speech with speech perception deteriorat-ing as speech rate increases (Calearo and Lazzaroni 1957; Konkle et al 1977). In addition, elderly persons may have difficulty discriminating pertinent sounds when there are background noises (Maurer and Rupp 1979). For example, a noisy air conditioner may exacerbate communication problems. Maurer and Rupp (1979, p 22) state, "Perhaps the epitome of unintelligibility for the typical aging ear is the soft-voiced speaker with a high pitch who delivers the message at a high rate of speech in a background of noise."

Compensatory teaching techniques

These findings indicate the utmost importance of assessing the elderly patient's visual and aural perception. Patients who have decreased sense perception in one area often compensate with an increased reliance on other senses. Therefore, the use of a multisensory approach in teaching will enhance learning. For example, in addition to auditory and visual materials to teach about low-salt diet, nurses need to have elderly patients taste low-salt food.

To compensate for a hearing loss of higher frequencies, the nurse giving instructions should speak clearly, concisely, and slowly in low tones, rather than in the loud, high-pitched voice that is commonly used with the partially deaf. Teaching should not be done in situations where there is loud background noise such as a running faucet or a blaring television set; teaching done in a noisy outpatient clinic may be useless. It is important to arrange for a quiet environment free of extraneous noises and distractions. It is recommended that teachers frequently check to ascertain that the patient understands the instruction. Finally, it is important for both the elderly patient and his or her teacher to be aware that some confusion and misunderstanding may be caused by a change in auditory function, and is probably not a sign of declining intellectual ability.

Memory

Age-related changes in memory affect both the ability to learn and to examine and judge the new information (Botwinick 1978). Although current research on memory is complex and the results are often contradictory, some information is available to guide the nurse's assessment of the elderly patient's memory capacity, as well as to guide development of effective teaching and evaluation techniques.

Much of the recent research on memory in the elderly has been based on information-processing models, which use concepts of primary and secondary memories. When a person is presented with a list of words, it is theorized that the words at the end of the list are recalled from the primary memory, and the words at the beginning are from the secondary memory (Craik 1977). A decline in secondary memory has been documented in the elderly in comparison with younger adults (Botwinick 1978; Craik 1977). Because most health-care learning involves secondary memory, elderly patients are more likely to have learning difficulties. However, Hulicka and Weiss (1965) report that when older (60–72 yr) and younger (30–44 yr) people are trained to an equal level of learning, the elderly may require more trials to learn, but once having learned the material to the same degree as the younger persons, they recalled the material equally well. Thus, initial learning is important in memory retention for the elderly; and some elderly may still need multiple repetitions of a task before it is learned.

It is a widely accepted notion that although an elderly person performs poorly on tasks of recent memory, his or her memory for events in the remote past will be unimpaired. Botwinick (1978) and Craik (1977) have presented a different view. They suggest that persons of any age are better able to remember events in the remote past that are considered to be important and are frequently recalled. The implication of these findings for teaching elderly patients is that the material will be better learned and remembered if the patient considers it to be important, the material is salient, and its contents are rehearsed frequently.

Some researchers have demonstrated the existence of a greater age-related decrement in recall memory than in recognition memory (Botwinick 1978; Craik 1977). However, when elderly persons were required to recall basic information that was learned a long time before, such as the names of fruits, little or no age differences for recall were found (Drachman and Leavitt 1972). Thus, difficulties with recall memory seem to involve primarily newly learned materials, and these findings have important implications for the evaluation of learning in old age. Evaluating new learning with recall tests (*e.g.,* sentence completion or "filling in the blanks") may not test the elderly patient's knowledge effectively, and by creating embarrassment and frustration, for the patient, may result in termination of the teaching–learning task.

For some elderly patients a more effective technique for evaluating learning may be a recognition memory task. Such a task (*e.g.*, multiple-choice or true–false test) is easier than a recall task, in part because there are cues present in the questions. These cues help in the active memory search for the answer that is correct. Cues also can help in recall tasks. For example, after instruction on calcium-rich foods, an elderly patient is more likely to give a correct answer to a cued recall question ("Name one kind of dairy product that is a good source of calcium.") than to a free recall question ("Name one food that is a good source of calcium.").

For patients with poor memories, it is particularly helpful to reinforce verbal instructions with a complete set of written instructions. This is a good way to reinforce learning and assist memory retention. In addition, suitable memory aids may be used. For example, a number of approaches have been recommended to help the elderly remember to take their medication: (1) the use of color codes (Freeman 1974; Gimble 1967); (2) the use of calendar packaging similar to that used for oral contraceptives; and (3) calendar sheets that provide a space for the patient to check off each medication as it is taken (Gimble 1967; Vestal 1978). Repetition of instruction is necessary to ensure initial learning, and periodic review of the material is also important. These memory aids may be used in combination, depending on the needs of the patient.

Intelligence

The first studies on intelligence suggested that adult intelligence begins to decline at an early age. However, more recent studies have shown little, if any, change in intelligence until much later in life (Botwinick 1978). Eisdorfer (1977) suggests that the cognitive processing of information is affected by factors such as education-level, apprehension, cautiousness, health status, and social and occupational experiences, thus changing the results of intelligence tests.

Nurses cannot modify a patient's intelligence or previous educational and life experiences; they can, however, assess a patient's cognitive functions and knowledge before instruction and adjust learning materials accordingly. A patient's knowledge in an area can be tested before instruction by asking questions about the subject that will be taught. Several instruments can provide an objective assessment of elderly patients' cognitive functioning. Commonly used tests are the Mental Status Questionnaire (Kahn et al 1960), the Mini-Mental State Examination (Folstein et al 1975), the Short Portable Mental Status Questionnaire (Pfeiffer 1975), and the Cognitive Capacity Screening Examination (Jacobs et al 1977). These easy and quickly administered instruments are used as screening tests of cognitive impairment—specifically of disorientation, impairment of recent memory, and impairment of new learning (Gurland 1980), and provide an index of the relative severity of cognitive impairment. None, however, is precise enough to be used for clinical decisionmaking. Although tests of cognitive impairment have not yet been perfected, when they are used in conjunction with clinical observation and personal judgment, nurses will find them a valuable aid in the assessment of the cognitive function of elderly patients.

Teaching considerations

Botwinick (1978) has drawn a distinction between learning as an internal process and performance as an external act. He states that we see only the act, and from the observation make judgments about learning ability, but it is possible to make incorrect inferences because "what may have made for poor performance may not be learning ability as such but the noncognitive elements surrounding the act." Poor learning performance of the elderly can be the result of factors that inhibit learning and problems in the ability to give appropriate responses, as well as any actual decrease in the ability to learn.

Researchers have identified several noncognitive factors that influence learning: pacing, the meaningfulness of the task, task difficulty, overarousal of the autonomic nervous system, cautiousness, and health status.

Pacing: speed of instruction and response time

Pacing concerns the speed of instruction, as well as the response-time condition (Arenberg 1965; Calhoun and Gounard 1979; Canestrari 1963, 1968; Eisdorfer 1965; Eisdorfer et al 1963; Hulicka et al 1967; Monge and Hultsch 1971). A number of studies of both healthy and hospitalized elderly showed that elderly learners benefited from slow-paced and self-paced instruction. Instruction that was delivered at a slow pace (106 words per min) was more effective than that given at a normal pace (159 words per min) (Kim and Grier 1981). Allowing more time for responding also had a beneficial effect (Kim 1985, 1986). Self-paced responses (the patient takes as much time as needed) were superior to those given in either slow-paced or fast-paced response conditions. Under self-paced response conditions, the time taken by elderly persons to give the correct answer varied considerably from person to person (Botwinick and Thompson 1968; Kim 1985; Pierson and Montoye 1958). Some patients took about a half-second to give a correct answer to a nurse's question, whereas others needed as long as 31 seconds for the same question (Kim 1985). Interestingly, however, the elderly patients who took a longer time to respond to one type of task also tended to do so in other types of tasks (Kim 1985).

Thus, speed of instruction and response-time condition are important factors in learning by elderly patients, and these findings suggest that instruction should be delivered slowly, particularly when presenting new information. Elderly patients' learning performances are better when they can work at their own speed. Because the pace in clinical practice is hectic, the pressures on nurses' time may conflict with elderly patients' need to work slowly. Therefore, it is important for nurses to remember that some elderly patients need a longer response time. If rushed, their learning performance may be poor, even though they know the material.

Task meaningfulness and difficulty

Hulicka (1967) studied responses by the elderly on word tasks that varied in personal meaningfulness. On tasks that were less meaningful, 80% of the older people terminated the task, stating they would not exert themselves to learn "such nonsense." If the exercise is made more meaningful, the task is easier to complete, it will be carried out more willingly, and the elderly will do relatively well with it.

Motivation plays a particularly important role in health-care learning because elderly patients must not only understand and remember health-care information, but incorporate the new regimen into their daily lives. The more that elderly patients participate in their learning, the more meaningful the task will be, and the better the learning outcome. The patient's family can be a valuable resource, and whenever possible, health-care teaching should involve both the elderly patient and family and friends. If family members understand health-care instruction, and have a caring attitude, they can help the patient to learn to manage his or her own health care. Family members can also help to shape the content so that it is more relevant to the patient's lifestyle, and help the elderly family member practice the new behaviors.

Nurses can take other steps to increase meaningfulness and decrease task difficulty. For example, nurses can guide the setting of easily attainable, short-term goals so that learning can be satisfying and meaningful. Assessment of the patient's educational and experiential background can help to determine the suitability of teaching materials. One way to adjust instruction to the patient's comprehension level is to use terminology and examples that are familiar to the person (*e.g.,* define unfamiliar medical terms). It is important to remember that word meanings often change over time, and it is essential for the elderly patient and nurse to share common definitions.

Printed material, used in conjunction with personal instruction, is an important factor in patient teaching. Unfortunately, a number of studies have indicated that the reading level of health-education materials is beyond the comprehension of some elderly patients (Doak and Doak 1980; Mohammed 1964; Taylor et al 1982; Vivian and Robertson 1980). Several readability formulas are available for estimating the reading level of written materials (Dale and Chall 1948; Flesch 1948; Fry 1968; Gunning 1968; McLaughlin 1969). These tools evaluate reading difficulty by measuring factors such as vocabulary difficulty and sentence length, and they indicate the level of schooling required to be able to comprehend the material. These formulas can provide only a rough estimate of the readability level; however, they can be helpful in guiding the selection of appropriate reading materials.

Irrelevant information

Irrelevant, uninformative materials can confuse the elderly patient and slow learning performance. A number of researchers (Hoyer et al 1979; Rabbitt 1965) have found that ability to ignore irrelevant information decreases with age. Rabbitt (1965) compared the actions of elderly and younger adults when performing a task that was related to problem solving. As the number of irrelevant variables increased, the elderly subjects were slower in performing the task than were the younger subjects. This finding suggests that nurses should avoid irrelevant details when teaching, because some elderly persons have difficulty sorting the relevant from the irrelevant (*e.g.,* visual material should contain only essential content). Any content not directly related to the learning material should be omitted.

Autonomic arousal level

Arousal of anxiety in the learning situation also influences learning in elderly persons (Eisdorfer et al 1970; Whitebourne 1976). Eisdorfer and coworkers (1970) report that the elderly are more anxious in learning situations than younger adults. When propranolol was used to block the autonomic end-organ response, the elderly's performance in learning improved. The study concluded that the heightened autonomic arousal of elderly learners may be responsible for some of their performance deficits.

Whitebourne (1976) measured test anxiety in elderly persons and younger adult college students and found that the elderly learners had higher levels of debilitating test anxiety than younger students, and test anxiety was related to memory performance among both groups. Thus, he suggests that an elderly person's performance on a cognitive task may be partly affected by test anxiety. A nonthreatening learning and testing environment, plus a great deal of reassurance from the teacher, should help to decrease high levels of anxiety.

Cautiousness

Cautiousness is a variable that has been found to influence the elderly's performance in learning tasks. In risk-taking situations older persons are more cautious than are younger adults (Eisdorfer 1965; Okun and Di Vesta 1976; Treat and Reese 1976). Fear of being wrong or fear of failure may cause the elderly not to respond in a doubtful situation. Generally, cautiousness is regarded as beneficial to learning; however, in fast-paced learning, older people tend to withhold answers, and therefore, perform poorly by not fully demonstrating what they know (Canestrari 1963; Eisdorfer 1965; Eisdorfer 1963; Taub 1967). Nurses should stay aware of this tendency toward caution in elderly patients.

Health status

Alteration of the physical health of the elderly can adversely affect their learning. Spieth (1964) found that a group of highly intelligent adults with untreated hypertension performed less effectively on psychological tests than a group of medi-cally managed hypertensive patients. Eisdorfer (1977) has reported that intellec-tual decline is highly associated with elevated blood pressure levels. He suggests that the intellectual decline among the elderly that has been reported by many researchers may be related to the fact that at an older age more people have car-diovascular or cerebrovascular disease. Mental health also influences the cogni-tive functioning of a person. For example, depression often leads to cognitive impairment (Kahn and Miller 1978).

Nurses need to consider the patient's comfort and level of available energy. Persons who are ill may have a shortened attention span. Therefore, teaching sessions must not be so lengthy that the patient becomes fatigued or distracted. These factors are also important in the assessment of the learning outcome through testing. For example, fatigue and poor concentration, or an overly long test, may result in a poor performance and produce inaccurate measurements.

Mediational techniques

Mediational techniques aid learning and memory (Botwinick 1978). These tech-niques link mental pictures to the concept or words to be remembered. For exam-ple, an elderly patient could remember the name of her drug, Lasix, by picturing the image of "a bird *lay six* eggs." Hulicka and Grossman (1967) have reported that elderly people, unlike young people, tend not to use mediational techniques. When older subjects were instructed on these techniques, their learning im-proved. Treat and Reese (1976) found that the elderly benefited from generating their own (thus more meaningful) images instead of using those suggested by the experimenter. However, self-generated images were useful in testing situations only when sufficient time was allowed for the patient to respond, not when the pace of testing was rapid. These findings demonstrate the value of training the elderly to use mental images to aid learning and memory, and the need for them to use self-generated images.

Summary

Health-care teaching is an important role for nurses. Nurses spend a large part of their time helping patients to understand causes of health problems, measures to prevent complications from disease, and ways to maintain optimal health status. As the number of elderly patients who require health care increases (Brehm 1980), nurses can expect that even more time will be spent in teaching this popu-lation.

Health education for the elderly is complex and challenging because of the many interrelated factors that affect learning. Age-related changes in visual and auditory perception, memory, cognitive functioning, and health status can make learning more difficult. Other factors associated with teaching and evaluation such as pacing, meaningfulness of the task, relevance of the information, and use of mediational techniques can hinder learning if not used in a manner appropriate for the elderly. Psychological factors such as high arousal level and cautiousness affect the ability to learn. Understanding these relevant factors should help nurses to develop better teaching strategies for their elderly patients. Given favorable learning conditions, the elderly should be able to gain significantly through health-care learning.

References

Arenberg D: Anticipation interval and age differences in verbal learning. J Abnorm Psychol 70:419–425, 1965

Botwinick J: Aging and Behavior, 2nd ed, p 262. New York, Springer, 1978

Botwinick J, Thompson LW: A research note on individual differences in reaction time in relation to age. J Genet Psychol 112:73–75, 1968

Brehm HP: Organization and financing of health care for the aged: Future implications. In Haynes SG, Feinleib M (eds): Epidemiology of Aging, Report of United States Department of Health and Human Services, Public Health Service, Publication No. 80-969. Washington DC, National Institute of Health, 1980

Calearo C, Lazzaroni A: Speech intelligibility in relation to the speed of the message. Laryngoscope 67:410–419, 1957

Calhoun RO, Gounard BR: Meaningfulness, presentation rate, list length, and age in elderly adults' paired-associate learning. Educational Gerontol 4:49–56, 1979

Canestrari RE: Paced and self-paced learning in young and elderly adults. J Gerontol 18:165–168, 1963

Canestrari RE: Age changes in acquisition. In Talland GA (ed): Human Aging and Behavior. New York, Academic Press, 1968

Corso JF: Sensory processes and age effects in normal adults. J Gerontol 26:90–105, 1971

Corso JF: Sensory processes and man during maturity and senescence. Adv Behav Biol 16:119–143, 1975

Craik FIM: Age differences in human memory. In Birren JE, Schaie KW (eds): Handbook of the Psychology of Aging. New York, Van Nostrand Reinhold, 1977

Dale E, Chall JS: A formula for predicting readability: Instructions. Educational Research Bulletin 27(Jan 21, Feb 17):11–20, 37–54, 1948

Doak LG, Doak CD: Patient comprehension profiles: Recent findings and strategies. Patient Counseling and Health Education 2:101–106, 1980

Drachman DA, Leavitt J: Memory impairment in the aged: Storage versus retrieval deficit. J Exp Psychol 93:302–308, 1972

Eisdorfer C: Verbal learning and response time in the aged. J Genet Psychol 107:15–22, 1965

Eisdorfer C: Intelligence and cognition in the aged. In Busse EW, Pfeiffer E (eds): Behavior and Adaptation in Later Life, 2nd ed. Boston, Little, Brown & Co, 1977

Eisdorfer C, Axelrod S, Wilkie FL: Stimulus exposure time as a factor in serial learning in an aged sample. J Abnorm Soc Psychol 67:594–600, 1963

Eisdorfer C, Nowlin J, Wilkie F: Improvement of learning in the aged by modification of autonomic nervous system activity. Science 170:1327–1329, 1970

Flesch RF: A new readability yardstick. J Appl Psychol 32:221–233, 1948

Folstein MF, Folstein SE, McHugh PR: "Mini-Mental State' a practical method for grading the cognitive state of patients for the clinician. J Psychiatr Res 12:189–198, 1975

Fozard JL, Wolf E, Bell B et al: Visual perception and communication. In Birren JE, Schaie KW (eds): Handbook of the Psychology of Aging. New York, Van Nostrand Reinhold, 1977

Freeman JT: Some principles of medication in geriatrics. J Am Geriatr Soc 22:289–295, 1974

Fry E: A readability formula that saves time. J Reading 2:513–526, 575–578, 1968

Gimble JG: Oral medications and the older patient. ANA Regional Clinical Conferences. New York, Appleton-Century-Crofts, 1967

Gunning R: The Technique of Clear Writing. New York, McGraw-Hill, 1968

Gurland BJ: The assessment of the mental health status of older adults. In Birren JE, Sloane RB (eds): Handbook of Mental Health and Aging. Englewood Cliffs, New Jersey, Prentice Hall, 1980

Hoyer WJ, Rebok GW, Sved SM: Effects of varying irrelevant information on adult age differences in problem solving. J Gerontol 34:553–560, 1979

Hulicka IM: Age differences in retention as a function of interference. J Gerontol 22:180–184, 1967

Hulicka IM, Weiss RL: Age differences in retention as a function of learning. J Consult Psychol 29:125–129, 1965

Hulicka IM, Stern H, Grossman J: Age-group comparisons of paired-associate learning as a function of paced and self-paced association and response times. J Gerontol 22:274–280, 1967

Jacobs JW, Bernhard MR, Delgado A, Strain JJ: Screening for organic mental syndromes in the medically ill. Ann Intern Med 86:40–46, 1977

Kahn RL, Goldfarb AI, Pollack M, Peck A: Brief objective measures for the determination of mental status in the aged. Am J Psychiatry 117:326–328, 1960

Kahn RL, Miller NE: Assessment of altered brain function in the aged. In Storandt M, Siegler HC, Elias MF (eds): The Clinical Psychology and Aging. New York, Plenum, 1978

Kim KK: Health Care Learning as a Function of Response Time in the Institutionalized Elderly. Ph.D. dissertation, University of Illinois at Chicago, 1984. Dissertation Abstracts International 46:85–04979, 1985

Kim KK: Response time and health care learning of the elderly patients. Res Nurs Health 9:233–239, 1986

Kim KK, Grier MR: Pacing effects of medication instruction for the elderly. J Gerontol Nurs 7:464–468, 1981

Konkle DF, Beasley DS, Bess FH: Intelligibility of time-altered speech in relation to chronological aging. J Speech Hearing Res 20:108–115, 1977

Maurer JF, Rupp RR: Hearing and Aging. New York, Grune & Stratton, 1979

McLaughlin GH: SMOG-Grading—new readability formula. J Reading 12:639–646, 1969

Mohammed MFB: Patients' understanding of written health information. Nurs Res 13:100–108, 1964

Monge RH, Hultsch DF: Paired-associate learning as a function of adult age and the length of the anticipation and inspection intervals. J Gerontol 26:157–162, 1971

Okun MA, Di Vesta FJ: Cautiousness in adulthood as a function of age and instructions. J Gerontol 31:571–576, 1976

Pfeiffer E: A short portable mental status questionnaire for the assessment of organic brain deficit in elderly patients. J Am Geriatr Soc 23:433–441, 1975

Pierson WR, Montoye HJ: Movement time, reaction time, and age. J Gerontol 13:418–421, 1958

Rabbitt P: An age-decrement in the ability to ignore irrelevant information. J Gerontol 20:233–238, 1965

Spieth W: Cardiovascular health status, age, and psychological performance. J Gerontol 19:277–284, 1964

Taub HA: Paired associates learning as a function of age, rate, and instructions. J Genet Psychol 111:41–46, 1967

Taylor AG, Skelton JA, Czajkowski RW: Do patients understand patient-education brochures? Nurs Health Care 3:305–310, 1982

Treat NJ, Reese HW: Age, pacing, and imagery in paired associate learning. Dev Psychol 12:119–124, 1976

Vestal RE: Drug use in the elderly: A review of problems and special considerations. Drugs 16:358–382, 1978

Vivian AS, Robertson EJ II: Readability of patient educational materials. Clin Therapeutics 3:129–136, 1980

Whitebourne SK: Test anxiety in elderly and young adults. International J Aging Hum Dev 7:201–210, 1976

Mildred Hogstel

Integumentary system

4

The skin, glands, hair, and nails rarely cause life-threatening problems for the elderly patient. Problems in the integumentary system, however, can cause severe physical discomfort and decreased self-esteem because changes and problems are so easily seen by others. As Kligman and co-workers (1985) state, ". . . the skin is a powerful organ of nonverbal communication. We estimate age, personality, status, race, and health merely by looking." Problems occurring in the skin, glands, or nails often cause discomforts and complications that can affect the total person. The nurse who cares for elderly patients is responsible for being knowledgeable about age-related changes of the integumentary system, how to assess changes, how to prevent possible problems, and how to care for abnormal conditions.

Age-related changes

All persons age at different rates, and the organs within a person age differently. Some age-related changes, however, are fairly common. According to Kligman and coworkers, 66% of persons over 70 years of age have skin problems. Of this group, 33% have three or more problems. They also note that "poverty and poor skin go together" (1985). It is important to understand the changes that occur in the skin, glands, hair, and nails during the aging process; and nursing care must be adjusted to those changes.

Skin and glands

Skin changes are probably the most apparent because the skin is the largest organ of the body and a large part of it is easily observable (*e.g.,* the face, hands, arms, and legs). The most common overall changes that occur are listed below.

Wrinkling of the skin, especially the face and neck

Thinning of the epithelial layer

Decreasing moisture, causing drying

Decreasing density, increasing rigidity, causing skin to be less flexible

Sagging of face, eyelids, ears, and jowls as a result of gravitational pull

Decreasing amount of subcutaneous fat

Decreasing activity of apocrine sweat glands (Oppeneer and Vervoren 1983)

Wrinkling, drying, thinning

The skin wrinkles during the aging process because collagenous fibers in the dermis become more stable and less flexible, because elastic fibers may fray with continued stress, and because the fluid content of the skin decreases, causing the skin to lose its elasticity and resiliency (Landau 1986). There is no specific treatment for wrinkles. Commercial products, although highly advertised, do not reduce wrinkling. Surgery will help and may be needed more than once.

The skin of women is thinner than that of men and therefore deteriorates more readily with aging (Kligman et al 1985). In a very thin 90-year-old woman, the size and position of the superficial blood vessels, bones, and ligaments can be seen through what appears to be paper-thin skin. The nurse must take special precautions to avoid traumatizing and bruising the skin while giving care to this type of patient.

Severe itching is a common result of dry skin. Pruritis is uncomfortable, painful, irritating, and it interferes with sleep. Itching usually causes scratching, which can easily introduce a bacterial infection (Kligman et al 1985), particularly if the patient's fingernails are long and soiled with food or feces. Scratching can further irritate other existing skin conditions such as a mole, wart, or skin cancer and can cause bleeding and additional skin damage. Drying the skin with a rough (Turkish) towel increases itching by stimulating the sensory nerve endings (Oppeneer and Vervoren 1983). The nurse must also determine if the itching is caused by food or drug allergies, or drug side-effects. Fissures of the heels, a very painful condition, can occur as a result of dry skin and sheet burn, and create the possibility of infection. A variety of nursing measures are available to soothe dry skin (see Nursing Care Plans, #1).

Subcutaneous tissue atrophies with age, primarily affecting the face, extremities, hands, and soles of the feet. Because subcutaneous tissue acts as a "shock absorber against trauma," these areas are more susceptible to trauma; the soles of aged persons lack subcutaneous fat, thus increasing the trauma of walking and magnifying the many foot problems of the aged (Kligman et al 1985). Kligman and coworkers (1985) described subcutaneous tissue as a "high calorie storage depot" that modulates conductive heat loss. Thus, elderly persons who lose substantial subcutaneous tissue are more prone to the dangers of hypothermia.

The skin is also less flexible because the collagen, a fibrous, insoluble protein in connective tissue, stiffens with age and causes tissue to lose its elasticity. The skin tissue of elderly patients does not "bounce back" like that of the young person. Because of this decreased skin flexibility and gravitational pull, conjunctivitis may occur when the lower eyelids droop and the eyes become dry. The ear lobes can be affected if heavy earrings have been worn regularly for years. The ear lobe often hangs up to 2 inches below the lower rim of ear cartilage. Sudden or severe loss of weight causes sagging of skin of the abdomen and arms, a problem related more to appearance than function.

Decreased gland secretion

Many factors cause the skin to become less moist with increasing age. The most important causes are presented here: (1) decreased secretion of sebum from the sebaceous glands, which normally provides a protective lipid film that retards evaporation from the stratum corneum; (2) thinned skin that causes moisture to escape; (3) decreased oral fluid intake; (4) inadequate nutrition; (5) long exposure to the sun; (6) low humidity (25%–40%); (7) harsh soaps; and (8) frequent hot baths (Kligman et al 1985; Oppeneer and Vervoren 1983).

Because of the decreased function of the apocrine glands, elderly persons perspire less. Women are especially likely to have less apocrine sweating in old age because of the decrease in androgen production after menopause. The elderly have less body odor from perspiration and have less need for deodorants; however, they are also at greater risk for hyperthermia during hot weather because they lose less heat through the evaporative process of sweating (Kligman et al 1985).

Decreased sensation for heat, cold, and pain

Because of decreased activity of the peripheral nerve receptors, the elderly often do not perceive and react to peripheral heat, cold, and pain stimulation as quickly nor as deeply as do younger persons (Potter and Perry 1985). For this reason, they are especially at high risk for injury from devices that are used to apply heat and cold for therapeutic reasons. They cannot monitor the amount of heat or cold produced and may not remove the treatment devices in time to prevent injury to the skin. Special precautions should be taken when applying heat and cold devices to elderly patients, especially those who have any type of peripheral vascular disease such as diabetes or arteriosclerosis, those who have had a cerebrovascular accident, and those who might have decreased peripheral sensation for any reason (see Nursing Care Plans, #2).

Senile lentigo

Senile lentigines are commonly called "age" or "liver spots," although they have no relationship to the liver. They are small, irregular-shaped light-brown patches that occur on the skin of both sexes, most frequently on the back of hands, forearms, and face. Various types of special creams and lotions will cover them temporarily, but will not remove them.

Seborrheic keratoses

Seborrheic keratoses are small, raised, flesh to dark pigmented and greasy lesions that occur mostly on the chest, back, face, and scalp (Oppeneer and Vervoren 1983). Sometimes they are round or oval in shape, and warty in texture. They are not caused by the sun and the degree of pigmentation increases with age. They may measure an inch or more in diameter and appear unattractive, but are considered to be harmless.

Actinic keratoses

Actinic keratoses are scaly lesions that range in color from yellow to brown and black. They have an irregular surface with sharp borders (Anders and Leech 1983). They may be scaling and red, and appear on areas that are exposed to sunlight (*e.g.,* scalp, ears; Malasanos 1986). They are considered to be premalignant, increase with age, and may lead to squamous cell carcinoma (Collier 1983a).

Acrochordons

Acrochordons are small flesh-colored skin tags that appear on the neck, trunk, axilla, and groin. They are harmless but can be removed for cosmetic reasons if desired (Oppeneer and Vervoren 1983).

Hair

The most common age-related changes of the hair are a decrease in the amount of body hair, and an increase in facial hair.

Alopecia or balding occurs most often on the vertex and frontal areas of men. Both graying and balding are inherited; the hair begins to turn gray at about age 40 (owing to decreased amounts of melanin) and thinning of the hair occurs about age 65. Traumatic marginal alopecia in black women is "caused by the use of hair curlers, Afro picks and from tight braiding" over a period of many years (Am J Nurs, 1979). Alopecia and hirsutism generally appear at the same age. Dark-haired women age 65 and over begin to grow dark, thick hair on their lips and chin; men have an increased amount of coarse, long hair on the lobes and rims of their ears, nostrils, and eyebrows. Both men and women in this age group have decreased body hair and loss of pubic and axillary hair as a result of hormonal changes (Kligman et al 1985; Oppeneer and Vervoren 1983).

Most of these changes of the hair have social significance, not functional, so there is no specific treatment or care except that hair colorings and conditioners may be used to change the person's appearance. To conceal hair loss, toupees and wigs are commonly worn, and hair transplants are another option. There is currently some experimentation with drugs that may help to grow hair. For the patient who needs assistance with daily grooming, the nurse should assist the female patient to remove unwanted hairs from the face (Hogstel 1983) and help the male patient trim long hairs on the ears, nostrils, and eyebrows.

Nails

With increasing age, the fingernails and toenails become hard, thick, and brittle. Thickening or hypertrophy of the nails is caused by trauma, psoriasis, fungal infections, and defective vascular supply. Brittleness is caused by anemia and decreased peripheral circulation. Nails grow about 0.1 mm to 1 mm per day, although growth slows with aging. It takes about 170 days for the full growth of a fingernail and one to one and a half years for a toenail (Malasanos 1986). The toenails especially become hypertrophied, opaque, and scaly, and are particularly prone to onychomycosis and infection.

Onychomycosis is a fungal infection that causes a thick, scaly substance to collect between the top of the toenail and the skin. It is difficult to treat, but causes no major problems except that it makes cutting and cleaning of the nails more difficult. If the patient cannot safely trim his or her fingernails, the nurse should do so about every two or three weeks. The nails should be cleaned daily, preferably soaked in warm water with the use of a superfatted soap to prevent further drying of the skin.

For several reasons many elderly people, especially those in their 80s and 90s, will not be able to trim their own toenails. They may not be able to reach their feet, may not see well, may be unable to manipulate scissors or clippers because of arthritic hands, and may have difficulty because of the extreme thickness of their nails. In many cases, the nurse also will not be able to trim the toenails because of difficulty cutting the nails with regular scissors or clippers. The patient should be referred to a podiatrist for safe and adequate trimming of the toenails.

Major skin problems

More severe and dangerous skin conditions that can occur in the elderly are

Pressure ulcers (decubitus ulcers)

Herpes zoster (shingles)

Basal cell carcinoma

Squamous cell carcinoma

Pressure ulcers

The prevention of *decubitus ulcers* is one of the basic components of nursing care of the immobile or partially immobile elderly patient. *"Decubitus"* is derived from a Latin word meaning "a lying down;" however, because decubitus ulcers can occur when patients are in other positions (*e.g.,* sitting in wheelchairs) the term *pressure sores* describes this condition more accurately (Phipps et al 1984). Ulcers or sores occur because increased pressure on the skin decreases circulation to the area, thus providing less oxygen and nutrition to the cells, preventing the elimination of waste products from the tissue, and causing the cells to die.

Destruction of the skin proceeds through several specific stages. Table 4-1 presents one method of describing ulcer staging.

Jones and Millman (1986) identified seven stages of pressure ulcer formation as follows:

* Stage 0:   skin intact; no pressure sore
* Stage I: skin red, blue, blistered
* Stage II: epidermal or dermal abrasion
* Stage III: subcutaneous tissue exposed
* Stage IV: muscle exposed
* Stage V: bone exposed
* Stage VI: unable to stage (sore covered with eschar)

Table 4-1. *Stages of pressure ulcer development*

Stage	Appearance
I	Skin is red and unbroken Redness disappears when pressure is relieved
II	Epidermis is broken Areas of redness, heat, induration Drainage may be present Pain may be present
III	Break in dermis and subcutaneous tissue, increasing depth of wound Drainage may be present Pain may be present Hard eschar or necrotic tissue present over wound
IV	Break through all of skin tissue, perhaps into muscle and bone Skin necrosis Drainage May be painful

(Phipps M et al: Staging care for pressure sores. Am J Nurs 84:999, 1984)

There are many predisposing causes of pressure ulcers. The more of these factors that are present, the greater the chance for the development of ulcers (Figure 4-1 and Table 4-2). The most common causes are

Immobility (in bed or chair)

Increased pressure against skin

Shearing force

Moisture, especially perspiration, urine, and feces

Wrinkled linen or clothing

Foreign objects between the patient and the bed or chair (for example, catheter tubing)

Poor nutrition, especially lack of protein and vitamins

Poor circulation because of disease (*e.g.,* diabetes and cardiovascular problems)

Table 4-2. **Assessment guide for risk of pressure ulcers**

Parameters	0	1	2	3	Score
General state of health	Good	Fair	Poor	Moribund	
Mental status	Alert	Lethargic	Semicomatose	Comatose	
			Count these conditions as double:		
Activity	Ambulatory	Needs help	Chairfast	Bedfast	
Mobility	Full	Limited	Very limited	Immobile	
Incontinence	None	Occasional	Usually of urine	Total of urine and feces	
			Usually of stools	Only of feces	
Oral nutrition intake	Good	Fair	Poor	None	
Oral fluid intake	Good	Fair	Poor	None	
Predisposing (diabetes, neuropathies, vascular disease, anemias, fever, infection, dehydration)	Absent	Slight	Moderate	Severe	

The higher the score, the greater is the potential to develop decubitus ulcers. Patients with scores above (12) should be considered at risk.
(Prepared for use at the VA Medical Center, New Orleans, Louisiana)

Weekly Pressure Ulcer Record

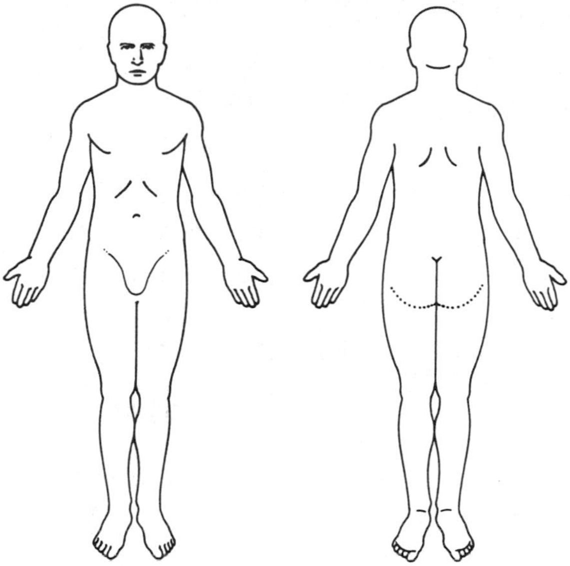

Stage I: Inflammation or redness of the skin

Stage II: Superficial skin break with redness of surrounding area

State III: Skin break with deep tissue involvement

Stage IV: Skin break with deep tissue involvement with necrotic tissue present, extending to muscle and bone

Location of skin breakdown: _____   Stage: _____

Date	Site	Size	Description (color, appearance, presence of exudate)	Odor if present	Physician notified (when)	Nurse's initials

Figure 4-1. Chart for keeping weekly record of development of pressure ulcers. (VA Medical Center, New Orleans, Louisiana)

The most common sites for pressure ulcers to occur are over the bony prominences.

The most important preventive nursing interventions include

Turning frequently (at least every two hours)

No * Gently massaging skin, especially around high-risk sites

Keeping skin dry and clean

Keeping a tight, well-made bed (free of wrinkles and foreign objects)

Adding a small amount of cornstarch on linens to facilitate movement

Maintaining a well-balanced nutritious diet (especially vitamins A and C, and protein)

Using sheepskin (decreases pressure and helps keep skin dry)

Using an egg-crate foam rubber mattress

Using a flotation mattress (with a soft gel consistency)

Using various types of electronic beds and devices (such as Stryker frame, CirColectric bed, Clinitron bed, Mediscus bed, water bed, sand bed) that help to relieve the pressure on the skin.

The most helpful preventive program in any institution is one that is specific, thoroughly known, and implemented by staff members. The work of preventing pressure ulcers cannot be a "hit or miss" activity. All staff members must work at prevention every day. According to Fowler (1985), "The most critical factor in prevention of skin breakdown is assessing the patient and determining the at-risk potential." Fowler suggests that all patients in acute-care, longterm-care, or home-health agencies be assessed upon admission on six variables: general physical condition, level of consciousness, activity, mobility, incontinence, and nutrition. A sample regimen or plan of prevention might be to take the actions presented below:

- Assess all patients and identify those who are high-risk (*e.g.*, those who are immobile, incontinent, and do not eat a sufficient amount of nutritious food)
- Carefully assess the skin of all patients upon admission
- Develop a position-change schedule for each immobile patient and ensure that staff on all shifts know it and follow it (*e.g.*, 8:00 am—back; 10:00 am—right side; 12:00 noon—prone; 1:00 pm—left side)
- Assess high-risk sites on high-risk patients every day
- Assess nutritional needs and plan a diet that includes all essential nutrients for high-risk patients
- Document any skin changes in high-risk patients every day, measuring and describing sites that are undergoing change (Phipps et al 1984)

Numerous products have been developed and used in the treatment of superficial pressure ulcers (Ahmed 1982). Generally, as Jones and Millman (1986) state, "use is based on personal preferences learned through clinical experience, on product availability, and on maintenance practicality requirements." Once pressure ulcers reach Stage III or IV, however, they are very difficult, if not impossible, to cure. Some traditional forms of treatment are

Cleansing with hydrogen peroxide or a mixture of hydrogen peroxide and normal saline

Whirlpool baths to prevent infection and stimulate healing

Ointments containing vitamins A and D, aloe vera, or antibiotics

Enzyme sprays

Granulated sugar

High concentrations of oxygen

Debridement

Skin grafts

Jones and Millman (1986) have proposed a systematic process of preventing and treating pressure ulcers; their recommendations include: (1) staging the ulcer; (2) assessing the specific cause of skin breakdown in high-risk patients; (3) applying a specific protocol based on the stage of the ulcer; (4) reassessing the skin status at least weekly; and (5) evaluating the effectiveness of the procedures.

Careful continuing documentation of preventive measures (turning schedule, skin hygiene, and nutrition intake), and evaluation of changes in the ulcers are essential. The condition of the ulcer should be recorded according to stage, site, size, edema, warmth, color, odor, eschar, slough, drainage, surrounding skin" (Jones and Millman 1986).

Herpes zoster

Herpes zoster (commonly called *shingles*) is a very uncomfortable skin condition that is caused by the varicella-zoster virus, the same virus that causes chicken pox. In fact, in order to develop herpes zoster a person must have had chicken pox already, probably because the organisms have remained dormant in the spinal ganglia or cranial nerve ganglia since the original varicella infection (Innes 1986). Herpes zoster is potentially contagious to anyone who has not had varicella or who is immunosuppressed (Collier 1983). It especially occurs in elderly persons whose immune systems have become less competent (Innes 1986). Herpes zoster can be very uncomfortable; the disease tends to be more troublesome in the elderly; healing is slower and complications are frequent and severe (Hallel 1985). In the elderly patient, the condition can last for more than a year.

The most common symptoms are fever, malaise, pain, burning, and tingling two to five days before a red rash occurs (Hallel 1985); the rash usually appears over some area of the trunk although it may occur over most of the body. The lesions tend to occur in a bandlike pattern along a dermatome, most frequently unilaterally on the thorax or face (Innes 1986). About 24 hours after the rash appears, vesicles with clear fluid develop. These vesicular eruptions occur along the distribution of the nerves from one or more posterior ganglia (Brunner and Suddarth 1986). About the third day the vesicles become pustules, which dry up in about five to ten days and form crusts that remain for about three weeks (Hallal 1985).

The major types of treatment and goals of care are

Analgesics and corticosteroids to relieve pain

Sedatives to reduce anxiety and increase rest and sleep

Antibiotics to reduce inflammation

Cool skin compresses for comfort

Creams applied to the rash

Dressings during the pustule stage

Decreased activity

Increased rest

Increased fluids

Cleanliness of skin and nails to prevent further infection (Hallal 1985)

Protection of the skin from friction and additional trauma

Wound and skin precautions (to prevent spread of organisms from drainage of lesions)

Basal cell carcinoma

Basal cell carcinoma is the most common and least dangerous kind of skin cancer. It can occur on the trunk and extremities, but most often is found on the face and areas that are frequently exposed to sunlight. Fair-skinned persons in their 60s, 70s, and 80s who have had extended exposure to the sun during their lifetimes are especially likely to develop this condition. The nurse should recognize when older patients fit this high-risk group and carefully assess their face and hands for sores that persist for several weeks without healing (Oppeneer and Vervoren 1983). The affected area may appear waxy and shiny, then ulcerated, and possibly bleed. This type of skin cancer can be removed fairly easily by curettage and cautery, surgical excision, radiation, and topical chemotherapy (Innes 1986).

Squamous cell carcinoma

Squamous cell carcinoma occurs less frequently and is more dangerous than basal cell carcinoma. The most common sites are the mucous membranes of the mouth and lips (owing to irritation from dentures and pipe smoking), the back of the hands, and areas that have been exposed to radiation or chronic infection. These lesions grow slowly, rarely metastasize, and they are usually removed through wide surgical excision (Innes 1986).

As was advised for basal cell carcinoma, the nurse should carefully assess the skin of older persons and refer patients to a dermatologist if a suspicious lesion changes in color or size and does not heal.

Assessment parameters

To determine specific nursing diagnoses of the integumentary system, the nurse must complete a thorough assessment, including nursing history and physical assessment. If the patient is being admitted to a hospital or nursing home, a careful assessment is especially important to determine the exact condition of the skin, establishing baseline data so that changes can be monitored and evaluated.

Nursing history

The most important parts of the nursing history that relate to the integumentary system are as follows

> Medical history
> Family history
> Drug history
> Diet history
> Sociocultural and environmental history

Medical history

It is necessary to determine if the patient has had prior problems of the integumentary system. Although the format of the history form will vary from institution to institution, some questions that should always be asked are

- Have you ever had any kind of problems of the skin before? If so, what sort of problems? When did they occur?
- Do you have any "unusual" or "ugly" moles? (Fraser and McGuire 1984)
- Have you ever been treated by a dermatologist or podiatrist? If so, for what reason? When?

- Have you had any kind of traumatic injuries to the skin, scalp, or nails? If so, what were they? When did they occur?
- Have you ever had any kind of surgery? If so, what type? When?
- Have you ever had problems with hair loss?
- Have you ever had an infection around the fingernails or toenails?
- Have you ever had any of the following conditions?
    Diabetes
    Decreased circulation
    Allergies
    Cancer

Family history

Areas related to family history that should be explored are

- Have any of your family ever had any of the following conditions? If so, who? When?
    Diabetes
    Blood problems (circulatory)
    Allergies
    Cancer (Collier 1983)

Diabetes, circulatory problems, allergies, and certain types of cancer have a familial tendency. Diabetes and circulatory problems can decrease the circulation to the skin of the lower extremities, causing the possibility of ulceration and infection. Meticulous foot care and toenail care is especially important if there is a possibility that either one of these conditions exists.

If the cause of skin allergic reactions is known in a family member, the same cause should be considered in the patient. It is also helpful to determine if a family member has had skin cancer in the specific location of the body at which it occurred.

Drug history

The following questions should be asked of the patient:

- What medicines are you currently taking? How much? When?
- Have you ever had any allergic reactions to medicines that affected the skin, hair, or nails?

Most unexpected drug reactions of the skin are minor, causing redness, rash, and itching, and disappearing when the drug has been discontinued. Some skin and hair reactions, however, are expected and severe. For example, many drugs used to treat cancer will cause loss of hair and discoloration of the skin.

Diet history

A well-balanced diet, and vitamins A, B, and C in particular, are important in maintaining normal integrity of the skin and mucous membranes. The foods listed below, which provide these vitamins, tend to be inadequate in the diets of older persons (Ebersole and Hess 1985). To assess a diet history, the following questions should be asked:

- Tell me about your appetite.
- Do you eat a well-balanced diet every day?
- Do you use dentures? How do they fit?
- Which of the following foods do you eat once or more a week?
  Vitamin A: carrots? squash? sweet potatoes? cantaloupe? spinach? greens? broccoli?
  Vitamin B: liver? vegetables? nuts? dried beans? peas? bran? whole grains? bananas? raisins?
  Vitamin C: oranges? lemons? tomatoes? grapefruit? strawberries? cabbage? baked potatoes?

Sociocultural and environmental history

Additional data that should be obtained in the nursing history include

- How often do you bathe?
- Do you usually take a shower or a tub bath?
- What kinds of soap do you use?
- Has the use of any specific cosmetic caused you any problems?
- Do you use any kind of lotions or creams on your skin? If so, what kind? How often?
- What kind of work do you do?
- Are you or have you been exposed to any kind of chemicals or radiation?
- About how many hours a day are you exposed to the sun?
- Have you been exposed to any harmful plants, such as poison ivy, or been bitten by any insects or ants?
- What kinds of shampoos, conditioners, rinses, tints, or dyes do you use on your hair?
- Do you use brush rollers? Blow dryers? Curling irons?
- Are you able to trim your own fingernails or toenails? If not, who does it for you?
- Do you wear shoes that do not fit well?

Many skin problems are caused by longterm, excessive exposure to harsh soaps, chemicals, wind, and sun. Harsh shampoos, tints, dyes, and certain mechanical devices that dry or curl the hair can contribute to hair loss.

Physical assessment

After the nursing history has been completed, it is important to assess systematically the patient's skin, hair, and nails by means of general observation, inspection, palpation, olfaction, and mensuration.

General observation

General observation means the overall observation of the client. It includes such factors as

Amount of skin exposed by clothing

General color of the skin

Any obvious abnormalities such as a skin condition that has distorted the shape of the face, head, ears, or extremities

Clothing that is intended to hide obvious abnormalities such as a wig, scarf around the head or neck, long-sleeved shirt, or long pants

Amount and grooming of the hair

Length and cleanliness of fingernails

Limping that could be caused by an infected toe

Inspection

The nurse moves from the general to the specific and inspects the exposed skin carefully, in a systematic manner so that no area is missed. The skin should be observed closely as each part of the total physical examination proceeds. For example, the nurse will assess the skin of the face while inspecting the eyes, ears, nose, and mouth. The hair and scalp will be assessed while inspecting the head, and the skin of the hands and arms will be assessed while taking the pulse and blood pressure. It is important to examine carefully the backs of caucasian males patients and the legs of caucasian female patients. With patients of other races, the nurse should be sure to observe the palms of the hands and the soles of the feet (Fraser and McGuire 1984). Specific points to note in inspection of the integumentary system are presented in Table 4-3.

Artificial light tends to distort skin color; any wattage less than a 100-watt lightbulb or fluorescent lighting will have an effect. Blue, yellow, or green walls, clothing, or sheets are also causes of skin color distortion. Indirect, natural, non-glare sunlight is best for inspection of the skin (Malasanos 1986), and it is always good to keep shades and curtains open in order to have as much sunlight as possible. A good penlight may be needed to observe the skin in areas that are not easily viewed, such as the genital and anal regions. A magnifying glass is helpful in visualizing the details of small skin lesions and other abnormalities. Also, it is important to use the principle of symmetry, comparing the color of one side of

Table 4-3. **Inspection of the integumentary system**

Criteria	Variations	Explanation or possible cause
Skin		
Color	White	Low pigment; genetic
	Pink	Infrequent exposure to sun; genetic
	Tan	Exposure to sun
	Bronze	Longterm exposure to sun
	Brown, black	High melanin, genetic
	Vitiligo	Areas of depigmentation
	Yellow	High carotene due to diet; jaundice; genetic; liver disease
	Dark, dusky, blue	High CO_2; $\downarrow$ 0, cold environment
	Bluish red	Low hemoglobin
	Bluish purple	Poor circulation
	Pale, pallor	Edema; low red blood cell count; anemia; shock
	Blanched	Edema
	Red, ruddy	High body temperature; embarrassment; infection; alcohol intake
	Gray	Malignancy, anemia, cachectic
General appearance	Translucent	Thinning of skin
Hair		
Amount	Full	Heredity; good nutrition
	Thick	Heredity
	Long	Preference; habit
	Thin	Heredity
	Sparse	Increasing age
	Short	Preference; convenience
	Absence	Infection; drugs; heredity
Distribution	Head	
	Face	Increases in women with age
	Axilla	Decreases with age
	Chest	Decreases with age
	Pubic	Decreases with age
Color	Blonde	
	Brunette	
	Gray	Decrease in melanocytes; heredity
	Red	
	Blue	Tinted; drugs
	Yellow	Sun exposure
Nails		
Length	Bitten, chewed	Anxiety
	Even with fingertips	
	Long	Preference

(continued)

Table 4-3. (*Continued*)

Criteria	Variations	Explanation or possible cause
	Long and curved	Inadequate grooming
	Cut straight across	
	Thick	Increased keratosis
Color	White	Low hemoglobin; anemia
	Pink	
	Blue	High CO; $\downarrow$ 0
	Yellow	Cigarette or pipe smoking
Grooming	Clean	Normal
	Dirty	Emotional depression
	Chipped polish	Poor eyesight

Skin

Temperature	Cold	Hypothermia; environment
	Cool	Normal
	Warm	Anxiety; embarrassment
	Hot	Fever
Texture	Soft	
	Smooth	Normal
	Leathery	Longterm sun exposure; increasing age
	Rough	Inadequate vitamins A and C
	Coarse	Longterm sun exposure, inadequate diet
	Flaky	Increased dryness from loss of secretions from sweat and sebaceous glands; low humidity in air
Moisture	Dry	Low humidity in air
	Moist, damp	Pain, anxiety
	Saturated	High body temperature
	Clammy	Pain, shock, nausea or vomiting
	Oily	Heredity; infrequent bathing
Turgor	Full	
	Flexible	
	Elastic	
	Supple	
	Resilient	
	Pliable	
	Peaking	
	Bouncy	
	Sluggish	Increasing age; dehydration; malnutrition
	Tented	Increasing age; dehydration; malnutrition

Hair

Texture	Fine	Increasing age
	Coarse	Heredity
	Brittle	Inadequate diet, especially of vitamins

(*continued*)

Table 4-3. (Continued)

Criteria	Variations	Explanation or possible cause
	Rough	Inadequate diet
	Dry	
	Oily	Lack of adequate shampooing; application of oil or vaseline
	Curly	Genetic; permanent-waving
Nails		
Texture	Soft	
	Hard	Increasing age
	Brittle	Increasing age
	Rigid	Increasing age, inadequate diet

the face with that of the other side of the face and one arm with the other arm, and so forth. Every abnormal lesion should be assessed for: color, anatomic distribution, configuration (pattern), and morphology (measurement) (Pfister and Bruno 1986).

Palpation

The second technique used in the physical assessment of the integumentary system is the use of palpation.

Skin. The fingertip pads should be used for palpation because their sensitivity best allows assessment of skin changes. The back of the hand or the inner aspect of the arm should be used to feel for temperature changes because these areas have more heat and cold superficial nerve receptors than the palm of the hand. The skin must be felt in order to determine its texture, whether it is smooth, rough, or flaky.

Excessive moisture or dryness may be obvious by visual inspection. Palpation, however, will be needed to assess the presence of mild degrees of moisture, clammy, or oily skin.

Turgor is assessed by pinching the skin slightly to determine its flexibility or pliability. The best location for testing skin turgor is over the sternum where subcutaneous tissue is minimal (Pfister and Brune 1986). This principle is especially true for the elderly because of their loss of skin elasticity. Table 4-3 outlines the classifications used in skin palpation.

Hair. Body hair can be inspected for amount, distribution, and color; however, hair growth on the scalp should be palpated for texture. A small amount of hair can be felt between the thumb and first finger to determine if the strands are fine or coarse, dry or oily, rough, brittle, or curly. These characteristics, with their possible causes, are listed in Table 4-3.

Nails.   Palpation of the nails consists of feeling them for texture. The normal age-related changes—the nails are hard, brittle, and rigid—are almost universal in the very old, especially in persons over 85 years of age. These characteristics and other possible causes are listed in Table 4-3.

Olfaction

The most obvious odors of the skin, hair, and nails are probably caused by inadequate cleansing. Because the apocrine sweat glands do not function well in old age, perspiration is diminished and, therefore, body odor from perspiration is not a major problem. There may, however, be body odor from food spilled upon the clothes, and urinary or bowel incontinence.

Infections of the skin or nails will produce odor, especially if there is a purulent drainage. When doing the total assessment, the nurse needs to be alert to any change in odor about the patient.

Mensuration (anthropometry)

Any lesions, marks, scars, sores, or other obvious abnormalities of the skin should be measured in centimeters (one inch = 2.54 centimeters), preferably with a clear, metric ruler.

Laboratory tests

Relatively few laboratory tests are used in the diagnosis of problems of the integumentary system because the history and physical assessment are most effective tools for these diagnoses. Table 4-4 summarizes some tests that are useful.

Table 4-4. **Diagnostic procedures**

Area	*Test*	*Rationale*
Skin	Biopsy and microscopic examination of tissue	Determine type of lesion
	Culture and sensitivity examination of drainage	Determine causative organism
	Wood's light test	Determine spore-producing microorganisms

Drugs

Table 4-5 details information about drugs that are used to treat conditions affecting the integumentary system.

Table 4-5. **Drugs used in the treatment of specific conditions affecting the integumentary system**

Drugs	Therapeutic response in elderly	Nursing implications
Hydrogen peroxide/normal saline mixture (half and half)	Effective cleansing agents for pressure ulcers and infected skin lesions. May cause some tingling discomfort on application.	As long as there is effervescence, there is no great destruction of bacteria because organic matter decomposes the solution. Store in a tightly sealed glass jar in a dark place.
Povidone-iodine (Betadine)	Can be irritating to thin, dry, fragile skin.	Used to clean skin, except on infected area.
Modified Dakin's solution (chlorine solution)	Effective, cleansing agent for infected skin ulcers. May cause bleeding because it dissolves clots.	May be diluted and used to irrigate wounds. Use only fresh solutions and store in dark bottles.
Acetic acid	Effective if pseudomonas is present. Could cause local skin irritation.	Vinegar contains 4% to 6% of this acid and is sometimes used as an antiinfective.
Tincture of benzoin	Acts as a skin barrier in prevention of ulcers but may irrigate aging skin.	Use sparingly.
Polymyxin B-bacitracin (Polysporin Ointment)	Effective as an antibiotic on minor skin infections. Available as an over-the-counter medication. Safe on aging skin. Less absorbable antibiotic.	Do not use if allergic to bacitracin.
Triamcinolone acetonide (Kenalog)	Low potency topical corticosteroid gives relief and promotes healing in herpes zoster.	If covered with an occlusive dressing, greater likelihood of toxic reaction in patients with impaired hepatic function. Assess for sensitivity to steroids. Apply with applicator or gloved hand.

(continued)

Table 4-5. (Continued)

Drugs	Therapeutic response in elderly	Nursing implications
Acetylsalicylic acid (aspirin)	Effective as an antipyretic if temperature is elevated owing to skin infection (*e.g.,* herpes zoster).	Should not be used for patients with GI problems.
Acyclovir (Zovirax)	Use with caution in patients who have impaired renal function, neurological abnormalities, and dehydration.	Administer intravenously slowly, and rotate injection sites. Keep patient well hydrated.
Vidarabine (Vira-A)	Metabolism and excretion may be prolonged in patients with hepatic or renal dysfunction.	Give intravenously in large amounts of fluids. Needs to be started early in the disease if it is to be effective.

Conclusion

The skin is the largest organ of the body. The appearance and condition of a person's skin is visible to himself or herself and to others. For this reason, natural changes that occur during the process of aging can affect self-concept and how the person relates with other people.

Normal changes during aging that affect the integumentary system are wrinkling, dry, and thin skin; decreased sebaceous and apocrine sweat gland secretion; decreased sensation for heat, cold, and pain; senile lentigo; seborrheic keratosis, actinic keratosis; acrochordons; alopecia; gray hair; decreased body hair in both sexes; increased facial hair in women; and thick, hard, and brittle nails. The most common skin problems that occur in older people are pressure ulcers, herpes zoster, and carcinoma.

The nurse is responsible for carefully assessing the skin, hair, and nails through the nursing history, which will help to determine past and present skin problems and related factors such as familial characteristics, use of drugs, diet, and sociocultural and environmental factors. Physical assessment of the skin, hair, and nails includes the techniques of general observation, inspection, palpation, olfaction, and mensuration.

Nursing care plans

Medical diagnosis: Xerosis

1. Nursing diagnosis: Impairment of skin integrity related to dry and thin skin

Goals

Skin will become less dry.
Skin will remain intact.
Skin will not itch.

Nursing interventions

1. Assess the skin of the high-risk patient daily; inspect for color.
2. Palpate for temperature, texture, moisture, turgor.
3. Limit total body bath to two times a week.
4. Bath face, hands, genital regions with warm water daily and after incontinence.
5. Pat or blot skin dry.
6. Use superfatted soap or bath oil.
7. Use no alcohol or powder on skin.
8. Massage back, arms, hands, feet with an emollient lotion.
9. Keep fingernails short and clean.
10. Touch skin and lift extremities gently with the palm of the hands rather than the fingers.
11. Encourage foods high in vitamins A, B, C (*e.g.*, carrots, bananas, orange juice).
12. Arrange for humidifier in the room or ask maintenance to increase the humidity to at least 60%.
13. Teach patient not to scratch skin or use powder on body.
14. Teach patient to limit exposure to direct sunlight to 20 min a day or less and to stay out of the sun from 10 am to 2 pm

continued

Medical diagnosis: Skin burns

2. Nursing diagnosis: Potential for injury related to decreased thermal perception

Goals

No skin injury will occur as the result of the therapeutic use of heat or cold.
Patient will be aware of the danger of excessive heat and cold.

Nursing interventions

1. Assess skin carefully for color, texture, and any abnormalities before applying any type of heat or cold.
2. Use the correct temperature for heating devices and bath water.
3. Check the skin every 5 min for the first 15 min of the treatment.
4. Apply heat or cold for the exact length of time ordered (not over one hour).
5. Observe and document any changes in skin color or texture and how well the treatment was tolerated by patient.
6. Remain with patient if he or she is in a sitz bath or whirlpool bath.
7. Teach the potential dangers from the use of heat and cold on the skin (*e.g.*, not to go to sleep with a heating pad touching the skin).

Medical diagnosis: Decubitus ulcers

3. Clinical nursing problem: Impairment of skin integrity: pressure ulcers

Goals

No infection will occur at the ulcer site.
Pressure ulcer will decrease in size.
Pressure will be reduced between skin and bed or chair.
No additional pressure ulcers will occur.

Nursing interventions

1. Assess the ulcer site(s) daily and categorize weekly according to stage and size.
2. Culture and sensitivity lab test of drainage if site is infected and tests are ordered.
3. Cleanse with hydrogen peroxide/normal saline mixture every 8 hr, if infected.
4. Whirlpool bath 3 times a week if condition permits.
5. Apply a medicated ointment if ordered.
6. Apply a sterile dry dressing if skin is broken. Use minimal paper tape and remove carefully toward ulcer.
7. Keep skin dry and clean.

continued

Nursing interventions

8. Massage, using lotion, over bony prominences at least every 8 hr.
9. Turn each 2 hr. Teach patient to turn self, if possible.
10. Use egg-crate, air, or Clinitron bed or mechanical pressure reducing bed if possible.
11. Obtain dietary consultation to evaluate protein. Increase protein, calories, vitamins intake, and minerals in diet.

Medical diagnosis: *Herpes zoster*

4. Clinical nursing problem: Impairment of skin integrity: herpes zoster

Goals

Areas of infection will not spread.
Skin will heal with no complications.
Minimal scarring will occur.

Nursing interventions

1. Assess location, severity, and progression of rash, vesicles, pustules, and crusts.
2. Keep skin clean and free of moisture and potential contaminants.
3. Keep patient's fingernails short and clean.
4. Discourage patient from scratching the skin.
5. Apply medicated ointments as ordered.
6. Prevent the spread of infected drainage to self or others by using wound precautions and careful handwashing techniques.
7. Teach patient to prevent the spread of the infection.

5. Clinical nursing problem: Alteration in comfort: the painful lesions of herpes zoster

Goals

Patient will be free of pain, burning, and tingling.
Patient will be free of fever.
Patient will be able to sleep 7–8 hr at night.

Nursing interventions

1. Assess amount and type of pain.
2. Assess degree of fever.
3. Assess patterns of sleeping.
4. Administer analgesics, antipyretics, and sedatives, as ordered.
5. Apply cool compresses, as ordered.
6. Encourage the use of clothing that will not cause pressure on the affected areas.

continued

Nursing interventions

7. Teach patient to limit activities after discharge and to get an adequate amount of rest and sleep.
8. Teach patient that pain may continue for several months and to seek assistance if it cannot be relieved.

Medical diagnosis: *Basal cell/squamous cell carcinoma*

6. Nursing diagnosis: Impairment of skin integrity related to basal cell/squamous cell carcinoma

Goals

Patient is free of skin carcinoma.
No additional skin cancers will occur.

Nursing interventions

1. Assess skin for ulcerated areas of 6 weeks' duration or longer.
2. Observe for changes in color or size of skin lesion.
3. Refer to dermatologist for diagnosis by scraping, excision, and biopsy.
4. Instruction to patient: use sterile pressure dressing for 24 hr after excision. Report abnormal bleeding to physician.
5. If incision site is 2 cm or larger, change dressing and cleanse site every day.
6. Teach patient to examine the skin every month (and to have a relative or friend examine the back of the trunk and legs).
7. Teach patient to limit direct exposure to sun to 20 min a day.

Medical diagnosis: *Pruritus*

7. Clinical nursing problem: Alteration in comfort: itching

Goals

Skin will stop itching.
Skin will remain intact, smooth, and flexible (Dunn 1986).
Skin will not become infected, red, or edematous.

Nursing interventions

1. Assess the skin for location, severity, and complications of itching. Especially note redness, rash, and edema.
2. Determine whether the contributing factors are pathophysiological or situational.

continued

Nursing interventions

3. Administer systemic and antipruritic medications as ordered, depending on the contributing factor(s) and degree of stress and agitation.
4. Bathe skin at least daily with tepid (not hot) water. Use soap only as needed. Rinse well; pat dry.
5. Apply cool moist compresses every 2–4 hr to relieve discomfort, if itching is severe.
6. Prevent the possibility of infection by using sterile or clean technique, depending on the severity of the skin damage.
7. If surgical tape must be used, choose a nonallergic type and apply it sparingly and lightly.
8. If not contraindicated, apply an emollient lotion several times a day.
9. Keep patient's fingernails short and clean.
10. Try to reduce patient's stress, if this is a contributing factor, by providing a calm, quiet environment.
11. Plan activities to help direct patient's focus away from scratching.
12. Administer sedatives as ordered, if scratching interferes with sleep.
13. Teach patient not to scratch the skin. If this is impossible, have him or her wear soft, clean, white cotton gloves. Use soft splints from the wrist to the most distal finger phalanges to prevent scratching, if absolutely necessary for the confused patient.
14. Teach patient to wear cool, soft, loose, nonirritating (*e.g.,* cotton and not wool) clothing.
15. Teach patient not to use bed covers while sleeping.

References

Ahmed MC: Op-Site for decubitus care. Am J Nurs 82:61, 1982

Anders JE, Leach EE: Sun versus skin. Am J Nurs 83:1015, 1983

Black skin problems. Am J Nurs 79:1092, 1979

Brunner LS, Suddarth DS (eds): Lippincott Manual of Nursing Practice, 4th ed. Philadelphia, JB Lippincott, 1986

Collier IC: Nursing assessment integumentary system. In Lewis SM, Collier IC (eds): Medical–Surgical Nursing: Assessment and Management of Clinical Problems, p 357. New York, McGraw-Hill, 1983a

Collier IC: Nursing role in management problems of the integumentary system. In Lewis SM, Collier IC (eds): Medical–Surgical Nursing: Assessment and Management of Clinical Problems, p 367. New York, McGraw-Hill, 1983b

Dunn LM: Nursing strategies for common integument problems. In Patrick ML, Woods SL, Craven RF et al (eds): Medical–Surgical Nursing, p 1385. Philadelphia, JB Lippincott, 1986

Ebersole P, Hess P: Toward Healthy Aging, 2nd ed. St. Louis, CV Mosby, 1985

Fowler E: Skin care for older adults. J Gerontol Nurs 85:44, 1985

Fraser MC, McGuire DB: Skin cancer's early warning system. Am J Nurs 84:1232, 1984

Hallal JC: Understanding herpes zoster and relieving its discomfort. Geriatr Nurs 6:74, 1985

Hogstel MO: Skin care for the aged. J Gerontol Nurs 9:430, 1983

Innes BS: Infectious and inflammatory skin disorders. In Patrick ML, Woods SL, Craven RF et al (eds): Medical–Surgical Nursing, p 1384. Philadelphia, JB Lippincott, 1986

Jones PL, Millman A: A three-part system to combat pressure sores. Geriatr Nurs 7:2, 1986

Kligman AM, Grove GL, Balin AK: Aging of human skin. In Finch CE, Schneider EL (eds): Handbook of the Biology of Aging, 2nd ed, p 104. New York, Van Nostrand Reinhold, 1985

Landau BR: Review of anatomy and physiology integument system. In Patrick ML, et al (eds): Medical–Surgical Nursing, p 1373. Philadelphia, JB Lippincott, 1986

Malasanos L: Health Assessment. St. Louis, CV Mosby, 1986

Mathewson MK: Pharmacotherapeutics: A Nursing Process Approach. Philadelphia, FA Davis, 1986

Oppeneer JE, Vervoren TM: Gerontological Pharmacology. St. Louis, CV Mosby, 1983

Pfister S, Bruno PM: Assessment of integument function. In Patrick ML, Woods SL, Craven RF et al (eds): Medical–Surgical Nursing, p 1378. Philadelphia, JB Lippincott, 1986

Phipps M, Bauman B, Berner D et al: Staging care for pressure sores. Am J Nurs 84:999, 1984

Potter PA, Perry AG: Fundamentals of Nursing. St. Louis, CV Mosby, 1985

Robinson JK: Moh's surgery for skin cancer. Am J Nurs 82:282, 1982

Spencer RT, Nichols LW, Waterhouse HP et al: Clinical Pharmacology and Nursing Management, 2nd ed. Philadelphia, JB Lippincott, 1986

Thomas CL (ed): Taber's Cyclopedic Medical Dictionary, 15th ed. Philadelphia, FA Davis, 1985

Suggested readings

Berliner H: Aging skin. Am J Nurs 86:1259, 1986

Boykin A, Winland-Brown J: Pressure sores: Nursing management. J Gerontol Nurs 12:17, 1986

Carpenito LJ: Handbook of Nursing Diagnosis. Philadelphia, JB Lippincott, 1985

Frantz RA, Kinney CK: Variables associated with skin dryness in the elderly. Nurs Res 35:2, 98, 1986

Fowler E: Skin care for older adults. J Gerontol Nurs 12:34, 1986

Tooman T, Patterson J: Decubitus ulcer warfare: Product US process. Geriatr Nurs 5:166, 1984

Virginia Burggraf

Sensory system

5

Sensation plays a central role in every person's response to the environment. The diminished ability to see, hear, taste, touch, smell, or maintain balance causes inordinate amounts of difficulty for the elderly. Nursing care for patients with sensory decline demands a great deal of sensitivity from caregivers.

The sensory decline that results from aging is a slow process, with changes in the sensory system frequently taken for granted or going unnoticed. The elderly themselves accept auditory and visual decline as normal and may not be able to distinguish a pathologic process until it has made significant progression.

The promotion of sensory integrity is a major responsibility of the nurse, which can be accomplished only if the nurse is aware of the past sensory environment of the patient, and the patient's lifestyle and coping patterns. When an abrupt change in environment occurs, and the elderly person is subjected to extremes in stimulation (deprivation or overload), the nurse can respond appropriately to the initial confusion and isolation that may be created and can provide the communication that is necessary to restore sensory integrity.

Age-related changes

With advancing age, all of the senses generally decline in acuity and function. Most elderly persons, however, continue to function well within their accustomed environment. Often it is when physical illness or psychologic loss occurs, that the diminished sensation becomes obvious to caregivers and family members. When the norms are compounded by diseases such as diabetes, neurologic impairments, otosclerosis, glaucoma, or cataracts, the nurse's work of presenting a stimulating environment becomes a significant challenge.

Visual

Multiple structural and functional changes occur in the aging eye. The eyelids atrophy and become wrinkled, a condition commonly referred to as "bags." It is this appearance that indicates that the individual is aged.

Eyelids invert (*entropion*) and the eyelashes can begin to rub against the eyeball. This condition is often found in elderly persons who blink frequently. The opposite condition is *ectropion,* or the outward turning of the eyelid, with the eyeball becoming reddened and congested.

Presbyopia, or old-age farsightedness, begins some time after the age of 40 and is attributable to loss of elasticity in the lens. Gioiella and Bevil (1985) compare the lens to an onion, with the oldest tissue in the middle and the youngest at the periphery. With increasing age, cellular growth slows, causing the lens to have a larger proportion of old to new tissue. The center yellows and becomes less flexible, and the ciliary muscle can no longer change the shape of the lens. An expression frequently heard from elderly persons is, "The older I get, the longer my arms become."

With advancing age, the lens becomes opaque and cloudy, causing cataracts and sensitivity to glare. Persons with less than 20/200 vision in one good eye are considered legally blind; 61% of such blindness in the elderly is caused by cataracts. Almost all persons over 70 years of age will have some degree of cataract formation. Certain diseases, diabetes in particular, can hasten cataract formation, as can certain cortisone ophthalmic preparations (McCoy 1981). Reading becomes a major problem, and the stresses caused by the loss of vision can lead to depression if not recognized. Fortunately, cataracts are a problem that can be alleviated.

In addition, research studies are fairly consistent in showing that the elderly have a loss of color sensitivity across the entire light spectrum, and a differential loss of discrimination at the blue end of the spectrum. In other words, the elderly have more difficulty discriminating colors of short wavelengths, such as green, blue, and violet. Degenerative changes in the retina have also been implicated in these changes (Sullivan 1983).

Darkness-adaptation time requirements increase because of the various changes that occur in the iris and pupil. Sclerosis of the iris results in a smaller pupil size, and thus limits the amount of light reaching the retina. The elderly have particular difficulty when driving at night, entering a dark room, awakening at night and then moving about the home, and going outside at night. Attention to providing good lighting conditions (*e.g.,* nightlights in the home), eliminating unsafe situations, and patient education can prevent problems before they begin.

Increased tearing is considered an abnormal finding; decreased lacrimation is the normal age-related change. Patients frequently complain about "dry eyes" and many require artificial tears to hydrate the cornea.

One primary ocular change with age is *arcus senilis,* a deposition of fat circling the cornea. However, little is known about the origins of this change.

The accumulation of elevated epithelial pigment deposits (*drusen*), seen only on ophthalmoscopic examination, is hereditary. This is the earliest clinical manifestation of senile macular degeneration (SMD), which causes the loss of central vision and eventual blindness in 25% of persons under age 80 and 40% of those over 80 years old (Lewis 1979). Senile macular degeneration is a leading cause of legal blindness in about 10% of the population. The cause is unknown, although it is thought to be related to a decreased blood supply to the sensitive nerve endings in this region. Central vision is lost, with major distortion in adaptation to any environment. This has important implications for the nurse/patient relationship. Nursing priorities are to reassure the patient that he or she will never become totally blind, and to train him or her in the use of peripheral vision. Consultation with an ophthalmologist is necessary to select appropriate patient education activities (Carnevali 1986).

Glaucoma is frequently identified with the elderly and must not be considered a normal age-related change. It is a disease process that can go undetected until symptoms occur (*e.g.,* eyestrain and morning headache). The chronic manifestation of this disease, *wide-angle glaucoma,* results from an obstruction in the normal flows of aqueous humor, causing fluid to back up, increasing intraocular pressure and damaging the optic nerve. All persons over age 40 should have yearly eye examinations, including tonometry testing for glaucoma.

The nurse's major responsibility with regard to vision is to realize that visual problems are normal in the elderly, occurring in 80% of this population. Patients should be asked about their glasses and their last eye examination. Glasses should be close at hand, and when the nurse gives written instructions, he or she must verify that the patient can read them. For a newly admitted hospital patient or a person who has been admitted to a nursing home, difficulties with navigation in the new and unfamiliar territory can make safety a problem. Light in the environment should be controlled to cut glare, and a nightlight should be left on in all bathroom areas. Three-way bulbs enable patients to adjust their own lighting situations. Appropriate colors (*e.g.,* bright yellows and pastels) will brighten the atmosphere. The addition of large-print books to patient libraries will facilitate reading as a source of pleasure.

Drugs

Table 5-1 lists some commonly used ophthalmic drugs, their side-effects, and their nursing implications.

Auditory

Presbycusis, the term frequently used to describe the normal hearing loss associated with age, is a sensorineural loss that progresses to an inability to hear sounds in the higher frequencies. Because consonant sounds are mostly composed in these frequencies, advancing age brings a generalized inability to comprehend the spoken word. This is caused by degenerative changes in the base of the cochlea, consisting of a decrease in the fibers that make up the auditory

Table 5-1. **Table of ophthalmic drugs**

Drug	Effect/response in the elderly	Nursing implications
Pilocarpine eyedrops (Ocusert)	Constricts the pupils (miotic) and is used in open-angle glaucoma to facilitate the movement of aqueous humor from the anterior chamber through the trabecular network.	Side-effects initially may include headache, eye redness, and blurred vision. Patient needs to be informed of this and told, if symptoms are prolonged, to inform physician. Atropine and any anticholinergic drug is contraindicated (*e.g.,* antihistamines, antiparkinson drugs, tricyclics and phenothiazines).
Carbachol eye drops	For patients allergic to pilocarpine.	
Timoptic eye drops (0.25%–0.5%)	Not a miotic, used to reduce elevated intraocular pressure. A beta-adrenergic blocking agent that is a myocardial depressant. Used in primary open-angle glaucoma.	Contraindicated in patients with asthma, dyspnea, cardiac problems. Visual system should be monitored every four hours and any abrupt changes reported.
Epinephrine (125–250 mg sequels, 500 mg) (Diamox)	A potent carbonic anhydrase inhibitor used for open-angle glaucoma to inhibit aqueous humor secretion.	Monitor patient for vomiting, diarrhea, and excessive urination. Acidosis can occur within 24 hours, as well as dyspnea, dermatitis, and tingling of extremities.
Echothiophate iodide (Phospholine Iodide)	Used to constrict pupil and increase outflow of aqueous humor. As a cholinesterase inhibitor, it may cause drying of mouth, or diarrhea.	This drug is contraindicated in the presence of asthma, peptic ulcer, parkinsonism, and recent myocardial infarction. Assess patient for cataract formation and blurring vision if drug used over long period. This drug must be stopped two weeks before surgery because it is systemically absorbed and can cause respiratory distress.
Hydrocortisone acetate (Epifoam)	Corticosteroid used as a topical steroid for lid infections. Has a definite antipruritic and anti-inflammatory response.	

nerve. Cerumen, if left to accumulate in the ear, can also cause a conductive hearing loss that is easily corrected. Cerumen, although secreted in smaller amounts with aging, contains more keratin and is more difficult to remove.

Because normal hearing loss is progressive, many elderly persons have "learned to live with it" and have compensated over the years by positioning themselves advantageously for hearing, lip reading, and restricting conversation. It is not uncommon to find that elderly persons are isolated and lonely because of the inability to comprehend their environment. When auditory loss is compounded with a visual loss, the resulting psychological depression and isolation can be profound.

Sometimes the older person, as a result of often feeling embarrassed and left out, becomes irritable and frustrated by the inability to comprehend and control the environment. Family members, friends, and staff fail to understand these feelings and behavior and frequently react with anger or frustration and label the person uncooperative, belligerent, or angry. The ability to understand the dynamics of auditory and visual loss, the two most common sensory losses, can make the difference between a socially interactive, happy environment or a socially isolated, depressed environment.

Taste and smell

The senses of taste and smell are interrelated. However, this may have direct implications for elderly persons because diminution in both these senses is equal in degree.

It is argued that changes in olfactory status are often attributed to disease, smoking, and the environment of the person rather than to normal age-related changes (Hall 1984). The average ability to identify odors reaches a peak in the third and fourth decades of life and then begins to decline gradually. *Anosmia,* the term used to refer to a diminished ability to smell, can have serious implications for the safety of an older person (*e.g.,* in detecting fire and gas or noxious chemical odors). Because of this, it is important to have fire detectors in the elderly person's home. A thorough safety check should be made for faulty appliances, electric outlets, and plumbing.

The mouth of the elderly person undergoes many changes, which include periodontal disease, gingivitis, and the loss of teeth and acquisition of dentures. All of these elements contribute to a lessening of taste sensation. Atrophic changes occur on the tongue, contributing to a decrease in taste sensitivity. Because taste is dependent on the sense of smell, the loss of a sense of smell alters the perception of taste. Usually it is the salty and sweet tastebuds that diminish in number, with bitter and sour remaining fairly constant (Witherly 1983).

A number of variables can contribute to oral problems. The flow of saliva diminishes with aging. Gingival tissue undergoes insult over time, becoming less elastic and more vulnerable to trauma. Atrophic changes in the buccal mucosa cause three-quarters of the tastebuds to be lost by the age of 70. It is not unusual for these atrophic tissues to cause *glossodynia,* a burning sensation on the tongue (Kopac 1983).

Two hundred to three hundred tastebuds are located on the soft palate, pharynx, and larynx. Three cranial nerves (facial, vagus, and glossopharyngeal) supply the afferent pathways for reception of taste. Investigation has shown that as a person ages most changes in taste are indirectly related to the function of these central nervous system (CNS) receptors. Although taste perceptions for salts and sweets naturally decrease with age, the decline also is involved with changes in the oral cavity. Both progressive alteration in the periodontal membrane and loss of teeth have marked effects on a person's oral environment and function of the tastebuds.

Nursing interventions center around maintaining a clean oral cavity, with the teeth being brushed at least once a day (an often-neglected area of hygiene). Some common-sense measure (*e.g.,* serving food while it is warm, and offering each item separately, rather than mashed all together) can help the patient to better taste the food. Dietitians can be consulted on the nutritional value of particular foods liked by the patient.

Touch

Much has been written about age-related changes in vision, hearing, and olfactory and taste sensation. However, changes in the sense of touch and the vestibular system are poorly documented. Neurologic insult over time and increased functional impairment are believed to cause many of the changes. All elderly persons experience a decreased reaction time and are slower to respond in comparison with younger persons; stronger neurologic impulses are required to produce the same response.

The sense of touch, which is allied with control of body position, relies on sensory input from sources such as the inner ear, eye, and receptors in the muscles and joints. These work together to maintain body orientation in space. Under normal circumstances, a person gives no conscious thought to controlling body position; however, in varying degrees, aging insults all the physical resources that are involved. Receptors are lost that affect gait, movement, response, and sensitivity. Disturbance in vestibular and kinesthetic sense may increase the likelihood of accidents. Although collagen and elastin on the skin surfaces decrease, no definitive evidence exists indicating major impairment in sensitivity to stimuli.

Sensitivity to pain is the most-investigated area of the cutaneous senses. Much has been written about decreased pain sensation with aging, but this theory is a still-debated issue. The experience of pain is an individual response. The nurse should be alert for physical signs that may indicate illness because the discomforts associated with severe illness may not be perceived by an elderly patient in the same degree as would be with a younger person. Any change in cognition, hydration, vital signs, or color should alert the nurse that a problem is imminent.

Touch, which is not only a means of sensory stimulation, but also an expression of warmth and caring, is frequently neglected by caregivers. Touch conveys the attitude of caring and should be made a priority intervention when performing all procedures.

Assessment variables

Elderly persons may minimize or eliminate data related to sensory changes, rationalizing, "I'm not important, I'm just getting older." The nurse is challenged to use interviewing skills to the fullest extent in order to elicit accurate information. The visual and hearing losses, readily apparent with age, are often taken for granted by health-care professionals. As a result, many problems are missed because of this *laissez-faire* attitude. Because the elderly person may accept these sensory losses as an inevitability of age, they may need to be coaxed to respond to in-depth questions during the health history.

The patient profile, begun initially in the history, reveals important data on living arrangements, activities, nutrition, and meal preparation that will indicate changes in sensory functioning. The person's present and past occupations are important as possible causes of sensory problems. For instance, members of our present-day elderly population once worked on railroads, in industry, and fought in wars. One aspect of these experiences is exposure to a high level of noise, a situation that will place any person at a higher risk for hearing impairment (Mezey 1980).

Activity patterns (*e.g.,* driving a car, walking daily, and leisure activities) can be limited by the patient's visual acuity. It is important to ascertain the reason for decreased attendance at social functions. Is the cause paranoia concerning "people talking about me," or an auditory deficit that needs further investigation? If the level of social interaction has been maintained, questions should be asked about satisfaction with health and life in general such as, "How would you rate your health—excellent, good, fair, or poor?" "Why did you choose this rating?" Shanas and coworkers (1968) have determined that people who are experiencing sensory deficits in hearing and vision are more likely to feel in poor health and to be less satisfied with their lives.

Nutritional changes, diet, appetite, food preference, and smoking habits all contribute to changes in taste, smell, dentition, meal interaction, and possible incidence of oral cancer. Certain vitamin deficiencies can cause visual disturbances and can be discovered only through an accurate diet history. It may be necessary to obtain a 24-hour history of food intake.

Past health history should not be neglected. Certain information relating to the last eye examination, visit to the dentist, or a hearing test will provide the practitioner with information about health maintenance practices, health status, and habits or diseases that may have caused sensory deficits. Mastoiditis was a chronic problem for many members of the present elderly population and can be the source of a hearing deficit from childhood. Past illnesses, treatment, and residual effects can elicit information on sensory and other problems. The presence of diseases such as diabetes, hypertension, arteriosclerosis, and stroke can suggest the value of looking for signs of sensory deterioration. A family history may reveal inherited diseases such as cataracts, glaucoma, or SMD. Many medications currently used to treat chronic illness will have an adverse effect on the eyes, ears, nose, and mouth. These drugs may be diuretics, aspirin, and certain antibiotics.

Physical assesment

Sensory-related aging changes impose many disadvantages for the elderly individual, including emotional devastation, social isolation, and a decrease in life satisfaction (Shanas et al 1968). Nurses who care for the elderly must maintain communication with them and invest time in the accurate history taking and assessment skills that lead to appropriate interventions to improve the sensory environment of the elderly patient. There can be no therapeutic relationship without communication; patience is also important. Following the taking of the health history, a relationship should exist that allows the patient to feel confident that the nurse has a caring attitude. Certain physical examination techniques are different for the elderly patient. Emphasis should be placed on the areas of the nervous system that were described in the history as being deficient. Eyeglasses, hearing aids, and any other prosthesis should be in place. The patient should not become fatigued during the physical examination.

While inspecting for facial symmetry, observe the eyelids for swelling, and note the direction of lash growth. Are the lacrimal ducts patent? Is there excessive tearing or redness? Note the vascularity of the conjunctiva while determining the color of the sclera. Arcus senilis, the opaque grayish ring encircling the iris, can be observed easily. The pupils should be tested for light and accommodation. They should contract to the same "small" size. Testing the extraocular muscles will demonstrate a slight-to-greater inability to converge, with some limitations in upward mobility, based on the degree of neurologic impairment. A test of visual acuity includes the Snellen Eye Chart, the Rosenbaum Card, or a newspaper. Make sure that patients with reading glasses wear them.

On ophthalmoscopic examination, the internal eye structure will mirror a picture of the health of the elderly person. If the arterioles are nicked, the structures of the internal eye may indicate hypertension. If loss of central vision is evident, the macula may be degenerating or the optic nerve may be damaged. A thorough discussion of the ophthalmoscopic examination is beyond the scope of this chapter. The nurse should determine if further examination is necessary using the results of the ophthalmoscopic exam as a guide. It is recommended that everyone over 40 have a thorough eye examination (Thompson and Bowers 1980).

When inspecting the ears, look for wax buildup, which can cause a conductive hearing loss. Removal of the cerumen can be time-consuming, but if impacted cerumen is present, it must be removed before the examination can proceed. An examination that involves use of the speculum is within the scope of the nurse's responsibilities. With a clean speculum on the otoscope, the appearance of the drum and the supporting landmark should be observed. Scarring from past infections, fungus, and any foreign bodies can be easily detected. Also, the nurse should be aware that it is not uncommon for confused elderly persons to place objects in their ears.

Carotenuto and Bullock (1980) caution practitioners against asking the elderly person to hold his or her nose and swallow as a means of visualizing the bones of the inner ear, because this action will compensate the equilibrium of the elderly.

Hearing can be tested with a ticking watch, the whisper test, or the tuning fork (Rinne's test and Weber's test). The watch should be held at a distance of 1 inch to 2 inches from the ear. If presbycusis exists, the ticking will not be heard. Normally, a whispered voice at a distance of 1 foot to 2 feet can be heard, but elderly persons will need for the sound level to be increased. Using the tuning fork will confirm air conduction, sound, and bone conduction; and air conduction is usually twice as long as bone conduction. These tests are simple to perform and short in duration.

The nurse's assessment of auditory ability can make the difference in improving communication and life satisfaction for many elderly patients. The Nursing Home Hearing Handicap Index (NHHI), presented in Table 5-2 is a handy

Table 5-2. *Nursing home hearing handicap index (NHHI)*

	Very often				Almost never
Staff version					
1. When this person is with other people does he or she need to hear better?	5	4	3	2	1
2. Do members of the staff, family, and friends make negative comments about this person's hearing problem?	5	4	3	2	1
3. Does this person have trouble hearing another person if there is a radio or television playing in the same room?	5	4	3	2	1
4. When this person is listening to radio or television, does he or she have trouble hearing?	5	4	3	2	1
5. How often do you feel life would be better for this person if he or she could hear better?	5	4	3	2	1
6. How often is he or she embarrassed because he or she does not hear well?	5	4	3	2	1
7. When he or she is alone does he or she need to hear better the everyday sounds of life?	5	4	3	2	1
8. Do people tend to leave him or her out of conversations because he or she does not hear well?	5	4	3	2	1

(continued)

Table 5-2. *(Continued)*

	Very often				Almost never
9. How often does he or she withdraw from social activities in which he or she ought to participate because he or she does not hear well?	5	4	3	2	1
10. Does he or she say "What?" or "Pardon me?" when people first speak to him or her?	5	4	3	2	1

Total: _____ × 2 = _____
                − 20 × 1.25 = _____ %

Self version for resident

	Very often				Almost never
1. When you are with other people do you wish you could hear better?	5	4	3	2	1
2. Do other people feel you have a hearing problem (when they try to talk to you)?	5	4	3	2	1
3. Do you have trouble hearing another person if there is a radio or television playing in the same room?	5	4	3	2	1
4. Do you have trouble hearing the radio or television?	5	4	3	2	1
5. How often do you feel life would be better if you could hear better?	5	4	3	2	1
6. How often are you embarrassed because you don't hear well?	5	4	3	2	1
7. When you are alone do you wish you would hear better?	5	4	3	2	1
8. Do people tend to leave you out of conversations because you do not hear well?	5	4	3	2	1
9. How often do you withdraw from social activities in which you ought to participate because you do not hear well?	5	4	3	2	1
10. Do you say "What?" or "Pardon me?" when people first speak to you?	5	4	3	2	1

Total: _____ × 2 = _____
                − 20 × 1.25 = _____ %

Categories and scores

Category	Scores (%)
No handicap	0–20
Mild hearing handicap	21–40
Moderate hearing handicap	41–70
Severe hearing handicap	71–100

After scoring, an objective hearing evaluation of the nursing home resident can be made.

(Schow R, Christensen J, Hutchinson J et al: Communication Disorders of the Aged: A Guide for Health Professionals, pp 138–146. Baltimore, University Park Press, 1978)

guide that can be used to assess accurately hearing loss (Schow et al 1978). The information obtained through use of this table cannot be considered a thorough examination, but is a useful guide to establish the degree of functional hearing loss.

Testing for olfactory sense is very easy and can determine physiological, nutritional, and safety interventions for the patient. Inspect the patency of each nares, occluding one at a time and asking the patient to inhale with a closed mouth. A narrowing or occlusion of the nares can indicate pulmonary obstruction. When checking for function of the olfactory nerve ask the patient (while his or her eyes are closed) to identify a smell such as coffee, or a sweet or aromatic scent from a bar of soap. Oil of wintergreen, frequently available in nursing homes and hospitals, should not be used. Because it is an irritant, the patient will respond to the irritation instead of the odor.

The oral cavity will mirror changes of age and any abuse to the gums and teeth. Ill-fitting dentures can be observed, along with the pale to bright-red gums that are indicative of disease, diminished vascularity, and a general deterioration in self-care practices. If visual deficiency is compounded by neurologic impairment, oral hygiene that requires good eyesight and manual dexterity is often neglected. This assessment component frequently is neglected by nurses and this neglect has serious implications for nutritional support, infection control, and disease prevention. Any abnormalities in color, the presence of white-gray patches on the buccal mucosa (*leukoplakia*), symmetry, and texture should be reported. Tobacco chewers, alcoholics, and pipe smokers are at great risk for oral cancer, the presence of which can be determined by a very brief inspection of the oral cavity.

Touch, kinesthesis, and vestibular sensation are tested on neurologic examination with light and deep touch and pressure to the skin, as well as observation of gait, posture, and stance. Persons who have had a stroke with resulting hemiplegia have lost position sense and must be spatially oriented when positioned. Touch used on the unaffected side is a very important form of communication because many stroke patients have lost verbal skills. To maintain a sense of continuity, attach a handy reference of tactile sensation to the care plan (Fig. 5-1). This will assist staff in caring for the patient and in making decisions about bathing temperature, safety, turning, and positioning. Neurologic impairments are discussed at length in Chapter 13. Refer to Table 5-3 for a more thorough tool for sensory assessment, which produces an index of sensory function. The higher the score on the area of assessment, the more profound is the loss.

Drug therapy

Many drugs currently being taken by the elderly to treat chronic illness will compensate the person further by causing sensory changes. It is important for the nurse to have a knowledge of these drugs. Among the systemic drugs implicated

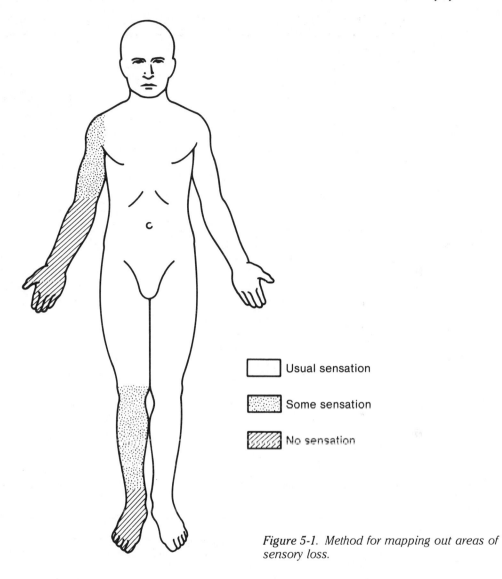

Figure 5-1. Method for mapping out areas of sensory loss.

in causing cataracts are corticosteroids and phenothiazines. Blurred vision can be caused by the antianxiety tranquilizers chlordiazepoxide hydrochloride (Librium), meprobamate (Equanil) and diazepam (Valium), as well as cardiac drugs in common use (digitalis and nitroglycerin). Aspirin, now widely used as a vasodilator, is taken daily in large doses (>3 g/day) by many elderly and can cause, in addition to visual problems, tinnitus and hearing loss. Narrow-angle glaucoma can be aggravated by the taking of many drugs, anticholinergics in particular. Cisplatin, an antineoplastic agent, can cause tinnitis.

Table 5-3. **Assessment of sensory function in the elderly**

Sense	Test	Scale	Ability
Vision	*Acuity* Have patient read newspaper print with one eye covered at a time. Corrective devices should be worn.	1 2 3	Reads all of the print Reads all except the fine print Unable to see the print (or only the headlines) 3 inches from the eye
	Color identification Put solid colored lines on a sheet of paper, using green, brown, yellow, red, violet, and orange crayons.	1 2	Identifies primary colors (red, blue, and yellow) Unable to identify any color
	Peripheral vision Place a colored block on each side of the patient at eye level outside the line of the patient's shoulder. Tell patient to look straight ahead.	1 2	Sees both blocks Sees one block or no blocks
Smell	Have patient identify the aroma of alcohol and coffee.	1 3	Able to identify both aromas Unable to identify aromas
Hearing	Speak to patient using a normal tone.	1	Responds to questions while assessor's back is turned
		2	Responds to questions while assessor is facing patient, but not when back is turned
		3	Does not respond to questions while assessor is facing patient

(continued)

(Adapted by A. Salway, RN, MN, from Bozian J and Clark H: Counteracting sensory changes in the aging. Am J Nurs 80:473–476, 1980)

Hearing will be further diminished in elderly persons who are taking thiazides (Diuril) and furosemide (Lasix) or some antiinfectious agents (*e.g.,* streptomycin, neomycin, kanamycin, and gentamicin; Dangel and Hovener 1983).

Quinine and chloroquine sometimes cause inner-ear damage. In the case of quinine, individual idiosyncrasy appears to be an important factor. Regional infusion has also caused deafness. Also, in some patients bleomycin in high dosage has caused sensorineural deafness.

Table 5-3. (*Continued*)

Sense	Test	Scale	Ability
	Snaps fingers lightly.	1	Able to hear snapping sound 12 inches from ear
		2	Unable to hear snapping sound 6 inches from ear
		3	Unable to hear snapping sound 2 inches from ear
Taste	Have patient taste salt and sugar at separate times. Give water between taste tests.	1	Able to identify both flavors
		2	Able to identify one flavor
		3	Able to identify neither flavor
Depth perception	Lay two pencils of the same length and color parallel on a table (one closer to patient than the other).	1	Able to correctly identify the closer pencil at 8 feet
		2	Unable to identify the closer pencil at 5 feet
		3	Unable to identify the closer pencil at 2 feet
Temperature	Touch patient's extremities with a warm cloth, then with a cool cloth.	1	Able to distinguish differences correctly
		3	Unable to distinguish differences correctly
Light touch	Touch patient with cotton-ball and tip of safety pin over extremities and forehead. (Have patient close eyes.)	1	Able to identify soft and sharp touches correctly
		2	Able to identify soft and sharp touches correctly on one side of body
		3	Unable to identify soft or sharp touches on either side of body
Position sense	Gently lift patient's extremities, followed by lifting fingers and toes (have patient close eyes).	1	Able to identify limb or digit being lifted.
		2	Able to identify limb lifted, but not digit lifted.
		3	Unable to identify limb or digit being lifted.

Decreases in visual acuity or blurred vision often occur after administration of antiviral agents, amantadine, and haloperidol (Haldol), the frequently used antipsychotic agent.

Taking the time to effectively teach the elderly patient the technique of administering eyedrops and ointment can mean the difference between compliance and noncompliance. Teach the patient or a significant other to instill eyedrops using the reference guide on page 90 for safe, efficient administration.

Administering eyedrops

1. Wash your hands.

2. Gently cleanse the eye of mucus or exudate with a gauze pad soaked in sterile normal saline (newly postoperative patient) or water (home use).

3. Ask the patient to tip his or her head slightly toward the side of the affected eye.

4. Pull the lower eyelid down and ask the patient to look up.

5. Place one drop of medication in the sac formed by the lower eyelid. Never drop medicine directly on the cornea because it is sensitive tissue.

6. Gently press on the inner canthus for 1 minute to 2 minutes, to prevent medication loss or absorption through the tear duct. At the same time, have the patient close the eye gently. Caution against squeezing the eye shut because this will force out the medication.

7. Gently wipe away any excess medication.

(Todd B: Using eye drops and ointments safely. J Geriatr Nurs 3:53–57, 1983)

Nursing care plans

Medical diagnosis: Presbyopia

1. Nursing diagnosis: Alteration in sensory perception related to decreased visual acuity

Goal

Patient will be able to communicate with the staff.

Nursing interventions

1. Face patient at all times when you are speaking.
2. Make sure patient's glasses are within reach at all times.
3. Touch patient while administering care to promote use of other sensory organs.
4. Assess the degree of visual deficit using the Rosenbaum Card or Near Card or any printed word from a newspaper.
5. Arrange for an ophthalmologic consultation if necessary.

2. Nursing diagnosis: Knowledge deficit of the effects of aging, related to lack of instruction

Goal	*Nursing interventions*
Patient will be informed of the visual changes that occur with age.	1. Explain that a regular pattern of diminished vision with aging is normal. 2. Discuss the visual changes that occur on the eye with aging. 3. Explain to patient the need to wear glasses for close work, reading, and driving. 4. Discuss the need for yearly visits to the physician to evaluate vision and prevent additional impairment.

Medical diagnosis: Cataract

3. Clinical nursing problem: Alteration in sensory perception–visual acuity: opacity of lens

Goal	*Nursing interventions*
Patient will have restoration of visual acuity that allows for performance of the functional activities of daily living (ADL).	1. Orient patient to the staff and surroundings of the environment. 2. Keep the call button within easy reach of patient. 3. Protect patient from injury by removing extraneous objects in his or her immediate path (*e.g.*, equipment, scatter rugs). 4. Provide a nightlight near bedside, leave light on in the bathroom, or instruct patient to call nurse if he or she needs to get out of bed. 5. Eliminate glare on floors. 6. Avoid sudden exposure to bright light. 7. Place food on tray or table in a consistent pattern—clock format is frequently used. 8. Provide diversional activity (*e.g.*, recorder, radio, conversation, and social interaction).

4. Nursing diagnosis: Anxiety related to impending surgery

Goal

Patient will experience a comfortable and informed hospitalization.

Nursing interventions

1. Allow patient to verbalize fears and concerns, and provide encouragement when fears are expressed.
2. Actively listen to patient, show interest by your acknowledgment, assess the verbal cues for predominant themes—acceptance, fears, depression, social isolation—that may have been caused by visual impairment.
3. Discuss the success rate of this surgery in improving vision.
4. Provide a relaxed atmosphere when talking with patient.
5. Orient patient to the environment, if hospitalized, to minimize disorientation.

5. Nursing diagnosis: Knowledge deficit of the disease process, surgical correction, and follow-up care related to lack of instruction

Goal

Patient will be informed about cataracts, their surgical removal, and the postoperative and discharge course.

Nursing interventions

1. Explain treatment procedures as indicated (*e.g.,* possible trimming of lashes, covering nonoperative eye, use of multiple types of eyedrops).
2. Explain the operative procedure to patient and significant others: length of time in surgery, use of preoperative medication and where the patient will be cared for immediately postoperative. Instruct the patient about sensation in the eye postoperatively and that analgesia is available on request.
3. Instruct patient and significant others on all postoperative and discharge instructions (*i.e.,* temporarily limit activities that will increase eye strain or pressure such as lifting, coughing, excessive reading, smoking,

continued

Nursing interventions

active sexual activity, showering, tub bathing, bending, and lifting).
4. Explain that patient will have distortion of
depth perception and light adaptation; and
that, in time, contact lenses or glasses can
alter these distortions.
5. Review drug therapy and side-effects, and
demonstrate eyedrop insertion.
6. Ask patient to perform a demonstration in
return. Encourage compliance and follow-up
visits.
7. Check on transportation plans to and from
follow-up appointment.
8. Teach patient and significant others to avoid
use of any substance that can cause sneez-
ing (*e.g.,* perfumed powders, sharp spices,
or astringents) (Duke University 1980).

6. Clinical nursing problem: Alteration in comfort: postoperative pain

Goal

Patient will experience a minimal amount of
uncomfortable sensations.

Nursing interventions

1. Provide analgesia with discretion, observing
for any signs of disorientation that may
mask pain.
2. Localize the area of discomfort; ask patient
to describe what type of pain is experienced. Provide alternate comfort measures
(*e.g.,* back rub, conversation, breathing relaxation techniques).
3. Have patient avoid straining at stool; obtain
an order for stool softener or laxative, if
appropriate.

7. Nursing diagnosis: Potential for injury related to decreased visual acuity

Goal	*Nursing interventions*
Patient will be protected from injury at all times while hospitalized and after discharge.	*1.* Remove extraneous objects in the immediate environment. *2.* Orient patient to any change in the environment. *3.* Home health nurse should perform a home safety assessment. *4.* Emphasize the need for slow careful movements for at least three weeks. *5.* Re-emphasize the importance of avoiding activities that can cause pressure. (See Nursing Care Plans, #5, item 3.)

8. Nursing diagnosis: Potential for infection related to surgical procedure*

Goal	*Nursing interventions*
Exhibit clean dressing without sign of exudate, and patient is free of severe pain.	*1.* Use sterile techniques at all times when changing dressings. *2.* Observe patient for any change in orientation and temperature change. *3.* Discuss with patient the need for hand washing, to avoid rubbing the operative area, and to report any severe pain, nausea, or vomiting.

* Refer to: Home Safety Checklist for Older Consumers. US Department of Health and Human Services Administration on Aging. Consumer Product Safety, Washington, DC 20207

Medical diagnosis: Glaucoma

9. Clinical nursing problem: Alteration in sensory perception–visual acuity: increased intraocular pressure

Goals

Patient will maintain visual acuity necessary to perform the functional ADL.
Patient will experience maximum therapeutic effect from compliance with medical regimen.

Nursing interventions

1. Provide for immediate medical attention if patient describes history of sudden cloudy vision, severe eye pain, and appearance of rainbow halos around lights.
2. Provide support during diagnosis and treatment, allaying fears and explaining all diagnostic tests.
3. Prepare for possible surgery (iridectomy) or longterm medical therapy.
4. Stress need for lifetime compliance in administration of eyedrops to control the disease.

10. Nursing diagnosis: Potential for lack of compliance related to self-care demands

Goals

Patient and family will prevent blindness through compliance with stipulated regimen.
Patient and family will understand and comply with treatment.

Nursing interventions

1. Emphatically explain that the disease is not curable but is controllable.
2. Assess patient's knowledge of glaucoma and teach in areas of deficit.
3. Discuss disease, its causes, which are not related to lifestyle (patient may feel guilty that he or she caused this condition and the family now has to suffer), and the limitations in vision that can occur if drug therapy is not observed (particularly, the potential for blindness).
4. Stress importance of continuous daily use of medications.
5. Advise patient to avoid all activities that may cause increased intraocular pressure (*e.g.,* emotional upsets, snow shoveling, lifting heavy objects, wearing constricting clothing, and straining in defecation).

continued

Nursing interventions

6. Teach patient and significant others insertion of eyedrops and have several return-
   demonstration practice sessions.
7. Stress the need for return visits to the clinic
   or physician's office and check on the transportation plans to and from these necessary
   appointments.
8. Make appropriate arrangements for home
   follow-up with a home health agency.
9. Recommend wearing a Medic-Alert bracelet.

*11. Nursing diagnosis: Potential alteration in family coping patterns related to patient's
loss of ability to care for self*

Goals

Patient will adjust through rehabilitation to
partial loss of vision and independence.
Patient and family will cope with limitation
imposed by decreased visual acuity.

Nursing interventions

1. Openly discuss with patient and family the
   adjustments necessary to maintain independence (*i.e.,* rehabilitation in ADL.
2. Arrange for an occupational therapy (OT)
   consultation to teach patient and family
   alternative methods to function in the home.
3. Make referral with discharge team for appropriate follow-up actions and, if necessary,
   referral to community agencies (Lighthouse
   for the Blind, and the local Lions Club).
4. Allow family to verbalize their fears and
   anxieties about the future, and stress need
   for medical compliance. If a support group
   meets nearby, refer the family to them.

Medical diagnosis: *Blindness*

12. Nursing diagnosis: *Powerlessness related to loss of vision*

Goal

Patient will adjust to limitations and loss of ability that is imposed by visual loss.

Nursing interventions

1. Observe for signs of depression, grief, self-pity, and withdrawal.
2. Encourage full participation in rehabilitation activities and allow patient to perform learned activities.
3. Allow patient to make decisions about care—bathing, dressing, and ADL.
4. Provide positive reinforcement when self-care activities are performed.
5. Suggest a psychiatric consultation if depression does not lift with rehabilitation.
6. Assist with interpretation of sensory stimuli in the environment.
7. Use alternative sensory stimulation: touch, speech, pleasant odors, foods of choice.

13. Nursing diagnosis: *Potential for injury related to blindness*

Goal

Patient will live in a safe environment

Nursing interventions

1. Keep environment uncluttered.
2. Teach family what to observe for at home that may cause an accident (*e.g.*, throw rugs, changes in furniture placement. See Nursing Care Plans, #7.)

Medical diagnosis: *Ectropion*

14. Nursing diagnosis: *Alteration in comfort related to atrophy of eyelid*

Goal

Patient will be comfortable.

Nursing intervention

1. Use lubricating medications to relieve dry eyes.

15. Nursing diagnosis: Potential for secondary infection related to ectropion

Goal

Patient will be free of infection.

Nursing interventions

1. Keep area clean at all times.
2. Advise patient to wash hands before applying medications.
3. Notify physician immediately if any redness, swelling, or pain exists.

Medical diagnosis: *Entropion*

16. Nursing diagnosis: Alteration in comfort related to inversion of lid margin

Goal

Patient will experience a decrease in pain and discomfort.

Nursing interventions

1. Pull skin below eyelid down toward the cheek by means of adhesive tape.
2. Prepare patient for surgery if planned as the definitive treatment.
3. Apply medication as ordered, giving patient instructions on administration of eyedrops.
4. Allay fears about surgery, explaining the short postoperative course and follow-up care.

Medical diagnosis: *Blepharitis/Keratitis*

17. Nursing diagnosis: Alteration in skin integrity related to infectious process

Goal

Patient will be free of infection.

Nursing interventions

1. Cleanse with a clean, soft cloth, using warm, moist compresses 3 times or 4 times daily for 5 minutes.
2. Apply antibiotic ointment as ordered, giving clear directions to patient to wipe away any loose crusts.
3. Instruct patient to keep hands clean and away from eyes.
4. Instruct patient to wear sunglasses when outside for photophobia.

Medical diagnosis: Macular degeneration

18. Nursing diagnosis: Alteration in sensory perception related to loss of central vision

Goal

Patient will maintain peripheral vision.

Nursing interventions

1. Assess the level of visual adequacy to determine nursing interventions.
2. Address patient from the side, making certain you can be seen.
3. Use alternative sensory modalities: touch, talking, pleasant odors.
4. Encourage use of low-vision aids: magnifiers, optocon, phone dial attachments.

19. Nursing diagnosis: Social isolation related to decreased visual acuity

Goal

Patient will engage in social interaction.

Nursing interventions

1. Encourage patient to participate in a group for the visually impaired or blind.
2. Assess degree of sensory deprivation and relationship to time, place, and person.

20. Nursing diagnosis: Knowledge deficit of the cause and prognosis of the disease related to lack of instruction

Goal

Patient will verbalize understanding of the disease process and treatment.

Nursing interventions

1. Use community resources for teaching (Lions Club and American Foundation for the Blind, 15 West 16th Street, New York, New York 10011).
2. Explain to patient that peripheral vision will remain intact and that familial tendencies play a role in the development of the disease.
3. Discuss photocoagulation therapy as an alternative treatment.

Medical diagnosis: Presbycusis

21. Nursing diagnosis: Alteration in sensory perception related to decreased auditory acuity

Goals

Patient will maintain auditory sensory acuity.
Patient will initiate communication when addressed.

Nursing interventions

1. Assess patient for hearing, using watch-and-whisper test, as well as normal speech.
2. Face patient directly while speaking.
3. Ask patient to repeat all instructions to ascertain hearing and learning.
4. Avoid use of the intercom and other auditory distractions; eliminate extraneous noises, particularly during patient teaching.
5. Clarify messages by asking for feedback, particularly in giving preoperative instructions. Include family and significant others when teaching.
6. Avoid labeling patient as belligerent, and so forth, without proper aural assessment.
7. Touch patient on hand or shoulder to provide sensory orientation and gain attention.
8. Make sure patient is wearing glasses, if necessary, so the most sensory information possible is provided and reading lips is a possibility.
9. Speak clearly in a normal tone and if necessary increase volume.
10. Avoid isolating patient. Speak directly to patient each time you are in the room.
11. Observe patient's response to interaction, noting any anger, paranoia, or hostility.
12. Assist patient in use of a hearing aid, reinforcing benefit of amplification.
13. Respect patient's right to turn off sound at times.
14. Arrange for aural rehabilitation if a profound hearing loss is suspected.
15. Assess patient medicines for possible ototoxic side-effects. (See section on Drug therapy, page 78.)
16. Communicate care plan to all staff to maintain continuity.

Medical diagnosis: *Impacted cerumen*

22. Clinical nursing problem: Alteration in sensory perception (auditory acuity): impacted cerumen

Goal

Patient will have improved hearing ability after removal of cerumen.

Nursing interventions

1. Inspect ears for cerumen.
2. Instruct patient to have ears checked and not to attempt to remove wax.
3. Remove cerumen as ordered, explaining the procedure to patient. If cerumen is hard and dry, a Water Pic can be used; however, it may be helpful to loosen wax with a few drops of mineral oil. Use a low-pressure gradient on the Water Pic, drape patient and run tap water at normal body temperature into the ear. Cerumen should be flushed out as patient tilts head. Dry the ear canal with tipped applicator. Re-examine ear with otoscope (Carnevali 1986).

Medical diagnosis: *Tinnitus*

23. Nursing diagnosis: Anxiety related to fear of incurable diagnosis

Goals

Patient will establish coping patterns and adjust to this problem during treatment.
Patient fears will be diminished.

Nursing interventions

1. On nursing history form, assess accurately the origin of problem, duration, and direct effect of lifestyle and ADL.
2. Explain during diagnosis that tinnitus is often a reversible symptom and reassure the patient that accurate information will be provided.
3. Allow patient time to verbalize anxieties about possible tumor, mental illness, or stroke. Reassure patient that feeling concerned is a normal response to a health problem.
4. Obtain a psychology consultation to teach patient relaxation and biofeedback techniques, if appropriate.
5. Distract patient from thinking about the

continued

Nursing interventions

   problem (*e.g.,* provide recreational activities).
6. Provide for a television or radio as a source
   of ambient noise to mask the subjective
   tinnitus (Haimovici 1979).
7. Keep family and significant others informed
   and make certain they do not compound
   anxieties.

24. Nursing diagnosis: Alteration in sleep patterns related to auditory paresthesia

Goal

Patient will experience normal sleep–wake
cycle.

Nursing interventions

1. Before bedtime make certain atmosphere is
   relaxed, visitors have gone, back rub has
   been given.
2. If patient is at home, set up a bedtime ritual
   (*e.g.,* sleep with music playing, drink warm
   milk).
3. Provide sedation if sleeplessness persists.

Medical diagnosis: *Cerebral vascular accident*

25. Nursing diagnosis: Potential for injury related to self-care deficits and risk of falling

Goals

Patient will be oriented to sensory stimuli in
the environment.
Patient will be free from harm and safe in his
or her environment.
Patient will be supported in rehabilitative efforts to regain ability to perform functional
ADL.

Nursing interventions

1. Assess patient for level of sensation.
2. Map out the sensory deficits in order to
   provide for accurate and continuous care
   (see Fig. 5-1).
3. Provide frequent tactile stimulation to patient on the unaffected side.
4. Reposition patient on a regular time schedule and align the body properly, giving an
   explanation to patient of location of body
   parts.
5. Arrange bed, personal objects, and furniture so that they are highly visible to the
   patient.

continued

Nursing interventions

6. Re-orient patient to sensory stimuli in the environment, speak in a normal tone and reassure patient.
7. In acute phase, make certain side-rails are properly placed, nightlights are kept on, and call button is reachable on unaffected side.
8. Do not alarm patient. Touch lightly, using proper name to call patient before beginning care.
9. Allot sufficient time for giving care. Be unhurried, remembering discussion is very important particularly if patient cannot speak. Use short sentences and a caring touch.
10. Protect patient from injury (avoid tight restraints during acute phase and try to eliminate clutter in the environment when patient is walking in convalescent stage).
11. Set up a risk protocol to alert other practitioners that the patient needs additional surveillance to prevent falls.

Medical diagnosis: Brain tumor

26. Nursing diagnosis: Potential for injury related to loss of ability to smell

Goals

Patient will be oriented to other sensory stimuli in environment.
Patient will exist in a safe environment.

Nursing interventions

1. Assess degree of sensory deficit.
2. Provide patient with sensory stimuli having a visual appeal (*e.g.,* flower arrangements, attractive food arrangement on tray).
3. Allow patient to choose foods that are appealing.
4. If patient is at home, be certain that smoke alarms are operating, that gas burners are off, and that spoiled food will not be eaten.
5. Ascertain what particular tastes and odors are appealing and attempt to have these incorporated into meals (*e.g.,* freshly brewed coffee, the crunch of corn flakes).

References

Carnevali D, Patrick M: Nursing Management for the Elderly, 2nd ed. Philadelphia, JB Lippincott, 1986

Carotenuto R, Bullock J: Physical Assessment of the Gerontologic Client. Philadelphia, FA Davis, 1980

Dangel M, Hovener W: Drugs and the Aging Eye. Geriatrics 38:133–140, 1981

Duke University Hospital Nursing Services: Guidelines for Nursing Care: Process and Outcome, p 219. Philadelphia, JB Lippincott, 1983

Gioiella E, Bevil C: Nursing Care of the Aging Client Promoting Healthy Adaptation. Norwalk, Appleton-Century-Crofts, 1985

Haimovici H: Peripheral vascular system. In Rossman I (ed): Clinical Geriatrics, 2nd ed, p 240. Philadelphia, JB Lippincott, 1979

Hall B: Mental Health and the Elderly. Orlando, Grune & Stratton, 1984

Lewis R: Macular Degeneration in the Aged. In Han SS, Coons DH (eds): Special Senses in Aging, pp 93–99. Ann Arbor, Institute of Gerontology, University of Michigan, 1979

McCoy K: Cataracts and intraocular lenses: From cloudy to clear. Nurs Clin North Am 16:405–414, 1981

Mezey MD, Rauckhorst LH, Stokes SA: Health Assessment of the Older Individual. New York, Springer Publishing, 1980

Schow R, Christensen J, Hutchinson J, Nerbonne M: Communication disorders of the aged: A guide for health professionals, Baltimore, University Park Press, 1978

Shanas E, Townsend P, Weedenburn D et al: The Psychology of Health. In Neugarten BL (ed): Middle Age and Aging, p 212. Chicago, University Press, 1968

Sullivan N: Vision in the elderly. J Geriatr Nurs 3:228–235, 1983

Todd B: Using eye drops and ointments safely. J Geriatr Nurs 3:53–57, 1983

Witherly S: Sensory response to food stimuli in the elderly and college-age subjects (abstr). Dissertation Abstracts International 44(3-B):741–742, 1983

Suggested readings

Bernardine L: Effective communication as an intervention for sensory deprivation in the elderly client. Topics in Clinical Nursing 6:72–81, 1985

Boyd-Monk H: Screening for glaucoma. Nursing 79A:42–44, 1979

Bozian J, Clark H: Counteracting sensory changes in the aging. Am J Nurs 80:473–476, 1980

Cohen S: Sensory changes in the elderly (programmed instruction). Am J Nurs 81:1851–1880, 1981

Kopac C: Sensory Loss in the Aged: The Role of the Nurse and the Family in Nursing Clinics of North America. Philadelphia, WB Saunders, 1983

Thompson JM, Bowers AC: Clinical Manual of Health Assessment. St Louis, CV Mosby, 1980

Mickey Stanley

Cardiovascular system 6

With advancing years, the heart and blood vessels change in several ways. Because the prevalence of cardiovascular disease is high in the United States, often it is difficult to determine which of the age-related changes of the cardiovascular (CV) system are due to disease and which are solely due to the aging process. In general, the onset of changes caused by the aging process is slow and insidious. For example, the symptom of dyspnea on exertion may occur progressively more frequently and in response to less strenuous activity as cardiovascular function declines. A sudden onset of dyspnea, however, associated with activities not previously known to be dyspnea producing is more likely to indicate a recent myocardial infarction (often silent) or episode of congestive heart failure (Hitzhusen and Alpert 1984; Lillington 1984). Therefore, an accurate nursing assessment of the CV system in an elderly patient demands both a thorough understanding of the effects of the aging process and a high index of suspicion for any recent or unexpected changes in behavior and function.

Age-related changes

Heart

In the absence of disease, the size of a person's heart increases slightly with advancing age, or remains proportional to body weight (Kennedy and Caird 1981). Some atrophy of the cardiac muscle has been noted on autopsy in sedentary persons (Wenger 1984b). Hypertrophy of the cardiac muscle, however, is not considered normal, but is a significant sign of cardiac disease (Gioiella and Bevil 1985; Harris 1983). The age-related changes in the heart muscle are associated with an increased density of collagen fibers and a loss of functioning elastic fibers (Chobanian 1983; Steffl 1984). Frequently, as a result of years of exposure to high-pressure blood flow, the endocardium thickens. The aging myocardium therefore becomes less distensible with a less-effective contractile force (Gioiella and Bevil 1985; Harris 1983; Kennedy and Caird 1981). As a result of these changes, the elderly heart is less able to handle the increased volume that accompanies such conditions as congestive heart failure or a rapid IV flow.

Within the heart, surface areas of the aortic and mitral valves thicken secondary to irritation from high-pressure blood flow with ridges forming along the valve closure lines (Gioiella and Bevil 1985; Weisfeldt 1980). This thickening process leads to an increased stiffness of the valves and may produce a common systolic ejection murmur. This characteristic murmur is soft, between grade 1 and grade 2, and may be difficult to hear because of changes in the respiratory system (Gioiella and Bevil 1985; Harris 1983). Similar changes may occur in the tricuspid and pulmonic valves, but to a lesser degree, principally because the right side of the heart has relatively lower pressures than the left. During times of increased heart rate (*e.g.*, fever, stress, and exercise) these stiff valves create an obstacle or impedance to blood flow through the heart. Incomplete ventricular emptying may result from the outflow obstruction and compromise coronary artery and systemic tissue perfusion (Wenger 1984b). Signs and symptoms of ischemia, transient ischemic attacks, confusion, memory loss, as well as falls frequently result from a drop in cardiac output that follows a decrease in systolic ejection time (Yurick et al 1984).

Conduction system

The resting heart rate changes minimally with aging. However, the maximal attainable heart rate, or the extent to which persons can increase their heart rate to meet increased body demands, does decline with advanced age (Wenger 1981). A number of physiological changes within the conduction system influence this decline. For example, the total number of pacemaker cells in the sinoatrial node (SA node) decreases. In addition, the bundle of His loses conduction fibers that carry the impulses to the ventricles (Weisfeldt 1980). Studies have demonstrated an increase in the level of circulating catecholamines in elderly subjects. Changes in the sensitivity of the receptor sites for these chemical mediators, however, lessen their ability to produce the necessary increase in heart rate during periods of stress or exercise (Chobanian 1983). In addition to being unable to maximally accelerate the heart rate, the elderly heart requires a longer time to return to baseline or resting rates after exercise or stress. Although these changes occur in the physically active as well as the sedentary, the effect is much more pronounced in the sedentary elderly (Wenger 1984b).

Cardiac output is also known to decline during the aging process. This loss may be secondary to the decreased distensibility and contractility of the ventricles, resulting from a loss of elastic fibers and increased collagen deposition, or the outflow obstruction from stiffened valves. Functionally, a decline in cardiac output prolongs the mean circulation time and predisposes to clot formation owing to sluggish blood flow (Wenger 1984b).

Because of the decrease in the number of pacemaker cells, the decline in the sensitivity to catecholamines, and the tissue changes associated with the aged heart, the inherent rhythmicity and conduction velocity of the myocardial conduction system also decline (Hitzhusen and Alpert 1984; Weisfeldt 1980; Yurick et al 1984). P wave notching, slurring, and a loss of amplitude are so common that they are considered normal (Rodstein 1977). These changes have correlated on autopsy with tissue changes and loss of muscle mass owing to the aging process. The P–R interval is frequently prolonged, with upper limits of normal being extended from 0.20 to 0.22 seconds (Hitzhusen and Alpert 1984; Rodstein 1977). This situation of a prolonged conduction time favors the development of re-entrant dysrhythmias. Decreased myocardial mass, obesity, senile emphysema, and increased A–P diameter may all contribute to the loss of QRS amplitude. The multitude of conditions affecting the R wave and S–T segment, including hypertension, left ventricular hypertrophy, digitalis, and tranquilizers, causes a loss of diagnostic specificity of these EKG changes (Michaelson 1983; Rodstein 1977). Harris (1983) notes

> *Some atrial dysrhythmias arise from focal thickening of the elastic and reticular nets, with infiltration of fat in and about the region of the SA node. These changes are unrelated to coronary artery disease or other known diseases of the heart and are considered the result of the aging process.*

The sick sinus syndrome frequently seen in the aged is due to the impaired function of the aging or diseased sinoatrial node and an abnormally unresponsive atrioventricular junctional pacemaker. Sinus dysrhythmias and sinus bradycardia are common and may result in periods of syncope, dizziness, palpitations, or feelings of weakness (Hitzhusen and Alpert 1984).

Although ventricular and atrial premature contractions are known to increase with age, cardiac dysrhythmias should be considered serious in the elderly because the uncoordinated and ineffective method of contraction compromises cardiac output and tissue perfusion (Gioiella and Bevil 1985). Falls or unexplained accidents in the elderly are frequently associated with cardiac dysrhythmias and should be thoroughly investigated (Rodstein 1977). Cardioversion for rapid dysrhythmias is dangerous in the elderly because it may produce a fatal sinus arrest. Cardiac pacing, however, allows for safe use of drugs to control rapid atrial rates and effective management of slow rhythms (Rodstein 1977; Schocken 1984).

Digitalis should be used with caution in the elderly patient. With the loss of lean muscle mass, and a decrease in glomerular filtration rate, plasma concentrations as well as half-life for the drug are increased. This situation leads to an increased incidence of digitalis toxicity and the development of dangerous dysrhythmias. The pediatric elixir of digoxin in doses as small as 50 μg/70 μg a day may be needed for toxic-free maintenance (Lowenthal and Affrime 1981; Rodstein 1977).

Blood vessels

With advanced age, the aorta and peripheral arterial system become tortuous and less able to respond to changes in pressure. Kennedy and Caird (1981) noted that these changes result from increased collagen and loss of elastic fibers in the medial layer of the arteries and not from atherosclerosis. Increases in pulse pressure and systolic pressure are common because arteries fail to stretch and accommodate the pressure delivered to them by the left ventricle. As a compensatory mechanism, the aorta and distal arteries progressively dilate to accept a greater volume of blood. As Chobanian (1983) states

The net result is an arterial system with diminished elasticity and distensibility and reduced ability to absorb pressure during cardiac systole or to recoil during diastole.

This stiffness of the arterial system further impedes left ventricular ejection during stress or exercise, and accounts for declines seen in cardiac output under these circumstances. Although changes in the systolic pressure are considered to be a result of the normal aging process, no change in diastolic pressure is considered normal.

As a result of the age-related changes in the arterial system, hypertension is a frequent problem in the elderly. The American Heart Association (1983) recommends the values of 160 mmHg systolic over 90 mmHg diastolic be considered the upper limits of normal for blood pressure readings in the elderly. These guidelines are used to established levels at which antihypertensive therapy should begin. Owing to a lack of convincing evidence of decreased mortality associated with treating isolated systolic hypertension of less than 180 torr, and increased complications associated with antihypertensive therapy, many physicians withhold treatment until systolic pressures reach 180 mmHg or diastolic pressures exceed 90–95 mmHg (Chobanian 1983; O'Brien and Pattee 1981). Common problems associated with antihypertensive therapy in the elderly include volume contraction, dehydration, and electrolyte imbalance from centrally acting agents; and increased incidence of heart failure and memory loss from vasodilators (Sheridan 1984). Blood pressure readings should be lowered slowly, with close attention to the development of unacceptable side-effects.

Many elderly persons have problems from hypotension caused by antihypertensive therapy. The baroreceptors located in the aortic arch and carotid sinus become blunted, or less sensitive, with advanced age (Wenger 1984b). Although increased amounts of circulating epinephrine and norepinephrine have been found in the elderly, changes in or reduced sensitivity of receptor sites to these stimulators decreases the ability of the vasculature to respond to changes in blood pressure (Wenger 1984b). A rapid change in position, therefore, frequently results in symptomatic orthostatic hypotension. Owing to the blood vessel's inability to adjust fully or quickly to changes in position, blood pressure levels should always be monitored with the patient either sitting or standing (Wenger 1981). This rule is especially significant when blood pressure is being monitored to determine the effectiveness of antihypertensive therapy. A drop in pressure of

20 mmHg when the patient changes position from lying to standing is not uncommon in the elderly. A fall of blood pressure of more than 20 mmHg or a fall to a systolic pressure of less than 100 mmHg is not considered to be within normal limits and may cause fainting, dizziness, or precipitate falls.

Kidney

Additional factors that influence the development of hypertension in the elderly are changes occurring in the kidney. Franklin (1983) notes

> *Beyond the fourth decade of life, the kidney undergoes vascular changes resulting in approximately a 20% reduction in glomerular filtration rate. The consequences of age-related loss of renal function are an inability to maximally concentrate or dilute urine, an inability to maximally conserve sodium on a low sodium diet or rapidly excrete a large sodium load.*

A high-sodium diet and a reduction in sodium excretory ability frequently lead to volume expansion and hypertension in the elderly (Kent 1981). In addition, aggressive use of diuretics without attention to fluid replacement may lead to a volume contraction and dehydration.

Musculoskeletal system

Changes in the musculoskeletal system also have impact on the ability of the CV system to accomplish its mission of delivering oxygenated blood to meet the metabolic demands of the body. Principal among these changes is a decline in the ability of the mitochondria of working muscles to extract oxygen from the blood (Wenger 1981). One contributing factor to this decline in oxygen uptake is the loss of lean muscle mass and increased fatty tissue that occurs with aging. When the working muscles are inefficient in their use of oxygen, the CV system is stimulated to provide additional oxygenated blood for the same or lower levels of activity. If the heart is unable to increase its cardiac output sufficiently to meet these increased demands, symptoms of dyspnea result (Wenger 1981).

Although these changes of loss of lean muscle mass, increased fatty tissue, and ineffective oxygen extraction are known to occur in every person, the effect is much less dramatic in those who remain physically active (Wenger 1984b). In addition, regular physical exercise in the elderly has been shown to increase the number of functioning mitochondria and to increase the body's ability to extract oxygen from the circulating blood (Blumenthal et al 1982). Recent research with patients who suffer from intermittent claudication has suggested that symptoms improve in this group because of this ability of working muscles to increase oxygen uptake after exercise training, rather than any increase in blood flow, as was previously believed (Blumenthal et al 1982).

Venous system

The venous system has been noted to have many of the same changes found in the arteries. Because of the lower pressure associated with the venous system, however, changes are not as pronounced as those in the arterial system. With age, the veins stretch and dilate. Structural changes in the valves contribute to a decreased venous return and increased venous stasis (Gioiella and Bevil 1985). As a result, varicosities, thrombophlebitis, and phlebothrombosis occur with increasing frequency. With aging, there is a redistribution of blood flow caused by changes in peripheral vascular resistance. Blood supply to the kidney, viscera, hands, and feet is especially reduced (Gioiella and Bevil 1985; O'Brien and Pattee 1981; Spittell 1984). This reduction in blood flow contributes to an inability of the elderly system to thermoregulate effectively during cold or hot weather. In addition, problems of arterial occlusion may occur, principally in the lower extremities.

Physical assessment

The standard physical-assessment techniques and questions used to elicit important data about the CV system may need to be altered for the elderly. The signs and symptoms of cardiac-related problems are often mistaken for the functional decline associated with aging, and treatment may be inappropriately delayed or neglected. Questioning elderly patients about the following areas will assist in more accurately determining their nursing needs:

Feelings of palpitations or a pounding in the chest

Difficulty catching the breath with usual activities

Description of usual daily activities

Weight gain unrelated to food intake

Clothes, shoes, or rings that have become too tight

Swelling in the feet and legs that decreases with elevation

A bloated feeling after small meals

Diuresis that begins 2 to 5 hours after going to bed or assuming a reclining position

Awakening with a smothering feeling during the night that is relieved within one hour by sitting up or walking

Increase in the number of pillows used at night

A nonproductive, irritating cough that occurs at night and clears during the day

Dizziness or black-out spells after a sudden position change

Episodes of memory lapses or periods of confusion

An assessment of the elderly CV system begins with a generalized inspection of the patient, who should be either lying down or seated. Specific attention should be focused on overall appearance, breathing pattern, and obvious signs of distress. Indicators of tissue perfusion such as color and temperature of the skin, amount of perspiration relative to room temperature, briskness of capillary refill, and level of alertness should be observed as a general indication of tissue perfusion.

Assessing the presence of edema related to CV dysfunction in the elderly patient requires discrimination among a number of noncardiac sources. All of the soft-tissue areas of the body should be observed and palpated for the presence of edema. Areas such as the medial maleolus, instep of both feet, knees, sacral area, abdomen, hands, and face should be closely observed. The edema associated with CV dysfunction is soft and pitting, symmetrical in distribution, and involves dependent body parts. Cardiac edema accumulates during the day and resolves with rest or the elevation of the dependent part. This type of edema is associated with feelings of fatigue and a heaviness of the extremities. For elderly persons who sit with their feet dependent most of the day, however, or who use garters to support their stockings, the dependent edema may be the result of the external obstruction to blood flow rather than CV dysfunction.

Nutritional edema, a frequent source of edema in elderly persons, is often mistaken for the edema associated with congestive heart failure. Edema associated with poor nutritional status or hepatic dysfunction involves all soft-tissue areas such as the abdomen, face, and eye orbits, and is not selective for dependent body parts. This type of edema is typically worse in the early morning and does not clear with elevation of the involved part (Michaelson 1983). Nutritional edema is not related to nocturnal diuresis or paroxysmal nocturnal dyspnea.

Other discriminating factors that should be considered when observing for edema are varicose veins or a history of vein ligation and stripping. The edema associated with varicose veins is usually asymmetrical, with prominent varicosities on the affected limb. Evidence of venous engorgement may be noted to decrease with elevation and refill with prolonged standing.

An important part of the CV assessment in the elderly patient is auscultation of the chest. Auscultation of the precordium should follow the same sequence as that used in the younger adult. Beginning either at the base (2nd intercostal space [ICS]), at the right sternal border (RSB), or at the apex (5th ICS, midclavicular line [MCL]), count the apical pulse for 1 full minute to allow for detection of irregularities of rhythm. Leaving the stethoscope in place, palpate a radial pulse while listening simultaneously to the apical pulse for an additional 60 seconds to assess for disparities or a pulse deficit. The most common sources of a pulse deficit in elderly persons are premature ventricular contractions and atrial fibrillation.

With the diaphragm of the stethoscope at the apex of the heart, concentrate on the two heart sounds. The first heart sound is best heard in this area. Listening here allows easy identification of *systole,* that interval between the first heart sound to the occurrence of the second heart sound, and *diastole,* that interval between the second and next first heart sounds. Auscultation of heart tones in the elderly is often difficult because of the senile emphysematous changes in the chest wall. If the heart tones are distant or difficult to hear, turn the patient onto his or her left side, with the left arm supporting the head. Place the stethoscope between the chest wall and the bed at the fifth intercostal space, midclavicular line and listen carefully for each heart sound. This position allows the heart to move closer to the chest wall and enhances the sound.

With the patient still lying on the left side, inch the bell of the stethoscope along the left sternal border and be attentive for the presence of murmurs. A low-intensity, systolic murmur, best heard at the base of the heart, that does not radiate toward the carotid arteries is considered normal in elderly persons (Harris 1983). A loud murmur, or one that occurs during the diastolic phase, is considered abnormal and indicates cardiac pathology.

Palpation for the point of maximal impulse (PMI) in the elderly may be difficult because of emphysematous changes in the chest wall or abnormal curvatures of the spine (Hitzhusen and Alpert 1984). If either of these conditions exists, the finding of an abnormal location of the PMI loses its diagnostic significance (Gioiella and Bevil 1985; Harris 1983). The PMI is palpated by laying the palmar surface of the hand over the apex of the heart and assessing for pulsations. The PMI is considered abnormal if it is located outside the MCL or below the 5th ICS (Harris 1983), a finding that is usually indicative of cardiac hypertrophy (Gioiella and Bevil 1985).

Because of the increased frequency of hypertension from the arteriosclerotic process, accurate assessment of blood pressure measurement is crucial to avoid the problems associated with the auscultatory gap. Inattention to such details as cuff size, activities preceding measurement, and consistency in technique may mean a misdiagnosis of hypertension and needless therapy for elderly patients. Therefore, the patient should quietly sit or remain lying down for 20 minutes before measurement of blood pressure. The cuff should wrap around the upper arm one and one half times, with good attachment of the Velcro closure. Palpate for the brachial artery and inflate the blood pressure cuff to about 220 mmHg. Slowly deflate the cuff while palpating for the first pulsation (Figure 6-1). After noting the level at which the first beat is felt, fully deflate the cuff. The cuff must not be re-inflated for 2 minutes, in order to allow for return of normal blood flow. After the 2-minute interval, place the bell of the stethoscope over the brachial artery and inflate the cuff 10 mmHg above the level of the first felt beat. Slowly deflate the cuff, auscultating for all three Korotkoff sounds (Figure 6-2). A period of silence frequently occurs between the first and third Korotkoff sounds and is known as the auscultatory gap. Preliminary determination of systolic blood pressure by palpation eliminates the mistake of beginning auscultation during this period of silence and erroneously recording low systolic pressures or high diastolic pressures (Franklin 1983; Knudson, 1984).

After assessment of the recumbent pressure, the patient is assisted to sitting, either with feet dangling or on the floor, remaining in this position for 3 minutes to 4 minutes. At this time, a second blood pressure is auscultated. If the patient is ambulatory, a third pressure is measured with the patient standing, allowing 3 minutes to 5 minutes for accommodation to the new position before measurement. This technique allows for accurate assessment of CV status and antihyper-

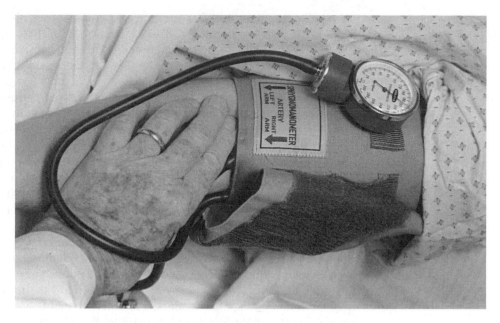

Figure 6-1. Palpating for the brachial artery (Photo by CJ Collins, photographer for University of Texas Health Science Center at San Antonio, San Antonio, Texas)

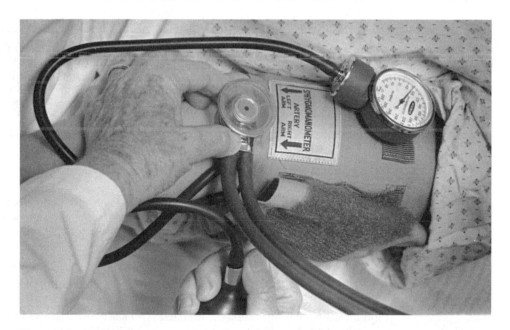

Figure 6-2. Auscultating the Korotkoff sounds (Photo by C. J. Collins, photographer for the University of Texas Health Science Center at San Antonio, San Antonio, Texas)

tensive therapy. In addition, it allows the nurse to evaluate for orthostatic hypotension, thus providing information that will allow him or her to plan appropriately for safety needs of the patient. After measurement of blood pressure in each position, the limb used for measurement and the position are recorded on the patient's record (Jessup 1984).

An important indicator of CV performance, that of renal perfusion, requires careful assessment in the elderly. Factors such as benign prostatic hypertrophy or cystocele may make urinary elimination difficult. Chronic or aggressive use of diuretics may have induced a state of dehydration and, therefore, decreased urine production. Patterns of nocturnal or rest-related diuresis are common in the elderly. An accurate fluid balance should therefore be assessed on a 24-hour basis. An even more sensitive indicator of fluid balance is the daily weight, with a weight gain of 1 pound per day or greater being indicative of fluid retention (McCauley and Burke 1984).

Knowledge of the normal aging process and important data from a thorough history and physical assessment will allow for accurate planning for the elderly patient with problems of the cardiovascular system. Table 6-1 gives information on the drugs commonly used with this patient population. Nursing interventions for many of the nursing diagnoses common to elderly patients with cardiovascular problems are detailed in the Nursing Care Plans in this chapter.

Table 6-1. *Drugs used in the treatment of cardiovascular diseases*

Drugs	Effect/response in the elderly	Nursing implications
Digoxin (Lanoxin)	Digoxin is excreted by way of the kidney. With a decrease in glomerular filtration rate, the plasma half-life is prolonged from 32 hr to 73 hr (Lowenthal and Affrime 1981). Signs of toxicity include: anorexia, cardiac dysrhythmias, halo or blurred vision, confusion, weakness and GI upset. Quinidine and verapamil raise the plasma level of digoxin (McCauley and Burke 1984).	Assess pulse rate 1 full min. Observe for signs of toxicity. Monitor serum K^+ levels. Teach patient to count pulse, report adverse effects, and take medication only as ordered. Monitor serum level of digoxin to determine therapeutic level.
Quinidine	Quinidine is detoxified by the liver. Conditions leading to decreased liver function (*e.g.,* caused by congestive heart failure or alcoholism) may result in a prolonged half-life. The interaction between quinidine and digoxin may lead to digitalis toxicity (Lowenthal and Affrime 1981).	Assess pulse rate 1 full min. Observe for signs of digitalis toxicity if used in conjunction.
Procainamide (Pronestyl)	Procainamide hydrochloride is excreted by way of the kidneys. The dosage should be reduced by 50% and administered q 12 h (Lowenthal and Affrime 1981).	Observe for signs of bradycardia or syncope.

(continued)

Table 6-1. (Continued)

Drugs	Effect/response in the elderly	Nursing implications
Lidocaine (Xylocaine)	Lidocaine is detoxified by the liver and excreted by the kidney. High blood levels of lidocaine may cause sedation, tremors, hypotension, and blurred vision (Lowenthal and Affrime 1981).	Administer bolus slowly (over 2–3 min). Begin with 25-mg bolus and increase as needed. Use IV controller to deliver lidocaine drip. Observe frequently for side-effects.
Propranolol (Inderol)	Propranolol hydrochloride is metabolized by the liver and is known to have a prolonged half-life in the elderly (Lowenthal and Affrime 1981). Owing to the beta-blocking action, propranolol decreases the force of cardiac contraction and may predispose the system to heart failure. Elderly patients are at risk for bronchospasm with propranolol because of age-related changes in the respiratory system.	Assess for signs of edema, decreased urine output, and rales. Monitor blood pressure and level consciousness. Monitor respiratory function.
Nitroglycerin	Nitroglycerin is metabolized by the liver. The effect may be prolonged in liver failure. Orthostatic hypotension, headache, tachycardia, and faintness may occur after administration (McCauley and Burke 1984). Long-acting nitroglycerin is known to increase intraocular pressure and should be avoided in elderly persons who have glaucoma (Gioiella and Bevil 1985)	Monitor blood pressure with patients sitting, standing. Teach patient to lie or sit with feet elevated when taking sublingual temperature. Teach patient to arise slowly, and to report faintness, dizziness, or falls.
Nifedipine (Procardia) Verapamil (Calan, Isoptin)	Nifedipine and verapamil produce vasodilation and a decreased peripheral vascular resistance. Hypotension, dizziness, faintness, or falls are potential side-effects. SA node depression and slowed atrioventricular (AV) conduction also occur (Sheridan 1984).	Monitor heart rate and blood pressure. Keep side-rails up. Teach patient to report faintness or falls.
Chlorothiazide (Diuril) Hydrochlorothiazide (Hydrodiuril)	Volume contraction, dehydration, and electrolyte imbalance occur frequently with the use of diuretics. Thiazides induce hyperglycemia, aggravate pre-existing diabetes mellitus, and may cause uric acid retention, precipitating an attack of gout (Sheridan 1984). Symptoms of electrolyte imbalance include: cardiac dysrhythmias, muscle weakness, confusion, GI disturbance.	Monitor blood pressure with patient lying, sitting, and standing. Monitor input and output q 24 h. Monitor urine color and appearance. Weigh patient daily. Schedule dose in morning to avoid nocturia or incontinence. Keep call bell within easy reach. Monitor electrolytes.

(continued)

Table 6-1. (Continued)

Drugs	Effect/response in the elderly	Nursing implications
Furosemide (Lasix)	Furosemide is more potent than the thiazide diuretics. Problems of dehydration and electrolyte imbalance occur with greater frequency. (See above for symptoms of electrolyte imbalance.) Problems of orthostatic hypotension, hemoconcentration, and vascular thrombosis may occur (McCauley and Burke 1984).	Assist to bathroom or have patient stand to void q 1h × 4 to avoid incontinence (see above for additional implications). Observe for Homan's sign.
Methyldopa (Aldomet)	Methyldopa is a sympatholytic drug frequently used with elderly patients. Problems of sedation, weakness, drowsiness, and nasal congestion may occur (Sheridan 1984).	Give first dose at night to avoid hypotension. Monitor blood pressure with patient sitting and standing. Teach patient to lie down if dizziness or faintness occurs, to arise slowly, and to report feelings of fatigue or weakness. Teach patient to avoid hot showers or steam rooms, standing for long periods, and exercising in hot weather.
Prazosin (Minipress)	Prazosin hydrochloride blocks alpha receptors, producing a lower peripheral vascular resistance. Problems of dizziness, weakness, and palpitations occur infrequently (Sheridan 1984).	See above for nursing implications.
Reserpine (Serpasil)	Reserpine is a sympatholytic drug that produces serious side-effects in elderly persons. Problems of depression, fatigue, impotence, and gastric distress are known to occur (Sheridan 1984).	See above for nursing implications.
Hydralazine (Apresoline)	Hydralazine hydrochloride is a vasodilator that has its greatest effect on the arterial system. Problems of reflex tachycardia resulting in angina, nausea, anorexia, and headache are known to occur (Sheridan 1984).	See above for nursing implications.

Nursing care plans

Medical diagnosis: Ischemic heart disease (angina pectoris)

1. Nursing diagnosis: Activity intolerance related to alteration in comfort

Goal

Patient will return to levels of independence or increased level of activity.

Nursing interventions

1. Do not allow patient to have prolonged bed rest—encourage chair rest during daytime.
2. Monitor heart rate and blood pressure during self-care activities.
3. Evaluate anginal episodes to determine precipitating factors.
4. Monitor vital signs before and every 15 min to 20 min after pain medication or nitrates are given until pain is relieved.
5. Use a calm, unhurried approach.
6. Remain with patient during anginal episodes.
7. Use deliberate touch and verbal reassurance to decrease anxiety.
8. Supervise ambulation and performance of range-of-motion (ROM) and stretching exercises at the bedside.
9. Encourage use of slow, repetitive movements to maintain muscle tone (*e.g.*, foot and arm circles, flexion/contraction of calf muscles).
10. Increase level of activity to tolerance.
11. Evaluate level of functioning frequently.
12. Offer realistic reassurance.
13. Use group activity and exercise to provide motivation
14. Caution patient to avoid extremes of heat or cold.
15. Caution patient to exercise only up to level of tolerance. Avoid excessive fatigue (*e.g.*,

continued

Nursing interventions

feeling tired 2 hr after exercise, or difficulty sleeping).

16. Instruct patient to wear a hat during hot and cold weather.
17. Instruct patient to cover mouth with a scarf during cold months.
18. Provide information regarding community centers with exercise/activity programs for senior citizens.
19. Evaluate patient concerns regarding sexual functioning.
20. Provide information on adverse effects/ signs of sexual intercourse, modifications of previous patterns to conserve energy.
21. Teach patient to report any history or development of glaucoma to physician.
22. Teach patient to avoid sudden changes in position.
23. Teach patient to sit with legs elevated or lie down when taking nitroglycerin for angina.

2. Nursing diagnosis: Knowledge deficit of disease, treatment, risk factors related to lack of instruction

Goals

Patient will verbalize symptoms of angina.
Patient should also be able to do the following
  • Give name, dosage, action, side-effects of prescribed medication
  • Enumerate activity restrictions
  • Discuss personal risk factors associated with ischemic heart disease (*e.g.,* smoking, diet, sedentary living, stress)

Nursing interventions

1. Identify concerns regarding condition and future lifestyle adaptations.
2. Evaluate home environment for daily physical exertional requirements, including: number of stairs climbed daily, current work status, preferred daily activities, laundry facilities, meal preparation and shopping, level of sexual activity, method of transportation, social interactions.
3. Teach patient and family the importance of rest periods before and after exertional activities.
4. Encourage regular exercise such as walking, golf, bicycling, and stretching and limbering exercises.

continued

Nursing interventions

5. Provide printed information on prescribed medications.
6. Provide a schedule of medication times that coincides with patient's daily routine.
7. Discuss with patient and family potential risk factors associated with heart disease.
8. Arrange for a dietary consultation if necessary.

Medical diagnosis: *Myocardial infarction*

3. Nursing diagnosis: Alteration in tissue perfusion related to decreased cardiac output

Goal

Patient will have adequate tissue perfusion to vital organs as evidenced by:
- Orientation to person and environment
- Vital signs within normal range for the patient
- Adequate urine output

Nursing interventions

1. Provide a quiet, unhurried environment.
2. Monitor heart rate and blood pressure response to activity (*e.g.,* chair rest, bathroom privileges, ambulate in hall).
3. Observe capillary refill, urine output, level of consciousness.
4. Elevate patient's feet when resting in chair.
5. Elevate head of bed during bedrest.
6. Count pulse one full minute to observe for dysrhythmias.
7. Palpate radial pulse simultaneously with apical to assess for pulse deficit.
8. Do not allow patient to have prolonged bedrest.
9. Give analgesics cautiously. Start with small doses and increase as needed.
10. Do not give patient sedatives.
11. Keep side-rails up at all times.
12. Massage patient's back and feet to promote rest.
13. Have patient maintain normal day/night sleep schedule.
14. Discourage the use of stimulants after 4 pm.
15. Have patient use bedside commode or stand-to-void position to avoid urinary incontinence or retention.
16. Apply antiembolic stockings.
17. Assess for Homan's sign every shift.

4. Clinical nursing problem: Alteration in comfort: pain secondary to ischemia

Goal

Patient will have decreased number and severity of pain episodes to allow for self-care and independence in activities of daily living (ADL).

Nursing interventions

1. Position patient for comfort.
2. Remain with patient during pain episodes.
3. Administer nitroglycerin and analgesics as ordered.
4. Monitor blood pressure and pulse every 5 min during pain episodes and every 15 min × 4 after pain relief has been achieved.
5. Position patient supine with head of bed elevated 45° during pain episode.
6. Observe and document precipitating events.
7. Encourage patient to resume self-care activities under supervision.
8. Encourage patient to perform stretching exercises and ambulation under supervision (Benison and Hogstel 1986).
9. Encourage group activities for diversion.
10. Instruct patient on relaxation methods (*e.g.,* deep breathing, progressive muscle relaxation, imagery) to be used during pain episodes.

5. Nursing diagnosis: Alteration in level of awareness related to hospitalization; medication; isolation

Goals

Patient will remain coherent and lucid during hospitalization.
Patient will enter into socialization with family and visitors.

Nursing interventions

1. Provide frequent, simple explanations of equipment for monitoring and care (*e.g.,* cardiac monitor, call bell, IV controller).
2. Orient patient frequently to surroundings (bathroom light switch, call bell)
3. Introduce self to patient frequently.
4. Address patient by proper name.
5. Provide clock, calendar, and personal articles within view and reach.

continued

Nursing interventions

6. Maintain normal day/night lighting and atmosphere.
7. Encourage stimulation (*e.g.*, recreational therapy, during day and quiet rest at night).
8. Encourage family members to discuss current events (personal and community) with patient.
9. Encourage patient to reminisce with family, friends, and staff.
10. Avoid giving patient sedatives.
11. Provide current reading materials.
12. Ensure patient has personal items such as glasses, hearing aid.
13. Massage patient's back and feet to promote rest.
14. Give smallest amount of narcotics/analgesics necessary to control pain.
15. Avoid use of intercom system.
16. Use nightlight or low-level lighting in room/bathroom at night to reduce confusion.
17. Keep bed in low position.
18. Administer diuretic during normal waking hours or at least 3 hr before sleep.
19. Provide bedside commode or bathroom facilities.

6. Nursing diagnosis: Self-care deficit related to fear; anxiety

Goal

Patient will resume previous level of independence of ADL.

Nursing interventions

1. Provide factual information regarding disdisease, treatment, and expected outcomes.
2. Encourage chair rest and increasing ambulation as soon as possible.
3. Supervise patient in performing personal hygiene as needed.
4. Allow patient choices where appropriate.

continued

Nursing interventions

5. Supervise stretching and range-of-motion exercises at bedside (Benison and Hogstel 1986).
6. Discuss home environment and ADL with patient.
7. Discuss methods to reduce energy expenditures for household chores.
8. Encourage participation in previous social activities.
9. Encourage participation in cardiac rehabilitation program.
10. Encourage patient to verbalize fears to family and friends.
11. Have other persons at more advanced stages of recovery demonstrate positive adaptation.
12. Allow patient time to verbalize fears concerning the "heart attack."
13. Dispel misconceptions patient may have about inability to resume regular ADL.

Medical diagnosis: *Dysrhythmias*

7. Nursing diagnosis: Decreased tissue perfusion related to dysrhythmias

Goal

Patient will have adequate tissue perfusion to vital organs

Nursing interventions

1. Maintain hydration status.
2. Weigh patient daily.
3. Monitor intake and output every 24 hours.
4. Monitor blood pressure and pulse with patient lying, sitting, standing, and after exercising.
5. Encourage chair rest and stretching exercises under supervision.
6. Teach patient to arise slowly to accommodate orthostatic changes.
7. Keep bed in low position.
8. Thoroughly investigate falls or unexplained bruises.
9. Assess radial and apical pulse simultaneously to detect pulse deficit.

continued

Nursing interventions

10. Observe for changes in level of consciousness, memory lapses, or restlessness.
11. Keep nurse call bell within easy reach.
12. Teach patient to lie down with feet elevated when dizzy or feeling faint.
13. Teach patient to report symptoms of dizziness, palpitations, or blurred vision.
14. Observe for side-effects of medications (see Table 6-1).
15. Arrange for a home call system ("life line") before discharge if patient lives alone.

Medical diagnosis: *Hypertension*

8. Nursing diagnosis: Alteration in tissue perfusion related to arteriosclerosis; treatment

Goal

Patient will not experience falls or accidents resulting from loss of consciousness.

Nursing interventions

1. Monitor blood pressure with the patient lying, sitting, and standing and observe for auscultatory gap.
2. Monitor blood pressure response to exercise and self-care activities.
3. Assess blood pressure response to medication (before and 2 hr after administration).
4. Teach patient to arise from a supine position slowly (dangle legs 5 min) to prevent orthostatic hypotension.
5. Encourage use of 2 pillows under head for sleep and use of support stockings before arising in morning to prevent venous pooling.
6. Teach patient to substitute appropriate spices for table salt.
7. Teach patient to avoid softened or conditioned water.
8. Encourage regular exercise such as walking, golf, dancing, cycling, and swimming.
9. Encourage patient to stop smoking (if applicable).
10. Instruct patient to avoid standing motionless for long periods (standing in line, shaving).

continued

Nursing interventions

11. Teach patient to flex and release muscles of legs or circle feet and arms.
12. Instruct patient to avoid hot baths, showers, or steam rooms.
13. Teach patient the signs of hypotension.
14. Observe for the side-effects of medications (see Table 6-1).

9. Nursing diagnosis: Knowledge deficit of disease or treatment related to lack of instruction.

Goal

Patient will be able to verbalize effects of uncontrolled hypertension and the recommended treatment.

Nursing interventions

1. Identify patient's concerns about his or her disease and its treatment.
2. See Chapter 3 on "Patient Education."
3. Prepare a medication administration schedule or aid.
4. Include information on generic drugs in teaching if applicable.
5. Caution patient never to stop taking medications abruptly.
6. Instruct patient on use of relaxation and exercise during stressful periods.
7. Caution against use of over-the-counter cold or cough remedies when taking antihypertension medications.

10. Nursing diagnosis: Potential for noncompliance related to side effects; asymptomatic nature of disease

Goal

Patient's blood pressure will be maintained within normal limits with minimal number of side-effects acceptable to the patient.

Nursing interventions

1. Develop rapport with patient by demonstrating a personal interest (Knudson 1984).
2. Use a professional approach to patient teaching. Address patient by proper name.

continued

Nursing interventions

3. Encourage patient to discuss feelings regarding longterm nature of disease.
4. Assess financial ability to purchase prescription medications. Make referral if needed for assistance.
5. Assess patient's willingness to comply with suggested regimen.
6. Allow patient choices when possible.
7. Reinforce how patient behavior affects disease progression.
8. Identify significant others to provide reminders or reinforcement for medication taking, diet, and exercise.
9. Simplify treatment regimen: combination drugs, fewer medication-taking times.
10. Use large labels that are easily read.
11. Use medication calendar or cups.

Medical diagnosis: *Congestive heart failure*

11. Nursing diagnosis: Alteration in tissue perfusion related to fluid excess

Goals

Patient will have adequate tissue perfusion. Patient will not have complications of pneumonia, decubiti, or thrombophlebitis.

Nursing interventions

1. Assess and record peripheral pulses, capillary refill, skin temperature, redness, and areas of breakdown.
2. Position with head of bed elevated 45°–60°.
3. Encourage patient to reposition self frequently. Assist with turning every 2 hr, if necessary.
4. Assess level of awareness frequently.
5. Keep side-rails up at all times.
6. Assess and record lung sounds every 4 hr.
7. Auscultate apical pulse 1 full min to identify dysrhythmias.
8. Inspect sputum for color, consistency, and odor.
9. Encourage deep breathing and coughing (Acee 1984).
10. Provide frequent explanations to decrease anxiety.

continued

Nursing interventions

11. Encourage chair rest, alternating with low-level activities during day (Knudson 1984).
12. Instruct patient to avoid prolonged bedrest.
13. Encourage active range-of-motion exercises at bedside and under supervision.
14. Apply antiembolic stockings.
15. Encourage patient to flex and contract calves q 1 h while awake.
16. Observe for Homan's sign every shift.
17. Weigh patient daily.
18. Measure circumference of edematous extremities daily.
19. Monitor intake and output every 24 hr.
20. Maintain fluid balance.
21. Limit fluids in the evening to prevent nocturia.
22. Provide ice chips as needed.
23. Provide frequent mouth care.
24. Provide foods low in salt.
25. Provide small, frequent meals.
26. Observe for side-effects or medications (see Table 6-1).

Medical diagnosis: *Arterial sclerotic obliterans*

12. Nursing diagnosis: Alteration in comfort related to arterial insufficiency

Goal

Patient's pain will be controlled to a level acceptable to the patient.

Nursing interventions

1. Encourage regular, low-level exercise.
2. Instruct patient to avoid vasoconstrictive substances such as tobacco and to avoid cold atmosphere.
3. Teach patient to stand or walk slowly to help relieve pain.
4. Teach patient never to sit with legs crossed.
5. Encourage use of lamb's wool to separate toes.
6. Teach patient to use wool socks that are clean and dry.
7. Encourage the use of well-fitting shoes.
8. Teach patient to avoid hot water bottles and heating pads.

continued

Nursing interventions

9. Teach patient to avoid going out in the cold without mouth and nose covered.
10. Encourage the layering of socks and use of insulated boots in winter.
11. Teach patient to avoid girdles, garters, and constricting clothing (Reich and Otten 1987).

Medical diagnosis: Varicosities

13. Nursing diagnosis: Decreased venous return related to venous engorgement

Goal

Patient will have adequate venous return.

Nursing interventions

1. Apply elastic or support stockings.
2. Teach patient to avoid sitting with feet dependent.
3. Encourage patient to exercise 3 or 4 times daily (Benison and Hogstel 1986).
4. Teach patient never to cross legs.
5. Observe for signs of thrombosis or phlebitis.
6. Teach patient to avoid standing for long periods.
7. Teach patient to exercise calf muscles.
8. Encourage patient to avoid hot baths, showers, or steam rooms.

References

Acee S: Helping patients breath more easily. Geriatr Nurs 5:230–233, 1984

American Heart Association: Heart Facts. Dallas, American Heart Association, 1983

Benison B, Hogstel M: Aging and movement therapy. J Gerontol Nurs 12:16–18, 1986

Blumenthal JA, Schocken DD, Needels TL, Hindle P: Psychological and physiological effects of physical conditioning on the elderly. J Psychosomat Res 26:505–510, 1982

Chobanian AV: Pathophysiologic considerations in the treatment of the elderly hypertensive patient. Am J Cardiol 52:49D–53D, 1983

Franklin SS: Geriatric hypertension. Med Clin North Am 67:395–413, 1983

Gioiella EC, Bevil CW: Nursing Care of the Aging Client: Promoting Healthy Adaptation. Norwalk, Connecticut, Appleton-Century-Crofts, 1985

Harris R: Cardiovascular disease in the elderly. Med Clin North Am 67:379–393, 1983

Hitzhusen JC, Alpert JA: The elderly heart: Special signs and symptoms to watch for. Geriatrics 39:38–51, 1984

Jessup LE: The chest, abdomen and genitourinary system. In Steffl BM (ed): Handbook of Gerontological Nursing. New York, Van Nostrand Reinhold, 1984

Kennedy RD, Caird FI: Physiology of aging of the heart. In Noble RJ, Rothbaum DA (eds): Geriatric Cardiology: Cardiovascular Clinics. Philadelphia, FA Davis, 1981

Kent S: How dietary salt contributes to hypertension. Geriatrics 36:14–20, 1981

Knudsen FS: Cardiovascular conditions in older adults. In Steffl BM (ed): Handbook of Gerontological Nursing. New York, Van Nostrand Reinhold, 1984

Lowenthal DT, Affrime MB: Cardiovascular drugs for the geriatric patient. Geriatrics 36:65–73, 1981

McCauley K, Burke K: Your detailed guide to drugs for CHF. Nursing 14:47–50, 1984

Michaelson CR: Congestive Heart Failure. St Louis, CV Mosby, 1983

O'Brien DK, Pattee JJ: Hypertension in older patients—What drugs to use and when. Geriatrics 36:111–120, 1981

Reich N, Otten P: What to wear: A challenge for disabled elders. Am J Nurs 87:207–210, 1987

Rodstein M: The ECG in old age: Implications for diagnosis, therapy and prognosis. Geriatrics 32:76–79, 1977

Schocken DD: Congestive heart failure: Dx and Rx in the elderly. Geriatrics 39:77–88, 1984

Sheridan ES: Drugs and the elderly. In Steffl BM (ed): Handbook of Gerontological Nursing. New York, Van Nostrand Reinhold, 1984

Spittell JA: Rehabilitative aspects of peripheral vascular disorders in the elderly. In Williams TF (ed): Rehabilitation in the Aging. New York, Raven Press, 1984

Steffl BM: Handbook of Gerontological Nursing. New York: Van Nostrand Reinhold, 1984

Weisfeldt ML: The Heart in Old Age: Its Function and Response to Stress. New York, Raven Press, 1980

Wenger NK: Rehabilitation of the elderly cardiac patient. In Nobel RJ, Rothbaum DA (eds): Geriatric Cardiology: Cardiovascular Clinics. Philadelphia, FA Davis, 1981

Wenger NK: Cardiovascular status: Changes with aging. In Williams TF (ed): Rehabilitation in the Aging. New York, Raven Press, 1984b

Yurick AG, Robb SS, Spier BE: The Aged Person and the Nursing Process, 2nd ed. Norwalk, Connecticut, Appleton-Century-Crofts, 1984

Suggested readings

Acee S: Helping patients breathe more easily. Geriatr Nurs 5:230–233, 1984

Alfano G: The older adult and drug therapy, Part II. Geriatr Nurs 5:28–31, 1982

Hudson HF: Drugs and the older adult. Nursing 14:47–51, 1984

Lonnerblad L: Exercises to promote independent living in older patients. Geriatrics 39:93–98, 1984

Pardini A: Exercise, vitality, and aging. Aging 344:19–29, 1984

Elizabeth Reed and Mickey Stanley

Respiratory system 7

Does the process of living and breathing lead to a decline in function of the respiratory system? In many areas of the United States and in the world, air pollution is thought to be a major risk factor with respect to the development of lung disease. Further complicating this question is the choice of many persons to smoke cigarettes. For elderly persons who live in areas of high pollution or choose to smoke, the process of living may indeed lead to a decline in respiratory function.

It is difficult to distinguish between pathologic changes associated with disease or with years of exposure to pollutants and age-related changes in the respiratory system. Regardless of the cause, however, structural and functional changes in the respiratory system known to occur with increasing frequency may limit an elderly person's ability to remain independent. A thorough understanding of the changes that have an impact on the respiratory system will allow the nurse to play a pivotal role in facilitating an optimal level of functioning for her elderly patients.

Age-related changes

If the physiological functions of a 30-year-old person and a 70-year-old person at rest were compared, few distinguishable differences would be found. If these same persons were stressed by exercise, however, physiologic dissimilarities would become apparent (Kenney 1985). The most common physiologic response to exercise in a sedentary, elderly person is the subjective feeling of breathlessness. This is related to decreases in vital capacity and diffusing capacity, and an increase in residual volume that occurs with aging. Pathologic conditions such as obesity, chronic pulmonary diseases, and heart disease serve to further increase the symptoms of breathlessness. Breathlessness, although frequently occurring with advanced age, often is not reported as a common symptom or complaint (Agate 1986). For many elderly people, shortness of breath is accepted as part of "getting old"; and they will diminish their activity to prevent this subjective feeling. Thus begins the destructive cycle of a declining ability of the respiratory system to meet the metabolic demands of the body during periods of increased need.

Structural changes

Study of the age-related biochemical changes in the respiratory system is difficult because of the ethical problems involved (Krumpe et al 1985). However, a recent study by Andretti and coworkers (1983) showed that collagen, a major structural protein, is reduced in the lung. In addition to a reduction of total collagen, rearrangement of the remaining structural collagen occurs, reducing lung elasticity and increasing compliance (Mahler et al 1986b). As compliance (the volume change per unit of pressure change across the lung) increases, less pressure is required to inflate the lung with a given volume. It might be assumed that it becomes easier to breathe as the body ages because the lungs become smaller and require less pressure to inflate. However, the stiffening of the thoracic cage, owing to increasing bone rigidity and loss of respiratory muscle mass, limit or offset the increased compliance. In addition, a decreased surface area of lung parenchyma, a decreased alveolar surface area, enlargement of the alveolar ducts, and flattening of the alveoli further compromise the elderly person's ability to perform the work of breathing during periods of stress or exercise.

Consistent with the entire skeletal framework, the bones of the thorax (ribs and vertebra) decalcify, resulting in a degree of kyphoscoliosis (Krumpe et al 1985). The costal cartilages also harden and calcify. These changes increase the anterior–posterior diameter of the thoracic cage while reducing the transverse thoracic diameter. Functionally, this anatomic change in the thorax causes an increased amount of oxygen to be diverted just to the activity of breathing. Upon observing an elderly person breathing it can be noted that, because of the stiffness of the rib cage, the use of abdominal and diaphragmatic muscles is increased. In the younger person, the abdominal muscles are used predominately in active expiration. With advanced age, the abdominal muscles contract, increasing intra-abdominal pressure and forcing the diaphragm up. This action, used in younger age groups as a means of increasing the force of expiration during times of stress, is a necessary part of normal breathing for elderly persons. As a result, the ability to increase the respiratory effort with exercise or stress is limited.

The pulmonary artery and its main branches undergo changes similar to those of the entire cardiovascular system (see Chapter 6). These changes increase vascular resistance to blood flow through the pulmonary vascular system. As a result, the pulmonary vascular response to hypoxia becomes less sensitive. This loss of sensitivity to hypoxia may be important clinically in situations such as pneumonia, atelectasis, and pulmonary emboli. In situations such as these, in which oxygen is unavailable to diffusion, blood will not be diverted away from the hypoxic regions of the lung (as it would be in a younger person), thus increasing the perfusion abnormality (West 1979). Therefore, the elderly person may be more at risk for the dangers of hypoxia, such as myocardial or cerebral ischemia, and confusion or falls during acute respiratory conditions.

Functional changes

One of the major functional age-related changes is a decline in respiratory muscle endurance. The development of a respiratory illness or disease may mean the difference between independence and institutional care for an elderly person. For example, when an elderly person with chronic obstructive pulmonary disease (COPD) contracts an upper respiratory infection or flu, severe disability may result from the added strain on the respiratory system. Therefore, patients should be taught to avoid large crowds (*e.g.*, crowded shopping malls) and persons with upper respiratory infections or flu. Most authorities recommend that all elderly persons, particularly those with a history of respiratory disease, receive annual vaccinations against influenza (Niederman and Fein 1986).

Additional functional age-related changes known to alter lung mechanics and ventilatory function include: loss of lung elastic recoil, increases in closing volume, alteration in lung volumes, and a decrease in maximum expiratory flow rates. A loss of lung elastic recoil is a hallmark of emphysema, secondary to the enlargement and destruction of the alveoli. Kenney (1985) noted that the aging lung undergoes similar changes. This loss of elasticity increases the distance over which gas exchange must occur, consequently diffusing capacity decreases. The loss of elastic lung recoil also reduces maximum expiratory flow. A diminished ability to cough results, posing a serious disadvantage when there is increased mucus production in the airways. Therefore, pulmonary hygiene is a crucial nursing intervention for every hospitalized or bedridden elderly patient. The nurse must be sure that the patient is able to effectively clear the airways without becoming exhausted in the process.

Lung volume changes result from the increased compliance of the lung and the decreased compliance of the chest wall. Little change occurs with the inhalation phase of respiration, thus total lung capacity changes little with aging. However, because of a decrease in muscle strength associated with exhalation, a decrease in elastic recoil, and an increase in closing volume, the volume of gas left in the lung at the end of a maximum expiratory effort is increased. This situation may put the person at increased risk of barotrauma if ventilating under high airway pressures, such as with intermittent positive pressure breathing (IPPB) or mechanical ventilation, or hypercarbia secondary to carbon dioxide retention.

Gas exchange in the lung presumes that ventilation (air getting into the lung) is matched to perfusion (blood circulating in the lung). During a normal respiratory cycle, a few alveoli collapse at the end of expiration and fail to expand with the following inspiration. In a young person, this situation of collapsing alveoli is compensated for by periodic sighs and yawns, or a deep breath (Risser 1980). In an elderly person, the loss of muscle mass in the intercostals, a stiffened thoracic cage, and the loss of elastic recoil within the lung tissue prohibit this normal process of re-expanding collapsed alveoli. As a result, areas of the lung may remain poorly ventilated. Perfusion of blood to this poorly ventilated area remains unchanged in most situations. Therefore, a mismatch of ventilation to perfusion occurs, resulting in poorly oxygenated blood circulating throughout the body (Figure 7-1).

Although any area of the lung is subject to alveolar collapse, the most common areas for collapse are the dependent areas (Brandstetter and Kazemi 1980). For the ill, elderly patients who are placed in a recumbent position, large areas of atelectasis may result. Nursing measures designed to prevent atelectasis, such as frequent turning, deep breathing, and coughing exercises, take on added significance. The importance of obtaining activity orders is critical to the prevention of further respiratory complications in this population.

The effectiveness of gas exchange is measured by assessing the gas tensions in an arterialized sample of blood. As a result of the ventilation–perfusion changes that occur with aging, determination of normal values for this population requires an adjustment. A number of formulae exist to determine the age-adjusted normal values for the elderly. A simple rule of thumb for estimating this change is a 4 torr decrease in PaO_2 per decade of life.

Often breathing patterns alter in the elderly person. Although absolute minute ventilation does not change, the respiratory rate increases as tidal volume decreases. Mahler (1986) suggests that this is an adaptive response to the decreased compliance of the thorax. Periodic breathing patterns such as Cheyne–Stokes respirations may be the result of decreases in cardiac output, metabolic abnormalities, or central respiratory changes. Any altered breathing pattern should

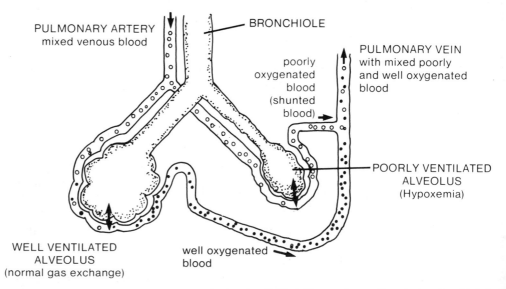

Figure 7-1. Comparison of well-ventilated alveolus (left) *with poorly ventilated alveolus* (right).

be noted. Careful attention is warranted when an elderly patient is receiving sedation. Oversedation may produce hypoxemia and hypercarbia secondary to further decreases in tidal volumes.

Elderly persons also have a diminished cardiopulmonary response to hypercapnia, resulting in an inability to meet metabolic demands during stress. Many researchers believe that response to central chemosensitive cells is reduced in the brainstem and peripheral chemoreceptors in the carotid bodies and aortic arch (Brandstetter and Kazemi 1980; Weitkamp and Aber 1984). One would expect to see an increase in heart rate and ventilation in response to hypoxemia or hypercapnia. This adaptive response is slowed or not seen at all in the elderly. As a result, the elderly person is more likely to experience tissue hypoxia and injury to vital organs such as the brain, heart, and kidneys during acute respiratory conditions (Lefrak and Campbell 1981).

Defense mechanisms

Pulmonary defense mechanisms are thought to decline with age. A major pulmonary hazard for the elderly related to this loss of defense mechanisms is the loss of airway protection. Many elderly persons have reduced cough strength, slowed mucus transport, and oropharyngeal dysphagia. This combination puts them at risk for aspiration. Aspiration may be avoided and swallowing enhanced by raising the head of the bed and avoiding drugs and foods that reduce peristalsis or esophageal sphincter contraction (theophylline, anticholinergics, beta-adrenergics, diazepam, alcohol, and fatty foods).

Defense mechanisms designed to clear the large airways of mucus and foreign bodies are the cilia that line the airways and the cough reflex. The cilia, or tiny hairlike projections, propel mucus toward the mouth where it can be expectorated. Advanced age, cigarette smoke, dehydration, air pollution, and respiratory infection are all known to reduce ciliary activity (Divertie 1981). See Figure 7-2. In

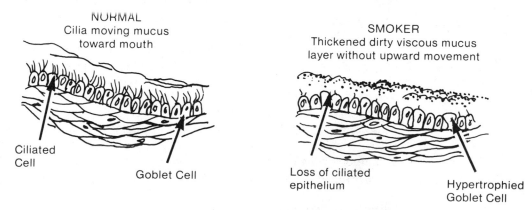

Figure 7-2. Normal bronchial mucosa (left) *and the changes that occur from chronic cigarette smoking* (right).

addition, the decline of respiratory muscle mass and stiffening of the thoracic cage inhibit an effective cough action. Therefore, nursing measures to aid in effective removal of secretions, such as adequate hydration and frequent oral hygiene, are most important.

Acute and chronic problems

For most elderly persons, respiratory function remains quite adequate under normal circumstances. But, as with many other systems, the ability of the respiratory system to meet the needs of the body during times of stress is limited. In addition, both the acute and chronic problems that occur with increasing frequency in the elderly person may limit seriously his or her ability to remain independent. The most prevalent of the acute and chronic conditions affecting the elderly are pneumonia, postoperative complications, and COPD.

Pneumonia

More than 50,000 Americans die of pneumonia each year. The majority of these deaths are among the elderly population (Weitekamp and Aber 1984). In view of the sophisticated antibiotic therapies that exist today, numbers such as these are staggering. To understand this problem, it is necessary to examine why the elderly are so vulnerable to pneumonia.

Pneumonia is usually a bacterial or viral lung infection. The pneumococcus organism is often a normal inhabitant of the upper respiratory system. The development of pneumonia in the elderly person depends on the number and virulence of the bacteria and the strength of the individual's defenses (Patrick 1986). Growth of the pneumococcus organisms is encouraged in a warm, moist environment such as exists in conditions of increased sputum production or poor mucus removal. Therefore, several disorders common to the elderly increase the risk of bacterial pneumonia: COPD, congestive heart failure, influenza, alcoholism, and any condition that results in prolonged immobility.

Several researchers have noted that cellular immunity, which is responsible for isolating and removing invading bacteria, is reduced with age (Weitkamp and Aber 1984; Brandstetter and Kazemi 1980). Defects in leukocyte and alveolar macrophage function for persons who smoke, or those undergoing chemotherapy or steroid therapy, are also cited as contributing to the increased susceptibility to pneumonia. Functional changes of a loss of ciliary action, poor cough reflexes, and oropharyngeal dysphagia contribute to the lack of natural defenses for the elderly person. These functional changes, together with the increased frequency of pulmonary disorders, and lack of cellular immunity, result in a vulnerability to acute respiratory infections such as pneumonia.

Nursing management

The primary goal of nursing management for the elderly patient with bacterial or viral pneumonia is early recognition, supportive care, and prevention of further complications. Recognition of pneumonia in the elderly is not always easy. Patrick (1986) noted that some display the classic pneumonia syndrome of a sudden onset of shaking chills, high fever, pleuritic chest pain, and a productive cough of purulent sputum. Many, however, present with an atypical picture of confusion, anorexia, lethargy, and weakness (Niederman and Fein 1986). Steffl (1984) noted that this atypical presentation may result in a delay in the initiation of necessary therapy. It becomes paramount, therefore, for the nurse to have a high index of suspicion for pneumonia for any elderly patient who is considered to be highly susceptible (see the boxed material below).

Supportive nursing care is directed at increasing the efficiency of breathing. Deep breathing is the most efficient and effective bronchodilator available (Acee 1984). Healthy persons normally breathe deeply through periodic sighs and yawns to achieve adequate alveolar expansion. The elderly patient with pneumonia requires a more concentrated effort to achieve these same benefits. Acee (1984) suggests the following steps for assisting an elderly person with deep-breathing exercises.

- Explain to the patient and family the importance of the exercises, what is to happen, and why it happens.
- Position the patient in as upright a position as possible.
- Demonstrate the following technique. The nurse should inhale slowly and deeply through his or her nose and exhale through pursed lips, tightening the abdominal muscles.
- Ask the patient and family members to practice the technique. If the patient is unable to inhale sufficiently through the nose, ask him or her to breathe in and out through the mouth.
- Allow the patient to rest after the practice session.
- Establish a log or checklist to assist the patient in remembering to practice the exercises every hour during waking hours.

Factors that increase susceptibility to pneumonia

Age

Immobility

Pre-existing respiratory problems

Immunosuppression

Steroid therapy

Recent anesthesia

Obesity

Smoking

Nasogastric feeding tube

In addition to promoting regular deep breathing, the nurse should also encourage effective coughing. Teach the patient to take three deep breaths to loosen any secretions that may have accumulated in the bronchial tree. After the third breath, have the patient contract the abdominal muscles tightly to increase the force of exhalation. Placing hands on the patient's abdomen and back may provide support and encouragement during the process. Consistent efforts to assist with deep breathing and coughing exercises should be carried out every hour during the patient's waking hours (Risser 1980). The use of a log or checksheet that lists the hours and a place for the patient to keep a record of the number of times each hour that the exercises are practiced may serve as a visual reminder. In addition, family members should be encouraged to participate in the regimen, assist the patient with the exercises, and to remind the patient to do them.

The nurse must recognize that the effort involved in simply breathing and coughing may consume a large portion of the elderly patient's energy. Attention to scheduling activities so as to avoid fatigue becomes especially important. Instead of performing all personal hygiene activities simultaneously, these activities may need to be spaced throughout the day to conserve energy. Many elderly patients find short nap periods during the morning and afternoon very restful. The well-rested patient will cooperate more with deep breathing and coughing exercises than will one who is fatigued.

Additional supportive measures to facilitate the work of breathing include adequate hydration, adequate nutrition, and frequent repositioning. For the elderly patient with pneumonia, fatigue and anorexia may limit the amount of oral fluids and food that can be consumed. A variety of methods may be required to ensure that the patient receives adequate food intake. Small, frequent meals that consist of cool foods are often tolerated better than large meals of spicy or heated foods. In addition, careful attention to oral hygiene measures after productive coughing activities enhances the taste and desire for food and drink. See Chapter 10, "The Gastrointestinal System," for suggestions on oral care.

The practice of repositioning a patient allows the work of breathing to be accomplished with less exertion. A frequent change of position prevents the pooling of secretions and alveolar collapse. If the pneumonia is consolidated in one side of the lung, the patient should be placed predominantly with the affected side down. Inspired air follows the path of least resistance, favoring the unaffected lung over the affected one. Therefore, with the unaffected side up, ventilation will be maximized. Turning the patient from side to side is recommended; however, the length of time the patient is positioned with the consolidated lung up should be minimized. A turning schedule for documentation, left at the patient's bedside or on the door, may serve as an effective reminder for this most important practice.

Efforts to prevent complications and foster rehabilitation must be initiated along with the initial phase of care. Existing chronic problems should be thoroughly assessed and a plan of care begun to prevent further decline in function. To prevent problems associated with disorientation, staff and family members should be encouraged to talk to the patient—not over them to another staff or family member.

Postoperative pulmonary complications

Some degree of impaired pulmonary function occurs in all patients post-operatively, regardless of the site of operation or type of anesthesia (Risser 1980, 51).

The functional and structural changes associated with aging that have been discussed render the elderly vulnerable to respiratory complications during anesthesia. For example, the loss of the protective laryngeal reflex predisposes them to pulmonary aspiration, which is aggravated both intraoperatively and postoperatively by central nervous system depressants (Stein and Hedley-Whyte 1986). For an elderly patient with pre-existing disease or altered function, the risk of postoperative pulmonary complications is increased. Close attention to nursing measures designed to maintain respiratory function and prevent complications may mean the difference between prolonged dependence or recovery for an elderly patient undergoing surgery.

Nursing management

Any number of factors may impact on a postoperative patient's ability to maintain good respiratory function. The amount of sedation the patient receives and the level of pain being experienced must be carefully assessed. Adequate relief of the patient's pain without oversedation is necessary if the patient is to cooperate fully in a respiratory regimen. See Chapter 14, "Pain in Elderly Patients," for more details.

Also, it is critical that the patient understand the importance of postoperative breathing exercises. Research findings on the effects of preoperative teaching on postoperative pulmonary status have been conflicting. Early studies demonstrated improved pulmonary status for those patients who received preoperative teaching. Recent studies have failed to replicate these findings. Hathaway (1986) suggested one reason for this contradiction is that patients do not do the postoperative exercises or do not do them correctly. Follow-up interviews have revealed a lack of sufficient understanding by the patient of both the purpose of the exercises and the suggested procedures to follow.

As the amount of time allowed for preoperative preparation is reduced, the nurse must be prepared to develop and use innovated approaches to preoperative teaching. For example, nurses working on a surgical unit may choose to develop a booklet that can be mailed to the patient's home, outlining exercises to be practiced before entry into the hospital. A question-and-answer session and return-demonstration session could be conducted either individually or in groups the evening before surgery. In addition, all members of the staff and family could assist in providing cues and reinforcing teaching during the postoperative period.

An effective respiratory program designed to reverse postoperative physiological changes is one that emphasizes maximal alveolar inflation and maintenance of adequate respiratory function (Risser 1980). In a research study designed to examine the effectiveness of different methods used postoperatively for respiratory care (*e.g.,* IPPB, blow-bottles, incentive spirometry, deep breathing), Bartlett and coworkers (1973) noted that high alveolar-inflating pressures exerted over a sustained period are required to achieve maximum inspired volume. Based on the results of their study, they suggested the use of deep breathing exercises with emphasis on holding during the deep inspiration phase. If additional aids are needed, the use of an incentive spirometry is recommended because of its use of inspiration, instead of predominantly expiratory measures such as blow-bottles.

A comprehensive respiratory regimen should begin with effective preoperative teaching that includes both the patient and significant others. After the surgical procedure, careful attention must be paid to the following areas:

- Relief of pain without oversedation
- Turning and positioning every two hours
- Deep breathing and coughing exercises every hour during the patient's waking hours
- Use of incentive spirometry every hour if the patient is unable to hold a deep breath for 3 seconds to 5 seconds
- Assessment for presence of crackles in dependent areas of the lung after coughing exercises

Chronic obstructive pulmonary diseases

Chronic obstructive pulmonary disease (COPD) is a progressive disease that is characterized by diminishing oxygen and increasing discomfort and disability. Unlike heart disease, mortality from COPD is increasing faster in women than men. COPD is a classification of diseases that all have obstruction to air flow in common. The three principal causes of COPD are chronic bronchitis, asthma, and emphysema. Frequently the person with COPD has a combination of more than one underlying disease (Mahler et al 1986a).

Chronic bronchitis.   The diagnosis of chronic bronchitis is made on the basis of patient history. Chronic bronchitis presents a history of a productive cough for at least three months of the year for the preceding two years. Other diseases that are known to cause a productive cough such as tuberculosis, tumors, and cardiac disorders must be ruled out. The patient frequently reports a long history of smoking or exposure to air pollutants such as coal dust (Patrick 1986).

Asthma.   Asthma is a reversible form of airway obstruction precipitated by reaction to noxious stimuli. During periods of reactivity, the trachea and bronchioles develop a generalized narrowing secondary to bronchospasm, mucosal edema, and hypersecretion of mucus (Patrick 1986).

Emphysema. Emphysema is characterized by destruction of the alve
resulting in an increased size of the air spaces. The dilation and destrι
the alveolar sacs decreases the surface area for gas exchange to take p
destruction can follow different patterns, but is usually more severe in t
lobes (Patrick 1986).

Assessment parameters

The quality of the first contact with the patient will affect the quality of the information obtained for the data base. As has been mentioned, breathlessness is
usually denied by the elderly because it is viewed as a normal consequence of
aging. Other signs of pulmonary dysfunction such as coughing may also be overlooked. The most frequent signs of acute respiratory failure—restlessness, confusion, and tachycardia—are frequently associated with mental deterioration or
having a cantankerous personality (Pierson 1982). If the association between
these symptoms and respiratory distress is not made, therapy related to correcting
the problem may be delayed or omitted.

Important gross observations that should be made include overall stature
and body size, posture, skin color, state of sensorium, speech patterns, and degree of ventilatory effort (Shapiro et al 1979). Most elderly are not aware of their
respiratory rate. A description of the breathing pattern and rate will provide clues
to any underlying problems.

Dyspnea is a subjective symptom and difficult to measure. Indices helpful in
assessing the state of breathlessness are the magnitude of the task that causes
breathlessness and the magnitude of effort required to compensate for the subjective response. Questions useful in eliciting a history of breathlessness are:

- Are you ever short of breath?
- Tell me about the last time you were short of breath.
- Is it ever hard for you to move air in or out?
- Do you get tired more easily now than six months ago? a year ago?
- Do you ever have the feeling of suffocation or tightness?
- If you couldn't tell anyone you were short of breath, how would they
  know? (Brown et al 1986)
- What events (name some examples [*e.g.*, crying, laughing, smoking, wind,
  bad weather, crowded places, fatigue]) cause you to become short of
  breath? (Brown et al 1986)

Many elderly who have diminished cardiopulmonary reserve from cardiac or
pulmonary insufficiency have learned to diminish their symptoms by changing
their ADL. It is helpful to ask specific questions about how their usual activities
have changed over the past month, year, or over several years. The nurse might
ask questions about activities the patient used to participate in that have been
given up because of breathing problems. In addition to slowing down his or her

activity level, are there any other practices the patient regularly engages in to help with shortness of breath?

While talking with the patient, note the use of the accessory muscles of ventilation. In the elderly, abdominal breathing is considered normal. Use of the sternocleidomastoid, trapezius, and pectoral muscles are not considered normal and should be documented and reported. Observe the ease with which the patient breathes, including the general posture, apprehension, and use of pursed-lip breathing. These observations will give clues to breathlessness.

The clinical picture of an elderly patient with emphysema is one of dyspnea, a barrel chest, and hyperresonant lung sounds. Most emphysematous patients will maintain adequate oxygenation with increased ventilatory effort until late in their illness. The patient with chronic bronchitis has excessive sputum production, moderate dyspnea with exertion, and a history of repeated respiratory tract infections. These patients frequently have cyanosis, hypoxemia, or right-sided heart failure. This is the picture of the "blue-bloater." Although the two diseases frequently coexist, patients with predominantly bronchitis are more compromised because of the pulmonary hypertension and right-sided heart failure.

Asthma in the elderly presents a mixed picture. Elderly patients with asthma usually have nonallergic or intrinsic asthma. The adage, however, that "all that wheezes is not asthma" is especially true for elderly patients. Wheezing may be secondary to congestive heart failure, aspiration, pulmonary emboli, and neoplasia (Braman and Davis 1986). Persons with asthma have intermittent wheezing, dyspnea, and a cough. The elderly who acquire asthma may develop severe disability similar to that of those people who have had asthma for many years. They frequently need continuous bronchodilator and corticosteroid therapy to control the symptoms. The unique feature of asthma that separates it from emphysema and bronchitis is that with treatment, the obstruction to airflow can be altered.

Nursing management

Although it is helpful for the nurse to understand the difference between the underlying causes of COPD and their typical clinical presentation, the focus of nursing care for all patients with COPD is to assist the person in managing responses to the disease process. Adaptation to a chronic, progressively debilitating disease such as COPD requires a great deal of understanding, support, and care. Comprehensive nursing management requires attention to all of the following areas:

Lifestyle changes

Education

Goal setting

Pulmonary rehabilitation

Prevention of complications

Lifestyle changes. The earliest response to the development of COPD is the forfeiture of activities that produce breathlessness. As the disease progresses, more and more activities will be relinquished. This gradual debilitation frequently results in anger, depression, and loss of self-esteem. A role reversal may occur, with the patient's husband or wife having to assume the responsibilities as bread-winner or homemaker. It is important for the nurse to carefully assess the meaning of these changes in lifestyle for the persons involved. To assume that all the changes are viewed as negative may be just as erroneous as to assume they are considered positive. Time should be provided for each person to reflect on how satisfying the current status is and what each perceives as his or her needs.

A long history of cigarette smoking is frequently reported for the patient with COPD. Although such patients are advised to quit smoking, many are unable or unwilling to stop. In many instances, the staff, spouse, and family members become angry and resentful toward patients because of their lack of concern or unwillingness to cooperate with the care being offered. Family members may choose to distance themselves from a person to avoid watching this slowly debilitating process. By viewing the response to a difficult situation such as this as a matter of personal choice and by realizing that the patient, by continuing to smoke, is making an effort to maintain some control over his or her life may help staff and family accept this seemingly wrong decision. Positive reinforcement for efforts made in other areas and the continued acceptance and support from those closest to the patient are critical.

The progressive nature of COPD causes it to eventually have an impact on all aspects of the patient's lifestyle. The one area of impact that is frequently overlooked by nurses is that of sexuality. Spennrath (1982) states that frequently nurses are uncomfortable when called on to discuss a patient's sexual needs. She notes that many health care providers still believe the following myths:

Sexual desire ceases with menopause.

Sex is only for the young.

Nothing can be done to treat impotence in older men.

"Sexuality is a basic human feeling and human right that persists from cradle to grave" (Spennrath 1982, 29). Even though the loss of sexual functioning may be of great concern, elderly patients rarely raise the topic themselves. The responsibility lies, therefore, with the nurse to assess carefully for any problems in this area and provide the appropriate information and counseling.

Education. The debilitating effects of COPD often occur slowly, over a prolonged period. Patients may not seek medical care until late in the course of the disease, having denied the severity of their breathlessness or attributing it simply to "getting old." As a result, patients may know surprisingly little about their disease, its progressive nature, or recommended therapy. Thoroughly assessing the level of understanding of both the patient and family members is the most important step in developing a teaching plan.

Although damage to the lung tissue cannot be repaired, improvements in functioning are possible with appropriate intervention. For example, the patient who is overweight will benefit from a weight-reduction program. All patients should be taught to use energy-conservation measures, such as using a pull-cart rather than carrying objects. In addition, the role of stress in acute attacks of breathlessness should be thoroughly explored. Stress management training, such as biofeedback or imagery, may be an effective strategy to control the frequency of acute problems.

Goal setting.   Assisting the elderly person who has COPD in setting realistic goals is a challenging, and sometimes difficult, task. This process may be hampered by the use of denial or anger as a coping mechanism. To help the patient begin to formulate some goals, questions such as "What do you see as your most troubling problem?" or "What would you like to be doing a year from now?" can be useful (Gioiella and Bevil 1985). The use of the life review or encouraging reminiscences may be beneficial to assist the patient and family to come to terms with what has gone before and what lies ahead. See Chapter 15, "Psychosocial Care," for more information on this nursing intervention. The process of working through the loss of physical abilities and dreams for the retirement years may aid adaptation and allow the direction of energies toward enjoying remaining time and opportunities to their fullest.

When attempting to help an elderly patient establish goals, a few guidelines may be of assistance:

- Goals should be aimed at compensating for irrevocable losses and slowing the disabling process.
- Goals must be attainable. Overly optimistic goals leave the person discouraged and decreases confidence.
- With a progressive disease, aiming for modest gains or maintaining the status quo may be all that is realistic.
- Goals should be mutually agreed on by patient, family, and nursing personnel.
- Goals should be written down and periodically reviewed and updated.

Pulmonary rehabilitation.   Outpatient pulmonary rehabilitation centers are growing in popularity across the country. Similar to cardiac rehabilitation centers, the pulmonary centers employ a multidisciplinary approach to help people with lung disease regain control of their lives. The emphasis in a rehabilitation program is to teach the patient to control symptoms, improve quality of life, increase confidence and self-esteem, and decrease the number of hospitalizations associated with the chronic lung condition. The principal strategies used in many of these centers are:

text continues on p 144

Table 7-1. **Table of drugs**

Drug	Effect/response in the elderly	Nursing implications
Beta adrenergic agents (oral, parenteral and inhalants)	Used for relaxation of bronchial smooth muscle/bronchodilation. Side-effects of increased heart rate, palpitations, nervousness, insomnia, headache, dizziness and urinary retention may occur. Serum glucose levels and serum potassium levels may be altered.	Observe for side-effects during initial administration. Monitor heart rate, blood sugar, K$^+$.
Methylzanthines (aminophylline, theophylline)	Used with adrenergic agents or alone to produce bronchodilation. Clearance is decreased in COPD, pulmonary, edema, CHF, hepatic dysfunction, renal failure and alcoholism. Clearance is reduced when used with macrolide antibiotics—erythromycin, troleandomycin, lincomycin, and clindamycin. Increased serum theophylline level is seen when theophylline is taken with cimetidine because of inhibition of hepatic metabolism of theophylline.	Monitor plasma theophylline levels (10–20 μg/ml therapeutic range). Signs and symptoms of toxicity include: nausea, vomiting, anorexia, nervousness, insomnia, and headache. Life-threatening toxic effects include: tachycardia, dysrhythmias, and seizure activity. Avoid rapid IV administration; use an infusion pump to provide a constant rate of administration. The liquid preparation is preferred for nasogastric use.
Chromosomes (disodium, chromoglycate, Cromolyn)	Variable response seen with intrinsic asthma; better in extrinsic asthma. Takes 2–4 wk before response is seen. Side-effects of throat irritation, nasal congestion, dryness of mouth, acute cough, and mild bronchospasm may occur.	Teach patient never to use cromolyn in an acute asthma episode—may provoke problem into becoming a more serious one. Only those elderly who can demonstrate ability to use a nebulizer or spinhaler should be discharged with this drug. Observe for side-effects.
Corticosteroids	May be used in severe reactive airway disease. Provides relief from dyspnea and a greater sense of well-being. Carbohydrate intolerance may be increased. Adverse effects include: development of cataracts, osteoporosis (see Chapter 8 on musculoskeletal system), decreased resistance to infection, gastric or duodenal ulcers, potassium loss.	Monitor closely patient who has other diseases that can be worsened by steroid therapy. Monitor blood sugar. Teach patient to see optometrist yearly. Teach safety precautions against falls (*e.g.,* eliminate waxed floors, throw rugs). Encourage patient to take flu shots. See Chapter 10 on gastrointestinal system. Monitor serum potassium levels.
Oxygen	Use of oxygen is based on ABGs, not the patient's appearance or degree of dyspnea. High liter flow eliminates the hypoxic drive to breathe in patients with COPD.	Assess for changes in arterial blood gases 20–30″ after a change in liter flow. Teach patient the prescribed schedule for use (*e.g.,* only at night, while exercising, continuous). Teach patient to avoid using oxygen for relief of dyspnea episodes.

Educating patients about the disease and its therapy

Assisting participants to stop smoking

Teaching stress management techniques

Improving exercise tolerance

Prevention of complications. The normal age-related changes, in addition to those disease-related changes previously discussed, leave the elderly patient with COPD vulnerable to additional problems. The incidence of upper respiratory tract infections is much higher among this patient population. Therefore, patients should be taught to avoid large crowds and persons with known upper respiratory infections or flu. Niederman and Fein (1986) recommend annual vaccinations against influenza and *Staphylococcus pneumoniae.* During flu and cold season special attention should be paid to maintaining a well-balanced diet and getting proper rest.

The incidence of peptic ulcer disease is also increased for this patient population. Emotional stress, increased acidity, and carbon dioxide retention are believed to contribute to the development of ulcers (Gioiella and Bevil 1985). The patient should be taught to recognize the symptoms of a peptic ulcer and be instructed when to seek medical care for this problem.

Drugs

Table 7-1 lists some of the drugs used in the treatment of respiratory distress, their side-effects, and nursing implications.

Nursing care plans

Medical diagnosis: Pneumonia

1. Nursing diagnosis: Alteration in respiratory function related to infectious process

Goal

The patient will not experience further complications and will return to previous level of function.

Nursing interventions

1. Begin deep-breathing exercise program.
2. Teach family and visitors how to assist patient with deep-breathing exercises.
3. Instruct patient and family in effective coughing exercises.

continued

Nursing interventions

4. Initiate log or record for deep-breathing, coughing exercises.
5. Avoid repetitive, nonproductive coughing with cough suppressant.
6. Schedule patient care activities to ensure adequate rest periods.
7. Encourage chair rest during the day for 1–2 h, 3–4 times per day.
8. Initiate a turning schedule for the patient on bedrest.
9. Provide a well-balanced diet in frequent, small meals.
10. Perform oral hygiene measures before meals.
11. Teach patient to avoid common sources of upper respiratory infections (see text).
12. Encourage patient to receive influenza shots.
13. Teach patient and family the signs of upper respiratory insufficiency. Encourage them to notify a physician promptly to avoid complications.

Medical diagnosis: Postoperative status

2. Nursing diagnosis: Alteration in respiratory function related to postanesthesia state

Goal

The patient will not experience complications and will return to previous level of function.

Nursing interventions

1. Elevate head of bed 30°.
2. Provide adequate pain relief without oversedation (see Care Plan on Acute Pain.)
3. Initiate deep-breathing exercise program.
4. Encourage use of incentive spirometry (IS).
5. Turn and reposition q 2 h.
6. Provide log or record at patient's bedside to record deep-breathing exercise performance, use of IS, and turning.
7. Assess lung sounds q 4 h.
8. Report the presence of crackles to physician.

Medical diagnosis: Chronic obstructive pulmonary disease

3. Nursing diagnosis: Impaired gas exchange related to chronic airway obstruction

Goal

The patient will maintain adequate gas exchange and be able to participate in ADL

Nursing interventions

1. Use a calm, unhurried approach with a positive and encouraging attitude.
2. Retrain patient in effective diaphragmatic breathing patterns to decrease the work of breathing and achieve relaxation.
   Instruct patient to
     • Relax jaw, shoulder, and neck muscles
     • Inhale using the intercostal muscle
     • Exhale through pursed lips
     • Follow exhalation with maximal inhalation
     • Perform this exercise while lying down, sitting, and while walking
3. Encourage the use of relaxation techniques (mental imagery, rhythmic breathing, selected muscle relaxation). Practice these exercises with patient.
4. Provide patient and family with appropriate educational materials related to disease process, medications, use of aerosal devices and home oxygen therapy, pulmonary hygiene, effective coughing, and deep breathing.
5. Provide patient and family with periodic review of techniques to be used at home.
6. Teach patient energy-conservation measures for ADL.
7. Encourage activities that position patient in upright rather than recumbent position.
8. Anticipate and provide for needs during periods of crisis.
9. Observe for and teach patient and family about changes in level of consciousness, such as complaints of headache, visual disturbance, or somnolence.
10. Teach patient benefits of oxygen therapy for chronic hypoxemia (<55 torr).

4. *Nursing diagnosis: Ineffective airway clearance related to reduced cough strength, slowed mucus transport*

Goal

The patient will not experience aspirations and will maintain a clear airway.

Nursing interventions

1. Teach patient energy-efficient methods of coughing (see text).
2. Avoid repetitive, nonproductive coughing with cough suppressants.
3. Keep head of bed elevated (at home, bed can be elevated on blocks).
4. Teach patient to eat slowly. Discourage talking while eating. Do not distract patient while he or she is swallowing.
5. Teach patient to avoid food and drugs that reduce peristalsis, or suppress cough reflex.
6. Encourage patient to stop smoking and to avoid air pollution and sources of respiratory infection.
7. Increase fluid intake to 2000 ml per day as tolerated.

5. *Nursing diagnosis: Activity intolerance related to dyspnea or fear of dyspnea*

Goal

The patient will accept breathlessness without excessive anxiety, fear, or depression.

Nursing interventions

1. Listen and encourage patient to express feelings and ask questions about disease.
2. Provide accurate information and realistic hope.
3. Organize the environment so activities can be performed that do not cause breathlessness.
4. Help family and significant others to understand their role in assisting with ADL.
5. Encourage patient to enroll in an exercise training program.
6. Provide information on location and person to contact for exercise program.
7. Discuss benefits and need for home oxygen therapy.

6. Nursing diagnosis: Alteration in nutrition (less than body requirement) related to fatigue, weakness, breathlessness

Goal

The patient will consume adequate food and fluids and enjoy mealtime.

Nursing interventions

1. Provide a balanced diet in small, frequent feedings.
2. Encourage patient to stop smoking.
3. Encourage patient to select cool, nonspicy foods.
4. Reinforce principles of good nutrition keeping patient's food preferences in mind.
5. Provide oral hygiene equipment before meals.
6. Encourage patient to eat when hungry, not at standard meal times.
7. Encourage the use of oxygen during eating to diminish fatigue and breathlessness.

References

Acee S: Helping patients breathe more easily. Geriatr Nurs 14:230–233, 1984

Agate J: Common symptoms and complaints. In Rossman I (ed): Clinical Geriatrics, 3rd ed. Philadelphia, JB Lippincott, 1986

Andretti L, Bussotte A, Cammelli D et al: Connective tissue in aging lung. Gerontology 29:377–387, 1983

Bartlett RH, Gazzaniga AB, Geraghty TR: Respiratory maneuvers to prevent postoperative pulmonary complications: A critical review. JAMA 224:1017, 1973

Braman SS, Davis SM: Wheezing in the elderly: Asthma and other causes. Clin Geriatr Med 2:269–283, 1986

Brandstetter RD, Kazemi H: Aging and the respiratory system. Clin Geriatr Med 2:419–429, 1980

Brown ML, Carrieri V, Janson-Bferklie S, Dodd MJ: Lung cancer and dyspnea: The patient's perception. Oncol Nurs For 13:19–24, 1986

Divertie MB: Changes in lung defense mechanisms associated with aging. In Gracey DR (ed): Pulmonary Disease in the Adult. Chicago, Year Book Medical Publishers, 1981

Gioiella EC, Bevil CW: Nursing Care of the Aging Client: Promoting Healthy Adaptation. Norwalk, Connecticut, Appleton-Century-Crofts, 1985

Hathaway D: Effect of preoperative instruction on postoperative outcomes. Nurs Res 35:269–274, 1986

Kenney RA: Physiology of aging. Clin Geriatr Med 1:37–40, 1985

Krumpe PE, Knudson RJ, Parson G, Reiser K: The aging respiratory system. Clin Geriatr Med 1:143–175, 1985

Lefrak SS, Campbell EJ: Structure and function of the aging respiratory system. In Gracey DR (ed): Pulmonary Disease in the Adult. Chicago, Yearbook Medical Publishers, 1981

Mahler DA, Rosiello RA, Loke J: The aging lung. Clin Geriatr Med 2:215–225, 1986

Niederman MS, Fein AM: Pneumonia in the elderly. Clin Geriatr Med 2:241–268, 1986

Patrick M: Respiratory problems. In Carnevali DL, Patrick M (eds): Nursing Management for the Elderly. Philadelphia, JB Lippincott, 1986

Pierson DJ: Respiratory care of the elderly. In Petty TL (ed): Intensive and Rehabilitative Respiratory Care, 3rd ed. Philadelphia, Lea & Febiger, 1982

Risser NL: Preoperative and postoperative care to prevent pulmonary complications. Heart and Lung 9:57–67, 1980

Shapiro B, Harrison RA, Trout CA: Clinical Application of Respiratory Care, 2nd ed. Chicago, Year Book Medical Publishers, 1979

Spennrath S: Understanding the sexual needs of the older patient. The Canadian Nurse, Jul/Aug, 25–29, 1982

Stein JM, Hedley-Whyte J: Anesthesiology. In Calkins E, Davis PJ, Ford AB (eds): The Practice of Geriatrics. Philadelphia, WB Saunders, 1986

Steffl BM: Handbook of Gerontological Nursing. New York, Van Nostrand Reinhold, 1984

Weitkamp MR, Aber RC: Nonbacterial and unusual pneumonias in the elderly. Geriatrics 39:87–100, 1984

West JB: Respiratory Physiology: The Essentials, 2nd ed. Baltimore, Williams & Wilkins, 1979

Sister Rose Therese Bahr

Musculoskeletal system 8

Aging brings many changes in the musculoskeletal system, a system that is often taken for granted. As a person ages, the potential increases for falls, fractures, and accidents; and mobility may be affected. When the mobility capacity is changed, the person has difficulty completing activities of daily living (ADL), resulting in a reduction of the quality of life (Kart et al 1978).

Generally, the onset of age-related changes in the musculoskeletal system is gradual and somewhat difficult to detect (Carnevali and Patrick 1986; Villaverde and Macmillan 1980). With advancing years, the age-related changes in this system and their effects on the physical state of the person provide the basis for understanding how disease processes in which mobility is altered can transform the lifestyle of a person from independence to dependency. Knowledge of these changes in an aging population is essential for the nurse. Assessing data on the status of the musculoskeletal system and incorporating appropriate nursing diagnoses regarding this system are integral components of the individualized nursing care plan. A thorough understanding of the musculoskeletal changes that accompany the aging process underlies the systematic nursing assessment needed to prevent high-risk problems and behaviors associated with this system.

Age-related changes

The musculoskeletal system is composed of muscle, bone structure, and joints that produce anatomic size and height. Each of these components is essential for a healthy functional musculoskeletal system. With advancing age, each of these components changes, resulting in difficulties in the assumption of a normal lifestyle.

Muscle

Muscles are composed of "postmitotic cells and are dependent on intact motor neuron innervation for survival" (Carnevali and Patrick 1986). A gradual and progressive loss of muscle mass and strength is a major characteristic of aging. Research studies have found that the decrease in the number of muscle cells with the onset of aging may exceed the loss of essential neural components in the muscle mass (Ebersole and Hess 1985; Gress and Bahr 1984). Some of the changes in the muscle mass may be masked by extracellular increases in fat, collagen, and interstitial fluid. These changes are both extensive and complex. The muscle cell may also become the depository for *lipofuscin,* the refuse of cellular function that is not removed efficiently from the cell. The muscle cells remaining are not capable of the high-level performance of normal cells. Density of capillaries per motor cell may also be decreased, leaving a less-functional vascular system in place for the muscle cell, with fewer nutrients brought to it by means of the blood vessels (Carnevali and Patrick 1986).

Use of oxygen per motor unit is unchanged in the older adult; however, the activity of the enzyme system is significantly reduced within the muscle function. Research studies have noted a prolongation of contraction time, latency period, and relaxation time of about 13% and the maximal rate of tension development decreases in the aging muscle. These processes are correlated with the decrease in the myosin ATPase activity within the muscle cell metabolism. The motor function decrease is compounded by deconditioning, malnutrition, endocrine changes, poor motivation, and normal involution occurring in the aging person. Exercise may improve muscle function and efficiency but the increment of function of the muscle performance decreases with age (Carnevali and Patrick 1986).

Muscle changes are caused by a decrease in the number of muscle fibers that result from muscle inability for regeneration and by fibrous tissue replacing the contractile elements of the muscle (Horwitz and Magee 1975). Muscle mass is lost, then, because the number and diameter of the muscle fibers decrease (Kart et al 1978). Extracellular water, chloride, and sodium are increased in the muscles of the elderly, whereas intracellular potassium is slightly decreased. Aging muscles may also have a lower reaction to stimulation. Muscle atrophy and denervation in the elderly have been suggested to result from a higher rate of protein breakdown rather than from protein synthesis. Muscle change during aging is an individualized process with a high degree of variability.

Hormones may also play a part in the aging musculoskeletal system. Alterations in the synthesis of thyrotropic and somatotropic hormones that involve protein metabolism may result in muscle atrophy (Yurick et al 1984). These changes may involve the muscle's ability to use the hormone effectively. In addition, neuronal changes may create muscle changes such as in the case of cerebrovascular accidents when the person moves from being an independent, active individual to one who is bed-confined for a considerable time. Muscular changes occur rapidly for elderly persons in such cases.

When the muscle mass is reduced, the elderly have difficulty controlling movement. The degree of mobility determines the level of independence. Mobility depends on the coordinated activity of nerves, muscles, and bones. Internal receptors in the muscles, tendons, and joints that measure the level of blood chemistry, hydration, and other body conditions affect the degree of control of movement (Yurick et al 1984).

Thus, the muscle mass in normal aging wastes with time, and correlates with the atrophy of tissues and organs (Burnside 1976; Palmore et al 1985). This change results in a decrease in the size of the muscles throughout the body (particularly in the upper and lower extremities), a reduction in strength of the muscles, and a diminution of functional ability. Elderly persons begin to notice the lessened availability of muscle strength for activities such as opening a heavy door or a tightly closed jar lid. Atrophy of the muscles in the hand make the hand look thin and bony, the muscles in the arms and legs of older adults appear flabby and small. Carrying packages and working around the home or garden become difficult and frustrating, and activities that once filled up the hours of the day become chores. The home-care nurse must be aware of the resulting social isolation that may occur.

In addition to muscle wasting and lack of strength, endurance and agility are also affected with aging. With lessened muscle strength, the ability to participate in extended periods of activity with flexibility of body movements diminishes and complaints of fatigue become common. Anderson (1971) notes that as aging changes occur, muscle power in the hand grip lessens. In the right hand of a man, the predicted power of the grip decreases from 44 kg pressure at 60 years of age to 32.1 kg pressure at 89 years of age. For women, the hand grip pressure changes from 32.4 kg pressure to 27.4 kg pressure. The left hand's grip is far less than the right hand for both men and women and the power in both hands remains greater for men than for women.

In aging persons, a condition called *senile muscular wasting* with resultant changes in posture is a common occurrence. In this condition the posture of the aging person tends to become one of general flexion, where the head and neck are held forward, the dorsal spine becomes gently kyphotic, the upper limbs are bent at the elbows and wrists, and the hips and knees are slightly flexed (Reichel 1978). This flexion is due to changes in the vertebral column and in the intervertebral disks, ankylosis of ligaments and joints, shrinkage and sclerosis of tendons and muscles, and degenerative changes in the extrapyramidal central nervous system (Reichel 1978; Villaverde and Macmillan 1980).

Disorders of movement are also present as a result of the decreasing function of muscles in aged persons. There may be an impassive facial expression, infrequent blinking of the eyes, and a decrease in spontaneous and associated movement. Movements of extremities are extremely slow. A resting tremor is also frequently present. The rigidity, infrequency and slowness of movement, tremor, and the flexion attitude, when intense, may be attributable to the degenerative state of the extrapyramidal system (Ebersole and Hess 1981, 1985; Gress and Bahr 1984; Hogstel 1981). This condition is identified as *parkinsonism*.

In assessing the needs of the person with a diagnosis of Parkinson's disease, the nurse must be aware of the patient's tendency to fall because of the rigidity of muscle movements. Clearing the path of the usual routes of travel (to bathroom, dining room, etc.) facilitates movement and is highly important. Because of slowness of movement, sufficient time must be given for executing any task requiring mobility (*e.g.,* getting into and out of bed to avoid incontinence, or facilitating the movements of eating by allowing sufficient time for adequate nutritional intake).

Tendon reflexes may be affected by muscular disorders of the aging process. Diminished tendon jerks such as in the ankle, arm, and knee may be observed in older adults. Frank extensor responses are regarded as an abnormal finding and possibly the indication of a lesion of the upper motor neuron (pyramidal tract or motor cortex) (Reichel 1978).

Muscular fasciculations or visible flickering movements of muscles may be present in the older adult as a result of muscular weakness and wasting and are manifestations of slowly progressive deterioration of anterior horn cells, cranial motor nerve nuclei, or nerve root motor nerves. These fasciculations may occur in the calf muscles, eyelids, hands, and feet, especially after fatigue or excessive loss of sodium chloride (Reichel 1978).

Cramps in muscle groups of the calf, foot, thigh, hand, or hip, especially after unusual muscular effort and occurring usually at night, may also be a disorder of the aging muscles. They may be the result of peripheral vascular insufficiency, sodium deprivation or loss, decrease in plasma concentration of calcium, hypoglycemia, certain toxins such as that of the tetanus bacillus, and rarely, anterior horn cell or peripheral nerve disease. Cramps may be terminated by passive stretch, hot bath at bedtime, or oral medication such as quinine sulfate, which lengthens the refractory period of muscle movement (Reichel 1978).

Another condition of the muscle groups is "restless legs," which relieves the paresthesias by motion of the legs after the legs have been quiet or motionless for some time. This disorder, which becomes troublesome as the person ages, may occur without any cause or as a result from neuropathy caused by diabetes, hypoglycemia, hypocalcemia, or alkalosis resulting from hyperventilation (Reichel 1978).

Skeletal muscle dysfunction may result from disease in the path taken by the stimulus for voluntary movement from the highest cerebral centers to the motor cortex, pyramidal tract, motor nuclei of the brain stem and anterior horn cells of the spinal cord, peripheral motor nerves, neuromuscular junction, and muscle fibers. Weakness occurs in almost all disorders and is the major presenting complaint. Weakness may be accompanied by stiffness, spasm, pain, or abnormal movements (Reichel 1978).

With muscle mass decreased, bony prominences become more evident. The bony parts of the elbow, bones in the upper and lower extremities, and the hip are much more evident when reduced muscle mass covers these regions. The skin over these bony prominences becomes highly vulnerable to breakdown because of loss of cushioning and padding. Alterations in skin integrity can occur.

Another muscular disorder, *myasthenia gravis,* is a chronic disorder of neuromuscular transmission characterized by weakness and abnormal fatigability

(Horwitz and Magee 1975; Kart et al 1978; Reichel 1978). Muscles innervated by the cranial nerves, usually those of the neck, trunk, and extremities, are particularly affected. Onset of the disease usually peaks in the third decade for women and the third and seventh decade in men. After the age of 60 the condition is more common in men (Palmore et al 1985, Reichel 1978). The disease becomes generalized, but may remain localized to the extraocular muscles. The usual symptoms are ptosis of the eyelids, diplopia, weakness of the legs, difficulty in swallowing, or generalized weakness of the musculature (Reichel 1978).

In managing the care of the patient with myasthenia gravis, the nurse should monitor the patient closely for rapid development of myasthenic crisis—sudden inability to swallow or maintain a patent airway for adequate respiratory exchange. Drug administration must be on a strict time schedule to reduce the potential for such crises. Because avoidance of any emotional upset is important, the nurse must control the environment as much as possible. Psychosocial needs of the person are a priority; the nurse should encourage the patient to express his feelings.

Bone

Bone undergoes specific changes in later life. Around the age of 40 and beyond, bone mass and density shift from increasing to progressively declining (Carnevali and Patrick 1986). Characteristic of this shift is the gradual reabsorption of the interior of the long and flat bones and a slower accretion of new bone on the external surface. As this condition advances, the long bones are enlarged externally but internally appear hollowed out, the vertebral endplates are thinned, and the skull is slightly enlarged. As this process occurs, trabeculae are also lost, making the bone weaker and prone to fracture.

A major change is the normal demineralization of the bone mass, resulting in a more porous substance. This normal demineralization occurs in the presence of age-related maintenance and inadequacy of dietary intake. Nutrients supply the body with minerals such as zinc, calcium, potassium, and cadmium. When these nutrients are inadequately provided by dietary intake, the body withdraws these minerals from organs throughout the body, including the bones. When the bones become porous and brittle the potential for fractures of the vertebrae, ribs, and hips is greater, especially in women (Burnside 1976; Palmore et al 1985). Fracture of the hips is the most serious condition, leading to immobilization and increased mortality (Carnevali and Patrick 1986). The removal or leaching of calcium from the bone matrix fosters the condition called *osteoporosis*, the most prevalent metabolic disease of the bone (Allen 1986; Miller 1985; Osteoporosis: The silent disease 1986).

Osteoporosis is observed with increasing frequency in women over 45 years of age and in men over 55 years of age. Bone loss in women is about 25% (750 g loss from the normal 3000 g) and in men the loss is 12% (450 g loss from the normal 4000 g) (Carnevali and Patrick 1986; Venglarik and Adams 1985). Studies have shown that persons in older age groups tend to have smaller amounts of bone and bone density. Studies have not demonstrated clearly if osteoporosis is a manifestation of a normal process of aging or if it is a distinct pathologic process (Reichel 1978). This disease has major implications in the cause of pathologic fractures. An elderly person may be healthy and functioning one day, and the next day be hospitalized with a fractured hip and become psychologically confused. The nurse should learn the circumstances that surrounded the fracture, and the independence level of the patient before hospitalization. Rehabilitation efforts should be toward maximizing the potential of the patient.

A major age-related change in the area of bone structure is the shortening of the trunk of the older adult as a result of the narrowing of intervertebral space. Vertebrae in the spinal column are a series of small bones connected by spaces that contain a cartilage substance to absorb shocks and jolts of walking and jumping. As a person ages, the spaces between the vertebrae narrow and flatten. This condition causes stooped posture and shortening of the trunk, resulting in a reduction in height (Kart et al 1978).

The nurse, in caring for persons with age-related changes in bone structure, should be alert to decreased area of vision that results from stooped posture. Clutter in the environment must be kept at a minimum to prevent injury from the patient's bumping into sharp edges on furniture. Limited mobility may also be caused by bone structures not functioning well in the later years. Walkers of various types may be needed to assist the person in walking short or long distances without having the tendency to fall as a major threat. Another area of concern for the nurse is the decreased lung expansion for the older adult suffering from a kyphotic or stooped posture. With the head and neck position close to the chest, the lungs are unable to expand to their fullest capacity. Consequently, proper oxygen intake is hampered and may create a hypoxic condition. Dizziness and slight confusion may result from the insufficiency of oxygen intake.

Joints

Joints, or articulating surfaces of joining bones, allow various body movements. Joints are covered with articular cartilage and encircled by a strong fibrous articular capsule. A highly vascular synovial membrane lines the capsule and produces a lubricant for smooth articulation. It is the articular cartilage and synovial fluid that allow for smooth, lubricated movement. The joint capsule and associated tendons and ligaments aid in stabilizing the joint (Kart et al 1978).

With advancing years, the joints of the body (*i.e.,* shoulder, elbow, knee, hip, ankle, and wrist) become less mobile, resulting in pain (Kart et al 1978). As a result of the lessened mobility, joints can tighten and possibly become fixed. When this condition is present, the muscles, on attempted movement, contract with much pain. Because the muscle mass is also lessened, the weakened muscles fail to support the joints properly, adding to the fixation of the joints (Kart et al 1978). Major deterioration of the joints can begin as early as the third decade and progress into the aging years. These changes are assumed to be the result of the accumulation of trauma during the lifetime and produce fraying and chipping of the cartilage and bone in and around the joints. As the cartilage becomes damaged and begins to erode, the bone makes direct contact with bone, and degeneration of the joint begins to be evident in the form of arthritis, with crepitation, pain, and limitation of movement (Carnevali and Patrick 1986). Another change is the loss of water from the cartilage, which causes the narrowing of the joint spaces, especially in the intervertebral disks, and contributes to the reduction in height (Carnevali and Patrick 1986).

Major degenerative joint disease, *osteoarthritis,* is evidenced by an irregular bony overgrowth at the edge of the joints, possibly resulting from previous trauma. When this condition occurs about the hip, for example, the femoral head becomes trapped, painful, and immobile. Osteoarthritis is the most common cause for hip replacements in older adults (Carnevali and Patrick 1986). When this condition occurs on the vertebrae, it impinges on spinal nerves as they penetrate the intervertebral foramina, causing severe pain.

Because of the changes in the vertebral column and loss of muscle strength and mass, the posture of the older adult may change and the condition known as *kyphosis* (a bending) of the spine may occur. Kyphosis brings a hump to the upper portion of the spinal column, which tilts the head forward. This condition occurs when intake of calcium is insufficient and the vertebral bone mass becomes porous and brittle.

When the joints become painful, stiff, or limited in movement, the range of motion for each joint becomes limited. That is, the full posterior, anterior, lateral, and medial motions that each joint should be capable of performing are reduced in range in terms of flexion, extension, abduction, and adduction. Chronic pain may be experienced and the nurse needs to assess its possible presence.

Major joint disorders evident in the later years include *arthritis, osteoarthritis, rheumatoid arthritis,* and *gout.* Arthritis is an inflammation or a degenerative change of a joint (Kart et al 1978), whereas osteoarthritis, a degenerative joint change that takes place in aging, is a gradual wearing away of the joint cartilage with resultant exposure of rough underlying bone ends that cause pain and stiffness but not inflammation (Kart et al 1978). Rheumatoid arthritis, a chronic, inflammatory disease that is more common in women than men, leads to bone dislocation, joint fusion, and great discomfort and pain (Kart et al 1978; Reichel 1978). An inflamed synovial membrane is the initial site of pathology in a joint with rheumatoid arthritis. This highly vascular structure becomes swollen and thickened. If the inflammatory condition persists, scar tissue and granulation tissue (new capillary formation and fibrous cells) are formed, extensively damaging the joint and its structures. Tendons may drift out of their normal position and shorten, causing joint deformity (Kart et al 1978). Gout is an inherited condition of abnormal purine metabolism characterized by excess blood levels of uric acid, usually excreted through the kidneys. Uric acid, if not normally excreted, can precipitate out to the joints to form sharp salt crystals and initiate an attack of gouty arthritis. This condition is characterized by sudden intermittent episodes of excruciating joint pain, swelling, and inflammation (Kart et al 1978).

Studies have shown that proper exercise and activity of the joints may maintain function of the joints for a longer time. Research has shown the positive effects of exercise on physical and mental status of the elderly population (Carnevali and Patrick 1986). Activity may be seen as central to the prevention of premature aging and a proper exercise program should be initiated to prevent limitation of mobility of the joints.

Anatomic size and height

With advancing years, the older adult may experience a reduction in body mass as a result of the total decrease in body protein and body water that occurs in direct proportion to the decrease in the basic metabolic rate (Ebersole and Hess 1985; Gress and Bahr 1984; Horwitz and Magee 1975). The slowing of the basic metabolic rate creates a decline in the use of calories. When this mechanism operates in the older adult, an increase in body fat becomes evident and the body becomes distinctly pear-shaped, with diminished fat in the arms and legs and an increase of fat in the trunk (hips and waist) area.

As discussed above, the vertebral column shortens, with an average decrease in height from one inch to four inches from young adulthood. On average, 1.5 inches of height is lost between ages 65 years to 74 years of age, increasing to 3 inches lost by ages 85 years to 94 years (Carnevali and Patrick 1986). Multiple factors cause this loss such as a decrease in the intervertebral disk spaces, vertebral osteoporosis and collapse, kyphosis resulting from both of these factors, and a characteristic knee flexion (Reichel 1978). Thus, the musculoskeletal system may have a great influence on the appearance of age in elderly persons.

Psychosocial manifestations of conditions

The conditions caused by changes in the musculoskeletal system often affect the psychosocial well-being of elderly persons. Problems can be observed in the older person when he or she faces surgical interventions, immobility, or hospitalization.

The self-image of the elderly adult may be altered as a result of loss of height or inability to move about freely. The nurse must encourage expression of feelings about this loss, and in whatever way possible, emphasize the patient's remaining strengths. These could include such positive situations as number of friends the patient has, or the degree of wellness that exists in the dimensions of physical well-being and the spiritual realm. Such acknowledgment of strengths often offsets the negative image the patient may have from the physical aspects of age-related changes.

When an older adult must have surgery as a result of a hip fracture, for example, many stressors are present (*e.g.*, possibly emotional reactions of fear; guilt; disruption in ability to trust; difficulty in maintenance of self-esteem, tolerating a major loss, or maintaining intimacy in close relationships [Barry 1984; Brunner and Suddarth 1974; Gress and Bahr 1984]). The older adult realizes that physically, he or she is not as strong and healthy as in former years and may fear that surgery will bring many inherent risks (cardiac arrest, respiratory difficulties) and a prolonged recovery period. The nurse should have knowledge of the psychosocial aspects of an illness and attempt to determine the possible effects on the patient. Eight factors upon which psychosocial adaptation depend when a major physical or traumatic event occurs provide an excellent format for data collection (Barry 1984; Brunner and Suddarth 1974; Gress and Bahr 1984). These eight assessment factors are

- Social history—information about the person's lifestyle, and the availability of persons who can support the elderly adult emotionally during the difficult event.
- Level of stress during the year before admission. What major stressors has the person experienced during the past year of life?
- Normal coping patterns.
- Neurovegetative changes. Are there changes in sleep patterns, appetite, bowel functioning, energy levels, and sexual functioning since the illness began?
- Mental status. Is there any dysfunction emotionally, intellectually, or perceptually?
- Patient's understanding of the illness. Does the patient fully understand what is happening? How long has he or she had to prepare psychologically for the effects of this illness upon the future?
- Personality style—the manner in which the patient interacts in normal life with other persons.
- Major issues of the illness. Obtain data on the manner in which the person perceives the psychosocial stresses of the illness.

Surgical intervention can be a frightening ordeal for the elderly adult with a bone, joint, or muscle dysfunction. The immobility caused by hip-replacement surgery, or any other type of orthopedic surgery can be of long duration with severe pain. The fear of losing part of one's body through surgery can be devastating to an older person's self-image and can contribute to a distorted view of the potential and capability for the future.

During the elderly patient's hospitalization, the nurse must be aware of any signs of depression or anxiety. The patient who has been extremely talkative and social will suddenly become less talkative, quiet, and withdrawn. These are danger signals that the psychosocial stresses of hospitalization are becoming too great to bear. The nurse should start supportive therapy immediately and alert the physician for possible medication regimen implementation. It is difficult for the elderly patient to be alone when facing an unknown future that may involve decreased mobility and increased dependence. Self-esteem is the crucial component for moving through the traumatic experience of hospitalization, and has been conceptualized as having four separate components (Barry 1984):

- The body self—the body image; how a person looks, feels, and functions; and the thoughts and feelings about the ability to perform basic functions.

- The interpersonal self—the person's thoughts and feelings about the manner in which he or she relates to others in both intimate and casual relationships.
- The achieving self—the person's thoughts and feelings about his or her ability to obtain goals in family, work, and school environments.
- The identification of self—abstract feelings and behaviors that are involved with moral and spiritual concerns.

The self perception of the elderly patient and the way others perceive him or her may have major implications for ego integration or despair. When faced with chronic pain or immobility, patients must be perceived as whole and capable so that achievement in the rehabilitative aspects of their care is possible.

By recognizing the impact any one of these components may have on the self-esteem of the elderly patient, the nurse can better appreciate the threat that hospitalization and musculoskeletal conditions can hold. Too often the incapacity, however temporary, of the elderly patient is seen by the family as a permanent disability; they create dependency in a situation in which fostering independence is so vital to a high level of self-esteem and self-maintenance (Hall 1984).

The psychosocial component and manifestations in conditions related to the musculoskeletal system in the older adult may take many forms. It is the nurse, with astute observations, who must quickly recognize the signs of an impending psychosocial crisis and implement a plan of care to ward off the crisis by early detection and nursing interventions.

Assessment parameters

A determination of the older person's level of incapacity may precede the actual physical assessment. Questions to be raised include the following list (Carnevali and Patrick 1986):

Can you go outdoors?

Can you walk up and down stairs?

Can you wash and bathe yourself?

Can you prepare your meals?

Can you get out of the house?

Can you cut your toenails?

Scoring for questions: 0 No incapacity

1 Does the task with difficulty

2 Unable to perform task

An assessment of the elderly musculoskeletal system begins with a generalized inspection of the person standing or sitting (as required by the movement that is being tested). Objective data that can be assessed by the nurse from casual observation include:

- General posture. Does the person have kyphosis, compensatory position of head and neck, flexion of extremities, or contractures?
- Stance. What is the distance between the feet when standing? Is there a toeing in or out to maintain the stance?
- Gait. When walking, what is the length of stride, the height the foot is lifted from the floor, are there shuffling movements?
- Normal speed in walking. Does the pace in walking decrease with the distance walked?
- Difficulty or ease in sitting down or standing. What type of furniture in the home is selected to sit on—easy chair, straight-backed chair?
- Support and balance. Is support for balance created by touching furniture, doorjambs, or railings as walking is attempted?
- Use of assistive devices (canes, walkers, crutches). What level of skill is demonstrated in using these devices? Is the skill correctly applied? Does the device fit properly in relation to the size of the person?
- Ability to climb and descend stairs. Can this be accomplished without difficulty or unsteadiness?

After these observations have been made, obtain objective measurements as baseline data for future evaluation. With the elderly person standing, take the weight measurement by having the person step on a well-calibrated scale. Document the reading in pounds or kilograms as directed by your health-care agency. Ask the client to step down from the scale and measure the height of the person in inches (*e.g.,* 63 inches).

Ask the patient to walk from one point (such as the examining table) to the door; stop the patient midway and ask that he or she hold the position of the feet in a normal walking stride. Measure the length of the stride (*e.g.,* 12 inches) and measure the height that the foot is from the floor when in a walking mode (*e.g.,* 3 inches). Note sizes of step if client shuffles so that contact with the floor is maintained. This information is significant in terms of identification of possible central nervous system pathology such as parkinsonism or some other motor involvement (Ebersole and Hess 1981, 1985). Also take note of the posture (degree of erectness) when the client is walking, width of base for maintaining balance, kind and condition of shoes worn, arm movements when walking (symmetry and length of arm swing), eye gaze while walking (Does the person watch foot placement?), evenness of walking pace, maintenance of balance, comfort while walking, and areas of discomfort while walking (Kart et al 1978; Tinetti 1986; William 1984; Yurick et al 1984).

Next ask the person to stand independently to measure proprioception. What is the balance with and without the eyes closed? What degree of sway is present (Romberg's Test for balance)? If a pronounced sway is present, be alert to assist the person to prevent a fall and injury (Hogstel 1981; Tinetti 1986; Uden 1985).

The patient should then be asked to stand in a relaxed position. Note the degree of erectness or forward-leaning flexion. Also take note of the curvature of the spine. Is it kyphotic? To what degree is kyphosis present? Is a "dowager's hump" present? Note the flexion at the elbows and wrists, hips, knees, and ankles. Ask the patient to sit. What is the normal posture in a sitting position? Assist the patient onto the examining table. What position does he or she naturally take when lying down—on the back? right side? left side?

With the client on the examining table, measure with a tape measure the size of each major muscle. Note the size of the calf, thigh, ankle, upper arm, and forearm on both the right and left extremities, and measure the size of the pelvis and chest. The measurement for each of these major muscle groups should be documented as baseline data for future evaluation. Since muscle mass is lost in aging, it is important for the nurse to have accurate data for future comparison.

Ask the person to move the legs away from the body, move the legs close to the body, raise each leg as high as possible and then lower it. Instruct the patient to lie on the stomach if possible and extend the legs as far as possible. Notice the differences in the right and left legs in terms of muscle weakness, strength, tone, tenderness, and coordination of movements. Ask the patient to lie on the back and assess the flexion of the hip and extension of the hip. Note any pain, limited movement, or jerkiness of movement. Document findings for the range of motion for the joints that have been assessed (Beland and Passos 1975; Burnside 1976; Yurick et al 1984).

Ask the client to come to a sitting position. At this point the spinal column should be examined for kyphosis. Where does the kyphotic curvature begin (cervical region, lumbar region)? What degree of kyphosis is present—mild, moderate, severe? Document the findings.

Next, the patient should grip the nurse's hands with his or hers. Is the grip equally tight in each hand? Are the hands arthritic (painful joints, difficulty in closing the hands completely because of pain or immobility of fingers or wrists)? The hand-grip measurement confirms whether potential muscle weakness of the arms is present. Note or document if any differences in strength of grip is evident in either hand.

While the patient is sitting, the nurse should ask him or her to open and close his or her mouth. Observe for any difficulty in this movement. In aging, mandibular joint changes may develop so that the opening of the mouth becomes a painful procedure. How widely can the patient open the mouth? Are chewing movements present? When the mouth is opened, is there a crepitus sound indicating arthritic changes in the mandibular joint? Does the patient complain of pain when this movement is initiated?

Finally, while the client is sitting, ask him or her to move his or her head in a rolling movement from side to side, and backward and forward. Assess the presence of any pain, limited range of movement, or crepitus sounds. Assess the movements, flexion, extension, adduction, and abduction of the shoulder, wrist, thumb joints, elbow, ankle, and toes. Is any limitation of motion present? Document your findings for the range of motion for these joints (Carnevali and Patrick 1986; Gress and Bahr 1984; Hogstel 1981).

Knowledge of the normal aging process and data from a thorough history and physical assessment allow for accurate planning of care for the elderly patient with problems of the musculoskeletal system.

Rehabilitation of the musculoskeletal system

Rehabilitation is the goal for an older patient who has muscle, bone, and joint injuries and diseases. The nurse, whose main focus is health, aids the patient in becoming as independent in living as possible. Rehabilitation concepts are to be emphasized in planning nursing care and are implemented on an individual basis, depending on the specific situation being experienced by the older person.

Forms of rehabilitation include range-of-motion exercises and activities to maintain joint functions of the wrist, elbow, shoulder, knee, ankle, and hip. Such exercises should be started as quickly as possible after an acute episode (*e.g.,* inflammation) to reduce the potential of loss of joint function.

Another form of rehabilitation is the use of crutch-walking to protect the weight-bearing joints from excess wear. Proper technique is essential and the patient should be instructed by qualified persons who understand the muscle, joint, and bone structures. Such instructors are physical therapists and nurses who have been educated in the use of crutch-walking.

Finally, physical therapy as ordered by the physician and executed by the professional physical therapist may take the form of heat applications to sore muscles, arm-stretching exercises on a wall-mounted wheel, bicycle riding to strengthen muscles, and other types of exercises to maintain independence of living. Physical therapy and rehabilitation are important components for inclusion in the nursing care plans of older patients who are experiencing changes in the musculoskeletal system.

Drugs

Some drugs commonly used in the treatment of problems with the musculoskeletal system are listed in Table 8-1.

Table 8-1. Drugs used in the treatment of musculoskeletal diseases

Acetaminophen and propoxyphene are almost always classified as mild (non-narcotic) analgesics that are used as adjunct therapy for musculoskeletal pain but are not considered specific drugs for use with musculoskeletal problems. Patients should be warned about using musculoskeletal drugs and anticoagulants together.

Nonsteroidal anti-inflammatory drugs (NSAID)

Drug	Effect/response in the elderly	Nursing implications
Aspirin (ASA, Bufferin, Ascriptin, Ecotrin, Empirin)	Exhibits analgesic, antipyretic and anti-inflammatory effects. No direct relationship between therapeutic response and blood concentration. Salicylate blood level of 20 mg%–30 mg% is therapeutic for anti-inflammatory effects; 3.25 mg–1.5 g daily for analgesia and fever; 2.4–3.6 g daily in divided doses needed for anti-inflammatory effect. Inhibits platelet aggregation and provides antithrombotic effect. Useful in reducing risk of transient ischemic attack (TIA), reduces risk of nonfatal recurrent myocardial infarction (MI) in patient showing an MI and microcirculatory thrombosis.	Monitor salicylates when blood level is greater than 30 mg%. Tinnitus is an unavoidable sign of toxicity and may be reversible. Monitor GI side-effects such as gastric ulceration. GI side-effects can be prevented by drinking a full glass of water or use of enteric-coated or buffered aspirin. Instruct patient to report symptoms of salicylism, ecchymosis, petechiae, bleeding gums, bloody or black stools. Monitor for potential drug interactions such as protein-binding-site displacement, which includes warfarin and potentiation of other NSAIDs on concomitant administration. Other protein-binding drugs, which include sulfonylurea, sulfonamides, hydantoins may be potentiated.
Salsalate (Disalcid)	Exhibits analgesic and antipyretic effects. May be used in patient with salicylate sensitivity. Useful in patients with GI intolerance to aspirin or when platelet functions should not be interfered with.	Caution patient about GI side-effects, including nausea, dyspepsia, pain, and diarrhea. Side-effects can be avoided when administered with food. Renal and hepatic side-effects are rare. Salsalate cannot be substituted for aspirin for the prophylaxis of thrombosis.
Diflunisal (Dolobid)	Possesses anti-inflammatory and analgesic effects. No tolerance or physical dependence on longterm therapy. Can cause gastric mucosal drainage. May inhibit platelet function. Can cause mild renal toxicity with high dosages or prolonged periods of use. 500 mg twice a day is as effective as acetaminophen 60 mg and codeine 60 mg.	Caution patient to space the administration of antacid with diflunisal because of a potential decrease in absorption. Instruct the patient to report any decrease in urine output. Advise patient to report any GI upset and bleeding. Observe for adverse effects from drug interactions by protein-binding site displacement of anticoagulant, salicylates, and sulfonylureas.

(continued)

Table 8-1. *(Continued)*

Nonsteroidal anti-inflammatory drugs (NSAID)

Drug	Effect/response in the elderly	Nursing implications
	May cause sodium and water retention and induce peripheral edema.	Avoid concomitant administration with other NSAIDs such as indomethacin to avoid GI side-effects. Have patient swallow drug whole and do not crush or chew tablets. GI side-effects could be prevented by taking it with a glass of water, milk, or food.
Fenoprofen (Nalfon)	Propionic acid derivative. Exhibits positive analgesic, antipyretic, and anti-inflammatory effects. Can cause gastric mucosal damage. Exhibits renal toxicity. Inhibits collagen-induced platelet aggregation and may prolong bleeding time.	Monitor patient for dyspepsia and constipation. GI side-effects may be reduced with meals or antacids. Monitor patient for potential drug interactions such as increased blood levels of warfarin, sulfonamide, sulfonylureas, salicylates, and phenytoin. Avoid taking aspirin or phenobarbital concomitantly, which may decrease plasma fenoprofen significantly. Educate patient to expect a fair degree of somnolence and avoid work requiring mental alertness (*e.g*, driving a motor vehicle). Assess patient for signs and symptoms of hemolytic effects, which include purpura, bruising, or hemorrhage. Monitor patient for renal effects including dysuria, cystitis, oliguria, or anuria.
Ibuprofen (Motrin, Rufen, Advil, Nuprin)	Possesses antiinflammatory, antipyretic, and analgesic properties. Administer 1200 mg–3200 mg daily for anti-inflammatory effect. Less than 1200 mg daily is used for an analgesic effect. Can cause fewer GI symptoms than aspirin in equally effective dose.	Optimal response occurs within 2 weeks. May administer with food or milk to reduce GI irritation. Monitor patient for dizziness and drowsiness. Instruct patient to report any reduction in urine output. For hematologic, renal, and drug interactions see section on ketoprofen.
Meclofenamate (Meclomen)	Pharmacological and clinical efficacies are similar to those of aspirin and other NSAIDs. Exhibits positive analgesic, antipyretic, and anti-inflammatory effect.	Inform patient that diarrhea is common. This may be dose-related. Instruct patient to report dizziness and headache to the physician.

Drug		
	Reported to have adverse renal effect. May cause gastric mucosal damage. Can transiently inhibit platelet aggregation.	May react with protein-binding drugs by enhancing warfarin anticoagulant effect. Avoid taking aspirin to prevent reduction of plasma level of meclofenamate.
Indomethacin (Indocin)	Structurally and pharmacologically related to Sulindac. Exhibits analgesic antipyretic and anti-inflammatory effects. May decrease renal function. Can inhibit platelet aggregation and increase bleeding time. Can cause gastric mucosal damage resulting in bleeding or ulceration.	Inform the patient that headache is common and that a dosage reduction may be necessary if the symptom is severe. Observe the patient for GI disturbances, including diarrhea, symptoms may be minimized by food or antacids. Assess peptic ulcer formation when given concomitantly with corticosteroid and other NSAIDs. Extended-release capsule of indomethacin should not be used in treatment of acute gouty arthritis. Monitor patient for renal insufficiency. Avoid cross-sensitivity in patients with aspirin-induced bronchospasm. Monitor patient for corneal deposits, retinal disturbances, and tinnitus.
Noproxen Naproxen Sodium (Naprosyn, Anaprox)	Pharmacological and clinical effects similar to fenoprofen and ibuprofen. The sodium salt contains 25 mg (1 meq) sodium and is more rapidly absorbed than naproxen. Half-life is 12 hr to 15 hr and possible for twice daily dosing.	May be given with food or antacids to reduce incidence of GI symptoms. May cause drowsiness and dizziness. Advise patient against performing potentially hazardous activities (*e.g.,* driving a motor vehicle). Advise patient to inform the dentist or surgeon before surgery that the patient is taking NSAIDs. May interfere with urinary assays of 5 HIAA. Monitor patient for central nervous system, otic, ocular, renal, and hepatic effects similar to those caused by other NSAIDs.
Phenylbutazone (Azolid)	Effective in short-term symptomatic relief of pain and inflammation. Inhibits leukocyte-release and migration or activity of lysosomal enzymes. Useful in the treatment of gouty arthritis and ankylosing spondylitis. May cause sodium and water retention.	Caution patient not to use this drug as a general analgesic or antipyretic. Drug is shown to be palliative for rheumatoid arthritis and does not alter the underlying disease process. May cause GI upset, nausea, dyspepsia; GI irritation may be minimized by taking with food. Can cause sodium and water retention. May aggravate pulmonary edema, pleural or pericardial effusion. Instruct patient to keep appointments for all follow-up blood studies because hematologic toxicities such as aplastic anemia or agranulocytosis may occur sud-

(continued)

Table 8-1. *(Continued)*

Nonsteroidal anti-inflammatory drugs (NSAID)

Drug	Effect/response in the elderly	Nursing implications
		denly or many weeks after drug use has been terminated.
		Can increase the action of warfarin, phenytoin, salicylate, and oral antidiabetic agents by displacement from protein-binding sites.
Piroxicam (Feldene)	An oxicam derivative structurally different from other NSAIDs.	Average plasma life is 50 hr, which allows once daily dosing.
	Exhibits anti-inflammatory, analgesic, and antipyretic activities similar to other NSAIDs.	Monitor for GI disturbance, bleeding time, and elevations of blood-urea nitrogen (BUN) and serum creatinine and renal functions. This is reversible on discontinuation of the drug.
	Can cause GI mucosal damage, resulting in ulceration or bleeding.	20 mg daily dosage is usually adequate. Dosage may go up 40 mg daily. It takes 7 to 12 days of therapy to achieve steady-state plasma concentration; therefore, adjustment of dosage should not be less than 2 weeks after initiation of treatment.
	May adversely affect renal function because of the inhibition of renal prostaglandin synthesis.	Monitor level, signs, and symptoms of lithium intoxication because of possible decrease in renal clearance of lithium. Initial manifestation of lithium toxicity includes confusion, coarse hand tremors and joint pain.
	As effective as phenylbutazone or indomethacin for symptomatic relief of ankylosing spondylitis and is better tolerated.	Like other NSAIDs, piroxicam enhances the effect of anticoagulants and antidiabetic agents.
Sulindac (Clinoril)	Structurally related to indomethacin.	Monitor patient for adverse nervous system effects, which includes headache and dizziness.
	Inhibits anti-inflammatory analgesic and antipyretic effects.	Caution patient who is already taking anticoagulant, thrombolytic agent (*e.g.,* salicylates) to report any bleeding.
	May have a lesser effect in inhibiting renal prostaglandins and may be the preferred NSAID in patients at risk with renal toxicity.	Potentially interacts with phenytoin and oral antidiabetic agents by enhancing their effect.
		Caution patient about adverse GI effects such as dyspepsia, nausea, and diarrhea.

Tolmetin (Tolectin)	Pharmacologic effect is similar to other NSAIDs. Exhibits antipyretic, analgesic, and anti-inflammatory effects. Like other NSAIDs, has adverse renal, GI, and hemorrhagic effects.	Each 200 mg contains 0.8 meq of sodium; should consider for sodium and water retention with compromised cardiac function. Caution patient on reduction in mental alertness or physical coordination (e.g., do not drive a motor vehicle). Monitor patient for enhanced anticoagulation, antidiabetic effects when adding tolmetin to the regimen. Encourage patient to administer tolmetin with meals or food to minimize GI effect.
Hydrocortisone (Cortex fluid)	Hydrocortisone is metabolically transformed in the liver into tetrahydrocortisone before excretion. Signs of toxicity include: production of Cushing's disease manifested by moon face, striae, hirsutism, acne, osteoporosis, muscle wasting, sodium and water retention, potassium, calcium, and phosphorus loss. Uses: anti-inflammatory for rheumatoid arthritis.	Observe the symptoms of Cushing's disease. Teach patient to supplement diet with potassium-rich foods (e.g., banana). Check patient's muscles for weakness and wasting. Monitor for toxicity.
Prednisone	Prednisone is metabolically transformed in the liver. Causes sodium retention and potassium loss. Serious toxic signs from high doses include: edema, Cushing's disease, hypertension, susceptibility to infections from lack of restraint of inflammation and interference with immune mechanism, insomnia, and psychosis. Uses: anti-inflammatory for rheumatoid arthritis and osteoarthritis.	There is a tendency toward gradual weight gain secondary to edema. Muscle wasting and weakness occurs from hypokalemia and anorexia. Warn patient he or she may feel faint and should lie down if this occurs. Encourage patient to counteract depression. Monitor weight closely.
Cortisone Acetate	Adrenocorticosteroid that is naturally occurring in the body. Should be used with caution in presence of diabetes mellitus, hypertension, congestive heart failure, chronic nephritis, osteoporosis, convulsive disorders, infectious diseases, natural hormone production by the adrenal cortex. Uses: anti-inflammatory for rheumatoid arthritis and osteoarthritis.	Assist patient with general hygiene with scrupulous cleanliness to avoid infections. Monitor blood pressure at least twice daily until stabilized on medication dosage. Observe for and report effects resembling Cushing's disease. Advise patient to report any symptoms of gastric distress so that antacids, special diet, and x-rays may be ordered by the physician.

Nonnarcotic analgesics

| Acetaminophen (Tylenol; see | Acetaminophen is well-absorbed by mouth and excreted in the urine as conjugated acetaminophen. | Monitor patient for signs of toxicity: rash, edema, wheezing. |

(continued)

167

Table 8-1. (Continued)

Nonnarcotic analgesics

Drug	Effect/response in the elderly	Nursing implications
Chapter 14, Pain in Elderly Patients)	Most serious toxic reactions include: blood dyscrasias such as leukopenia, thrombocytopenia and pancytopenia. Effects can be developed by persons who have taken this drug for a number of years. A rare side-effect can be gastric irritation. Uses: analgesic to relieve mild to moderate pain; antipyretic.	Teach patient drug is to be discontinued and physician notified if patient has skin reactions, fever, sore throat, or ulcerated mucous membrane. Administer before or after meals with a glass of milk to minimize gastric irritation.
Propoxyphene (Darvon)	Propoxyphene is metabolized and excreted in the urine rapidly; partly conjugated in the liver and about 30% appears in the urine within 12 hours. Signs of toxicity: dizziness, nausea, vomiting, depressed respiration, or constricted pupils. Uses: analgesic to relieve mild to moderate pain.	Advise patient that the drug may impair performance of activities such as driving a car or operating machinery. Advise patient to lie down if dizziness, nausea, or vomiting occurs. Monitor patient for early signs of toxicity and depressed respirations.

Narcotic analgesics

Drug	Effect/response in the elderly	Nursing implications
Meperidine (Demerol)	Meperidine is a shorter-acting narcotic analgesic, rapidly metabolized in the liver. Dependency on the drug is possible. Signs of toxicity include: respiratory depression, dizziness, sweating, dry mouth, vomiting, weakness, drop in blood pressure. Uses: analgesia for severe pain.	Monitor patient for signs of toxicity. Assess blood pressure, pulse, and respirations often during use of drug. Check liquid input and output and for bladder distention because urinary retention may occur.

(Adapted from Brunner LS, Suddarth DS: The Lippincott Manual of Nursing Practice. Philadelphia, JB Lippincott, 1974; Cutting WC: Handbook of Pharmacology: The Actions and Uses of Drugs, 5th ed. Norwalk, Connecticut, Appleton-Century-Crofts, 1972; Loebl S, Spratto G, Wit A: The Nurse's Drug Handbook. New York, John Wiley & Sons, 1977)

Nursing care plans

Medical diagnosis: Rheumatoid arthritis

1. Nursing diagnosis: Self-care deficit related to inability to perform functional ADL

Goal

Patient will perform self-care activities within physical limitations and activity restrictions imposed by treatment.

Nursing interventions

1. Teach patient that the primary goal is to maintain function of all joints.
2. Discuss patient's usual ADL before onset of illness and actual or potential changes now anticipated.
3. Maintain mobility, pain control, and exercise program (Benison and Hogstel 1986).
4. Modify personal hygiene items: large grips on combs and brushes; raised toilet seat; safety bars in bathroom; special aids to assist in dressing. Assist patient to learn to use new or changed devices.
5. Assist significant others by giving instruction on modifying the environment and assisting the patient to be independent, (e.g., no scatter rugs, avoid clutter).
6. Allow patient sufficient time to complete tasks.
7. Provide for sexual counselling if necessary.
8. Arrange visiting nurse evaluation before discharge with follow-up later.
9. Arrange for consultation with and referral to other agencies as necessary.

2. Nursing diagnosis: Knowledge deficit of disease process, treatment, and risk factors related to lack of instruction

Goal

Patients and significant others will verbalize possible causes of disease, risk factors, treatment, and expected progression.

Nursing interventions

1. Discuss the disease, possible causes, necessity for treatment and longterm progression with the patient and significant others.
2. Discuss medication regimen prescribed as treatment program, possible side-effects, signs of toxicity, precautions while taking drugs.
3. Discuss activity restrictions and rationale for such actions.
4. Discuss diet recommendations and rationale.
5. Discuss possible complications during the disease process.
6. Emphasize importance for reporting to physician any signs of disease progression (*e.g.*, increasing stiffness or deformity of the affected areas) or possible exacerbation of disease process.
7. Encourage patient and significant others to raise questions of concern.
8. Use visual aids with large print and appropriate colors to aid learning.
9. Pace instructions to patient's speed of learning.

3. Nursing diagnosis: Alteration in self-concept related to deformities

Goal

Patient will verbalize increased confidence in ability to deal with illness, changes in lifestyle, and possible limitations.

Nursing interventions

1. Encourage verbalizations about fears of disease process.
2. Take time to sit down and talk with the patient.
3. Do not appear rushed or in a hurry during conversations.

continued

Nursing interventions

4. Deal with behavioral changes in the patient.
5. Discuss with the patient what behaviors are acceptable. Reinforce positive behavioral changes.
6. Be supportive but firm in dealing with patients and their behaviors (*e.g.*, self-care behaviors).
7. Give positive reinforcement for tasks accomplished.
8. Reinforce explanations of disease process, expectations, and limitations.
9. Discuss patient's perceptions of how significant others perceive limitations.
10. Maintain a therapeutic nurse and patient relationship.

Medical diagnosis: Osteoarthritis

4. Nursing diagnosis: Impaired physical mobility related to disease process

Goal

Patient will perform optimal functioning at acceptable level for patients.

Nursing interventions

1. Help patient protect joints from undue strains and trauma.
2. Keep joints and muscles warm with blankets as necessary.
3. Encourage patient to rest involved joints with splints, braces, and traction, as prescribed by physician.
4. Instruct patient in the use of assistive devices such as canes, crutches, and other mechanical aids.
5. Instruct the patient in correct posture and body mechanics.
6. Provide information about and encourage the use of range of motion and isometric exercises to maintain function of joints.
7. Discourage vigorous activity.
8. Assist the patient to make realistic plans for activity to allow for performance of optimum functioning at acceptable level for the patient.

5. Nursing diagnosis: Self-care deficit related to inability to perform functional ADL

Goal	*Nursing interventions*
Patient will perform self-care activities within physical limitations and activity restrictions imposed by treatment plan.	1. Discuss patient's usual ADL before onset of disease, potential changes the patient anticipates, or actual in which he or she presently experiences difficulty.
	2. Monitor stiffness of joints, especially in distal joints of fingers, knees, hip, vertebrae, and occasionally the ankles.
	3. Allow patient sufficient time to complete tasks.
	4. Maintain mobility, pain control, and exercise program (Benison and Hogstel 1986).
	5. Instruct patient on proper diet to maintain weight without increase to alleviate stress on weightbearing joints.
	6. Monitor range of motion for all joints to maintain optimum functioning.
	7. Assist patient to be as independent as possible.

6. Nursing diagnosis: Alterations in self-concept related to deformities

Goal	*Nursing interventions*
Patient will verbalize increased confidence in ability to deal with illness, changes in lifestyle, and possible limitations.	1. Establish therapeutic nurse and patient relationship.
	2. Refer to Nursing Care Plans, #3, in this chapter.

7. Clinical nursing problem: Activity intolerance: painful and limited knee and shoulder joint motion

Goal

Patient will be able to move all joints in extremities within normal range of motion.

Nursing interventions

1. Identify patient's concerns about activity intolerance and joint motion limitation.
2. Instruct patient on comfort measures for painful joint(s).
3. Protect joints from undue strains and trauma.
4. Maintain patient's functional capacity as much as possible.
5. Carefully perform range of motion with all muscle groups to maintain function and prevent atrophy.
6. Control pain through use of analgesics or other medications prescribed by physician.

8. Clinical nursing problem: Alteration in comfort: pain

Goal

Patient's levels will be maintained within zone acceptable to patient.

Nursing interventions

1. Apply heat to affected joints; try cold if heat is ineffective.
2. Encourage patient to use elasticized gloves for pain in hands or wrist during the night.
3. Provide patient with realistic assessment of the condition and alleviation of pain.
4. Refer to Chapter 14, Nursing Care Plans, #2 for further nursing interventions.

Medical diagnosis: *Osteoporosis*

9. Clinical nursing problem: Potential for injury: porous bones

Goal

Patient will be protected from injury.

Nursing interventions

1. Encourage a high-calcium diet (*e.g.*, milk products, cheese, and broccoli) to ensure 1500 mg daily.
2. Recommend multivitamin pills (for vitamin D).
3. Be aware that compression fractures of the vertebrae are complications of this disease process and the patient should be instructed not to attempt activities that will produce jarring motions (*e.g.*, as jumping or jogging).
4. Instruct patient to sleep with bedboard under mattress.
5. Encourage patient to keep physically active (*e.g.*, walking, swimming) to prevent disuse atrophy and further bone destruction.
6. Teach the patient to weigh himself or herself periodically (indicator of the stabilization of the disease).
7. Use bracing and other supportive devices to protect the joints as much as possible.
8. Instruct patient to remove all scatter rugs and other potentially hazardous environmental item (*e.g.*, no waxed floors).

Medical diagnosis: *Gout*

10. Clinical nursing problem: Alteration in comfort: pain related to inflammation of metatarsophalangeal joints

Goal

Patient's pain will be relieved or controlled.

Nursing interventions

1. Maintain bedrest for 24 hr after acute attack.
2. Place foot cradle over bed to remove pressure from toes.
3. Instruct patient to avoid high-purine foods in diet such as sardines, anchovies, and organ meats (*e.g.*, liver, kidneys).
4. Weigh patient weekly.

continued

Nursing interventions

5. Encourage loss of excess weight.
6. Encourage patient to drink large amounts of fluid.
7. Give medications with milk or meals.
8. If diarrhea occurs, instruct patient not to take colchicine.
9. Refer to Chapter 14, Nursing Care Plans, #1 for further nursing interventions.

Medical diagnosis: *Myasthenia gravis*

11. Clinical nursing problem: Activity intolerance: fatigue

Goal

Patient's fatigue will be reduced with proper rest and medication.

Nursing interventions

1. Be certain that the patient receives the anticholinesterase drugs according to a fixed schedule (exact time) to control symptoms (a delay may result in inability to swallow).
2. Give the drug with milk, crackers, or other buffering substance.
3. Be alert for side-effects of the medication—abdominal cramps, nausea, and vomiting.
4. Monitor closely for rapid development of myasthenic crisis—inability to swallow or to maintain a patent airway for respiratory exchange.
5. Give patient a tap bell to be used in an emergency situation.
6. Give neostigmine methylsulfate immediately if severe symptoms develop.
7. Support respirations when muscles of respiration and swallowing become severely involved.
   - Suction patient—aspiration is a common problem.
   - Prepare for tracheostomy.
   - Place patient on assisted mechanical ventilation.
   - Give appropriate antibiotics as indicated by physician.

continued

Nursing interventions

8. Determine the time of onset of symptoms in relation to the last dose—is patient undermedicated or having a mild cholinergic reaction?
9. Crisis may be precipitated by physical activity or emotional upset.
10. Allow patient to rest daily to avoid becoming too fatigued.
11. Begin light exercises after patient's medication is regulated.
12. Ensure proper diet and fluid intake.
13. Instruct patient to chew food well so that swallowing is less difficult.
14. Assist the patient with activities that foster independence.

12. Nursing diagnosis: Self-care deficit related to inability to perform functional ADL

Goal

Patient will perform self-care activities within physical limitations imposed by treatment plan.

Nursing interventions

1. Discuss patient's usual ADL before onset of disease and actual or potential changes in performance the patient anticipates or now experiences.
2. Modify personal hygiene habits to accommodate impairment of function.
3. Encourage patient to become independent in performing ADL.
4. Instruct patient to maintain muscle strength by an exercise plan daily.
5. Counsel the patient to express fears and anxieties about the illness.
6. Assist significant others by giving instructions about the disease.
7. Teach patient the importance of strict medication schedule.

Medical diagnosis: Fractures and falls

13. *Nursing diagnosis: Impaired mobility related to pain and edema of extremity*

Goal

Patient will be able to move all extremities within normal range of motion without pain or swelling.

Nursing interventions

1. Refer to Nursing Care Plans, #4, in this chapter.

14. *Nursing diagnosis: Anxiety related to fear of accidents*

Goal

Patient's anxiety and fear will be reduced.

Nursing interventions

1. Encourage patient to express the source of anxiety and fear.
2. Assess the environment for hazards (*e.g.,* scatter rugs, slippery houseshoes, clutter, poor lighting).
3. Remove all hazards so that pathways to various areas are clear.
4. Explain how bone fractures are repaired through use of surgery or casting.
5. Teach how ADL can be carried out while fracture is healing.
6. Perform actions to reduce pain such as elevating leg on chair, or arm with pillow beneath it.
7. Assist patient to gain confidence in walking so that fear of accident is reduced.
8. Encourage adequate lighting day and night to prevent falls when going from an area with adequate light to one with less light.

15. Nursing diagnosis: Social isolation related to immobility

Goal

Patient will have increased social contact with significant others.

Nursing interventions

1. Encourage patient to express feelings from own perspective about social isolation and its causes.
2. Establish a therapeutic nurse and patient relationship.
3. Assess the relationships that were important to patient before the fall and fracture.
4. Design a plan with the patient for social contacts within the clinical setting or home, with the patient assuming responsibility for the initial contacts.
5. Encourage patient to continue to confidently include friends in a regular social calendar during the period of immobility required for healing.

Medical diagnosis: Total hip replacement

16. Nursing diagnosis: Impaired mobility related to bedrest

Goal

Patient will achieve maximum physical mobility within limitations imposed by total hip replacement.

Nursing interventions

1. Explain to patient the use of the trapeze, pillows, and traction preoperatively.
2. Provide information about proper use of bedpan.
3. Instruct and practice exercises to be performed postoperatively: quadriceps and gluteal muscle setting, osmetrics, leg lifts, dorsiflexion, plantar flexion of the foot.
4. After surgery, instruct patient to remain on bed rest with bed flat, elevating the head no more than 45° for meals.
5. Encourage and assist patient in doing exercises as practiced preoperatively.
6. Turn patient on unoperated side, maintaining operated hip in abducted position supported by pillows.

continued

Nursing interventions

7. Encourage patient to use trapeze to lift body and change position frequently.
8. Instruct patient to avoid marked flexion of the hip.
9. Observe patient for increased pain and shortening of limb.
10. Massage skin on coccyx, heels, and elbows and observe for skin breakdown.
11. Maintain proper diet and fluid intake.
12. Monitor closely for any signs of bleeding postoperatively or signs of infection around surgical site.

17. Nursing diagnosis: Alteration in thought processes related to sensory deprivation and sensory overload

Goal

Patient will resume complete control over thought processes based on realistic perception of condition.

Nursing interventions

1. Encourage patient to verbalize about feelings and thoughts.
2. Monitor drug intake closely to detect if problem stems from overmedication.
3. Evaluate the patient's dietary and fluid intake to ensure adequate hydration and nutrients for mental alertness.
4. Note time of day or night when confusion occurs and document.
5. When possible, encourage patient to sit in chair or walk for sensory stimulation and increased oxygen intake.
6. Promote social contact with other patients in the clinical setting.
7. Encourage patient to listen to radio or television to obtain sensory stimulation and contact with reality.
8. Encourage social contact with relatives and friends on a regular basis.

(References for Nursing Care Plan Section: Brunner and Suddarth, 1974; Carnevali and Patrick, 1986; Doenges et al, 1986; Duesphol, 1986; Iyer et al, 1986; Ulrich et al, 1986; Williams, 1984.

References

Allen LH: Calcium and osteoporosis. Nutr Today 21:6–10, 1986

Anderson WF: Practical Management of the Elderly, 2nd ed. Oxford, Blackwell Scientific Publication, 1971

Barry PD: Psychosocial Nursing Assessment and Intervention. Philadelphia, JB Lippincott, 1984

Beland IL, Passos JY: Clinical Nursing: Pathophysiological and Psychosocial Approaches, 3rd ed. New York, Macmillan, 1975

Benison B, Hogstel MO: Aging and movement therapy. J Gerontol Nurs 12:16–18, 1986

Brunner LS, Suddarth DS: The Lippincott Manual of Nursing Practice. Philadelphia, JB Lippincott, 1974

Burnside IM: Nursing and the Aged. New York, McGraw-Hill, 1976

Carnevali DL, Patrick M: Nursing Management for the Elderly, 2nd ed. Philadelphia, JB Lippincott, 1986

Doenges ME, Jeffries MF, Moorhouse MF: Nursing Care Plans: Nursing Diagnoses in Planning Patient Care. Philadelphia, FA Davis, 1986

Duespohl TA: Nursing Diagnosis Manual for the Well and Ill Client. Philadelphia, WB Saunders, 1986

Dychwald K: Wellness and Health Promotion for the Elderly. Rockville, Maryland, Aspen Publication, 1986

Ebersole P, Hess P: Toward Healthy Aging: Human Needs and Nursing Response. St. Louis, CV Mosby, 1981

Ebersole P, Hess P: Toward Healthy Aging: Human Needs and Nursing Response, 2nd ed. St. Louis, CV Mosby, 1985

Gress LM, Bahr RT: The Aging Person: A Holistic Perspective. St. Louis, CV Mosby, 1984

Hall BA: Mental Health and the Elderly. Orlando, Florida, Grune & Stratton, 1984

Hogstel MO: Nursing Care of the Older Adult: In the Hospital, Nursing Home and Community. New York, John Wiley & Sons, 1981

Horwitz O, Magee JH: Index of Suspicion in Treatable Diseases. Philadelphia, Lea & Febiger, 1975

Iyer PW, Taptich BJ, Bernocchi-Losey D: Nursing Process and Nursing Diagnosis. New York, WB Saunders, 1986

Kart CS, Metress ES, Metress JF: Aging and Health: Biologic and Social Perspectives. Menlo Park, California, Addison-Wesley, 1978

Miller G: Osteoporosis: Is it inevitable? J Gerontol Nurs 11:10–15, 1985

Osteoporosis: The silent disease. Calcium Currents 1:1–2, 1986

Palmore E, Busse EW, Maddox G et al: Normal Aging, Part III. Durham, North Carolina, Duke University Press, 1985

Reichel W: Clinical Aspects of Aging. Baltimore, Williams & Wilkins, 1978

Sullivan RJ: When the get up and go has got up and went. J Am Geriatr Soc 34:323, 1986

Tinetti ME: Performance-oriented assessment of mobility problems in elderly patients. J Am Geriatr Soc 34:119–126, 1986

Uden G: Inpatient accidents in hospitals. J Am Geriatr Soc 33:833–841, 1985

Ulrich SP, Canale SW, Wendell SA: Nursing Care Planning Guides: A Nursing Diagnosis Approach. Philadelphia, WB Saunders, 1986

Venglarik JM, Adams M: Which client is a high risk? J Gerontol Nurs 11:28–30, 1985

Villaverde MM, Macmillan CW: Ailments of Aging: From Symptom to Treatment. New York, Van Nostrand Reinhold, 1980

Williams TF: Rehabilitation in the Aging. New York, Raven Press, 1984

Yurick AG, Spier BE, Robb SS, Ebert NJ: The Aged Person and the Nursing Process, 2nd ed. Norwalk, Connecticut, Appleton-Century-Croft, 1984

Grace Olmsted and Virginia Burggraf

Hematology and the immune system

9

Remarkably little age-related change has been reported for the blood and its components. Despite a decrease in cell mass, blood volume remains fairly stable until the eighth decade of life. Although anemia is common in the elderly, no specific anemia is characteristic of old age. When anemia is present, it is often a secondary symptom. Most immune functions, however, decline with age and this decline in the immunologic competence may herald the emergence of numerous disease entities. Cancer is the disease that is commonly thought of when discussing the failing immunologic system. The longer a person lives, the more likely it is that he or she will develop cancer (Gioiella and Bevil 1985). It is precisely the high mortality from cancer in the elderly that challenges nursing to develop strategies to educate the younger and middle-aged generations in prevention and warning signs, while being empathetic in caring for the terminally ill.

Age-related changes

With advancing age, there are small, subtle changes in the red blood cells. Survival time of red blood cells remains the same. Any delay in replacement after bleeding may be the result of iron depletion. Serum iron and iron-binding capacities, as well as iron absorption, are moderately decreased. Anemias, common in old age, often present as a symptom of something else (*e.g.,* a gastrointestinal dysfunction or beginning malignancy or leukemia). Normally the bone marrow replaces 1% of circulating erythrocytes, 10% of platelets, and three to four times the number of circulating blood granulocytes daily. The bone marrow also produces a large proportion of the circulating lymphocytes. When normal bone marrow is replaced by a tumor, bone marrow failure occurs. In elderly persons, prostate and breast cancers cause extensive marrow depletion.

Rossman (1979) describes a study of healthy nursing-home residents in whom hemoglobin and hematocrit values fell below the previously accepted norms. He concludes that this finding might be compatible with the general health in this population, but warns against being lulled into a false sense of security about the individual patient by this information. If a doctor or nurse anticipates finding major problems (*e.g.,* occult bleeding, malignancy), anemias associated with chronic disorders may be overlooked. Therefore, anemia and related disorders require the same assessment for the elderly patient that one would do for a younger one.

The recommended daily allowance (RDA) of iron for the elderly is about 10 mg/day, whereas the general population has an RDA for iron of 10 mg to 20 mg/day (Walsh 1983). If an elderly person consumes a normal diet, the iron content should be adequate. Researchers do not agree concerning the physiology of iron metabolism and absorption in the elderly (Marcus and Freedman 1985).

Normal events occurring in the gastrointestinal tract can contribute to the development of pernicious anemia. Pernicious anemia and chronic atrophic gastritis, causing an iron deficiency anemia, are often associated with the elderly population. With the diminished secretion of pepsin and hydrochloric acid, as well as a diminished production of intrinsic factor needed for B_{12} absorption, elderly patients are at significant risk. Atrophic gastritis has also been associated with a higher-than-normal risk of gastric carcinoma (Carnevali and Patrick 1986).

The changes occurring in the immune system with aging are so comprehensive and predictable that they have been termed an immunodeficiency state. These changes include defective cell-mediated (T cell) and antibody-mediated (B cell) responses. The B-lymphocytes develop in the bone marrow and are responsible for humoral antibody responses. B cells possess binding sites for foreign antigens. The B-lymphocyte cells leave the bone marrow and travel through the cardiovascular and lymphatic systems to lymphoid tissue. The lifespan of the B-lymphocyte is about 16 days. With aging, the number of B-lymphocytes remains stable (Gioiella and Bevel 1985). Once in the lymphoid tissue, the B-lymphocyte can be activated by antigens, causing them to differentiate further. The mature B-lymphocyte is called a *plasma cell* and manufactures antibodies or immunoglobulins. The B-lymphocytes' response to stimulation from certain antigens decreases markedly with aging (Gallucci and Rokosky 1986).

The T-lymphocyte cell precursors are also located in the bone marrow. The T-stem cells leave the bone marrow and migrate to the thymus. In the thymus the T cells mature and acquire molecules on the cell surface that identify them as T-lymphocytes. T-lymphocytes do not secrete antibody; they merely grasp it. They are believed to have three functions: effector, helper, and suppressor (Gioiella and Bevel 1985). The age-related involution of the thymus gland and its diminished function also suppresses the already-decreased lymphocytes.

The increased incidence of infections, both viral and bacterial, in elderly persons also has been explained on the basis of declining immunity. The increased risk of virus infections is attributable to the decrease in T-cell function. When infection of any type strikes an elderly person, erythropoietic activity is diminished and anemia can result (Rossman 1979). Signs and symptoms may be less pronounced (*e.g.,* symptoms of pain may be absent, fever may be absent or low-grade). It may be difficult to localize the patient's signs and symptoms to sites of infections.

Caution should be used when interpreting the significance of the immune changes of aging. It would be wrong to assume that the immune systems of all elderly persons undergo similar changes. Although aging is considered commonly as a degenerative process, not all age-related changes need have degenerative effects. Our nation's elderly are survivors—those who have successfully adapted to their internal and external environments. The professional must be skilled in assessment techniques, both physical and functional, to be able to contribute to the quality of life for all elderly patients.

Assessment parameters

History

When assessing the elderly for hematologic alterations, it is important that the nurse ask questions about nutrition, particularly dietary intake. If the patient appears undernourished, the nurse should ask if the patient lives alone, and how he or she prepares meals and shops for food. Questions that require only a "yes" or "no" response (*e.g.,* "Do you eat well?") are ineffective for gathering data because a patient may report eating well but may actually have a low level of hunger that leads to an inadequate dietary intake. Additionally, does "eating well" have the same meaning for nurse and patient? It is important to note if there has been any recent weight loss. Nutritional iron deficiency is a common problem. Elderly persons who live alone and have reduced incomes may subsist on tea and toast, which contain virtually no iron. Achlorhydria, seen in 30% to 40% of elderly persons, may be an additional factor contributing to a nutritional iron deficiency. Habits such as caffeine ingestion or smoking are also important to investigate for their negative effect on the altered gastrointestinal system. The patient with a longstanding anemia will be chronically fatigued, by dyspneic on exertion, and have sensitivity to cold. Note the physical presentation of the patient. Is he or she wearing a sweater? Does he or she ask for additional blankets on the bed? A blood dyscrasia in the elderly person presents the same symptoms as in a younger adult. Therefore, questions about recent bruising, bleeding tendencies, and observance of blood in the stool should be asked, and medication intake (particularly aspirin) should be assessed. Elderly persons may take it for granted that an infection that fails to heal is a normal situation of aging (Mezey et al 1980).

Of all the anemias distinctively associated with old age, pernicious anemia invariably is the first to come to mind. Although far outranked in frequency by iron-deficiency anemia, it deserves consideration when taking a hematologic history.

In contrast to an iron-deficiency state, pernicious anemia presents differently; on history, the nurse should ascertain from the person if there have been any neurologic disturbances (*e.g.*, loss of vibratory sense in the toes, numbness and tingling in fingers and toes). Because of the loss of the intrinsic factor necessary for vitamin B_{12} absorption, the integrity of the myelin sheaths is disrupted. This condition is a defined vitamin B_{12} deficiency disease, and can be corrected with intramuscular injection. It usually develops over a period of years, with the patient becoming increasingly debilitated before diagnosis (Rossman 1979).

Symptomatic anemias are yet another category of hematologic disorders. They are related directly to some other, underlying, disease process. Of these processes, cancer is the most feared, and this fear may cause the patient to delay seeking medical attention. When carcinoma of the colon and breast occur in elderly persons, they frequently produce metastases to the bone. The patient may complain of joint pain, similar to arthritis. It is important to ascertain when the pain began, how diffuse it is, and when it occurs. This information is important because polymyalgia also presents with pain and stiffness in the shoulders and hips, but is usually more aggravated at night. Polymyalgia is usually associated with giant-cell arteritis that occurs after a period of steroid treatment. When the steroids are withdrawn, the patient complains of rheumatismal-like pain.

Leukemias, lymphomas, and myelomas are caused by varied degrees of host resistances, as well as disruptions in the surveillance mechanism of the immune system. History-taking must include, in addition to the seven warning signs of cancer (see box, below), documentation of any painless areas of swelling, which may go unnoticed by the person and be first discovered by physical examination. In addition, asking about vaginal discharge is important because it is frequently taken for granted by postmenopausal women. Chronic lymphocytic leukemia takes years to develop and has a higher incidence in men over the age of 60 (Rossman 1979). It is difficult to develop a good clinical picture of these diseases without thorough examination and laboratory findings.

When elderly patients see their physicians, treatment is generally limited to the acute complaint, and may be palliative and temporary. Unfortunately, the complaint is frequently not investigated from the gerontologic perspective of an interdisciplinary team. The nurse in any facility is equipped to elicit a holistic

---

Cancer's seven warning signs

Change in bowel or bladder habits

A sore that does not heal

Unusual bleeding or discharge

Thickening or lump in breast or elsewhere

Indigestion or difficulty swallowing

Obvious change in wart or mole

Nagging cough or hoarseness

picture of the patient's condition and to work as a part of an interdisciplinary team to provide, if cure is not possible, answers and treatment that are acceptable to the patient. Disorders of the blood-forming organs and the immunologic system present as complex problems. Obtaining an accurate history takes time, effort, and commitment to the patient. Once the history is obtained, however, the picture becomes more focused as the physical assessment begins.

Physical assessment

The nurse should inspect for the common signs of anemia: pallor of the nail beds, conjunctiva, and buccal mucosa, and cracking around corners of the mouth. Inspection of an elderly patient's palms will give the nurse a better indication of the hemoglobin level (Mezey et al 1980). If the normal red lines can be seen in the folds of the palms when the hands are slightly stretched, anemia is unlikely.

Table 9-1 shows the hematologic values for the 60+ age group that have been determined by current research (1983–1984). Although these values are demonstrably valid, medical practitioners have shown hesitancy about changing their accustomed methods. It is common to feel comfortable working with the old values, which may not necessarily be the true ones for elderly patients. Some laboratory forms differentiate values for elderly persons. Therefore, it is wise to rely on other diagnostic criteria in addition to laboratory values (Carnevali and Patrick 1986).

Many of the immunodeficiency diseases, chronic lymphocyte leukemia, myeloma, lymphoma, arteritis polymyalgia, and malignancies affect on a multiplicity of other systems, which, because the presenting symptoms are nonspecific, make diagnosis difficult. Over 25% of elderly patients are asymptomatic, and that they have a disease is often discovered through a routine physical examination or blood test. A thorough evaluation of the musculoskeletal system, assessing bone pain and mobility, is necessary because lytic lesions can present as pathologic fractures. Because the pain associated with multiple myeloma in elderly patients is intermittent, it is easy to assume wrongly that it is the result of the arthritis

Table 9-1. *Hematologic values for the 60+ age group*

	Male	Female
Red blood cell	4.2–5.5	3.7–5.6
White blood cell	45 or 11,000	
Hemoglobin	15–17	13.8–15.6
Hematocrit	42.6–48	39.7–44.7

(Adapted from Carnevali D, Patrick M (eds): Nursing Management for the Elderly, 2nd ed, p 104. Philadelphia, JB Lippincott, 1986)

associated with old age (Cohen 1985). Renal disease can also be a manifestation of myeloma. Polymyalgia rheumatica first appears as asymmetrical pain in the shoulders, with stiffness that often mimicks arthritis; the only difference in symptoms is that night stiffness is more evident. The condition is also frequently related to giant cell arteritis (Rossman 1979).

Giant cell arteritis, also known as temporal arteritis, is an inflammatory disorder that affects the temporal and occipital arteries, with most cases appearing in Caucasians (both men and women). The disease is rarely seen in other races (Stromberg 1982). Since the disease involves the carotid and cranial arteries directly, headache pain is one of the presenting manifestations, occurring particularly in the temporal area. The patient may complain of dimness or loss of visual acuity with, if the arteritis is widespread, accompanying pains in the shoulders and hips. The temporal arteries are always tender, sometimes lose their pulsation, and occasionally stand out as thickened cords under the red, heated, overlying skin. On funduscopic examination, retinal hemorrhage is evident, with some degree of optic atrophy or thrombosis of the retinal artery in half of the patients (Rossman 1979). When palpating for areas of tenderness, the nurse should observe for swelling. It is critical that the nurse take care in communicating with the patient in order to avoid inadvertently alarming him or her. Always maintain a calm manner, and bear in mind that the patient probably has had considerable facial or eye pain for weeks and may have been going from physician to physician "shopping" for relief. A feeling of caring can be conveyed by allowing the patient sufficient time to talk and by the touch of a hand.

When assessing for possible cancer, the nurse should be aware that many cancers appear more frequently in older age groups; colon and rectal cancer rank among the three most-frequent kinds of cancer for persons over 55 years of age. Each patient should be weighed and particular attention paid to recent instances of weight loss, and changes in bowel habits. Over age 55, men experience nocturia, which can be a normal response to an enlarged prostate, heart failure, or insomnia. Because prostate cancer is common in this age group, it is extremely important to stress the need for yearly examinations. The same is true for pap smears and breast examinations for women. Some older women are so embarrassed by the procedure required for a pap smear that they are reluctant to have one made. In these cases, it may be helpful to suggest seeing a female gynecologist. The nurse should reinforce the need for this examination because a common fallacy is that once menopause has begun, these examinations are unnecessary.

The nurse who works in an outpatient department or in a hospital must remember that the patient who presents with insidious symptoms may be convinced he or she has a dreaded disease. An elderly patient may have delayed seeking care while settling his or her personal and financial situations in preparation for a serious, possibly fatal illness. Nurses need to be aware of this tendency, and of the patient's feelings of powerlessness, anxiety, and fear of impending death. Be an attentive listener, allay fear, and promote communication with patient and family.

The nurse must be aware of the complications of bleeding and infection, of the resulting anemias, and of diarrhea. It is imperative to examine for hemorrhage under the skin, gingival bleeding, and tarry stools, as well as decreased white blood cells. Any sudden changes in temperature or drop in blood pressure can precipitate tachycardia, heart failure, and respiratory complications.

Infection, one of the most serious complications of chemotherapy, further complicates an older person's life because of the required protective isolation. Nurses, although aware of the reasons for this type of isolation, often treat the patient as if he or she were contaminated. Explaining to the patient and family the rationale for this type of isolation and giving them support during this crisis may reduce psychological damage. The nurse should talk with the patient, observe for any signs of depression, and allow the patient to vent his or her feelings. Many patients wish to discuss their fears and anxieties and will do so if given a chance to talk.

Quality of life

In planning nursing care for the elderly patient with cancer, the nurse's major role is to assist in initiating strategies to maintain quality of life. This can be done by assisting the patient in accomplishing life tasks while balancing illness demands with coping resources.

In the past too little has been said about quality rather than quantity of life for patients who have cancer. Elderly patients with cancer, especially if debilitated by disease and compromised physiologically, tolerate aggressive radiation and chemotherapy poorly. Value judgments made by the health professionals who are caring for the elderly patient frequently influence decisions to treat or not to treat. The decision to treat or withhold treatment must be given careful consideration for all age groups. Both the patient's and family's wishes must be explored and understood. The potential for quality time after treatment must be assessed realistically and explained to the patient. The importance of informed consent has an added significance for health-care professionals caring for an elderly patient with cancer.

An excellent tool for assessing quality of life in elderly patients is the Spitzer Scale. This scale is simple to use: the higher the score, the better the quality of life. Based on five measurements (activity, daily living, health support and outlook), the scale is subjective and will allow the nurse to develop a care plan with realistic goals (Table 9-2). Tools such as this have a place in making determinations for patient care. Criteria obtained from them should be shared with the patient and family and goals for the patient should be communicated.

Drugs

A list of the drugs commonly used in the treatment of hematologic disease is found in Table 9-3.

Table 9-2. **Quality of life index**

Activity	Score
1. I work full-time (or nearly so) in my usual occupation, or study full-time (or nearly so), or manage my own household, or take part in as much unpaid or voluntary activity as I wish, whether retired or not.	2
2. I work or study in my usual occupation or manage my own household or participate in unpaid or voluntary activities, but I need a lot of help to do so or I work greatly reduced hours.	1
3. I do not work in any capacity nor do I study nor do I manage my own household.	0

Daily living

1. I am able to eat, wash, go to the toilet, and dress without assistance. I drive a car or use public transport without assistance.	2
2. I can travel and perform daily activities only with assistance (another person or special equipment) but can perform light tasks.	1
3. I am confined to my home or an institution and cannot manage personal care nor light tasks at all.	0

Health

1. I feel well most of the time.	2
2. I lack energy or only feel "up to par" some of the time.	1
3. I feel very ill or "lousy" most of the time.	0

Support

1. I have good relationships with others and receive support from *at least one* family member or friend.	2
2. The support I receive from family and friends is limited.	1
3. The support I receive from family and friends occurs infrequently or only when absolutely necessary.	0

Outlook

1. I am basically a calm person. I generally look forward to things and am able to make my own decisions about my life and surroundings.	2
2. I am sometimes troubled and there are times when I do not feel fully in control of my personal life. I am anxious and depressed at times.	1
3. I feel frightened and completely confused about things in general.	0

(Developed by Professor Walter O. Spitzer, MD, Chairman Department of Epidemiology and Biostatistics McGill University, Montreal, Canada. In Spitzer WO, Dobson AJ, Hall J et al: Measuring the quality of life of cancer patients. J Chron Dis 16:590, 1981)

Table 9-3. **Drugs used in treatment of hematologic diseases**

Malignant lymphoma*

Drug	Effect/response in the elderly	Nursing implications
Corticosteroid prednisone (Deltasone)	Fluid retention, GI ulceration, and bleeding. Mood changes. Osteoporosis. Hypertension. Hypokalemia immunosuppression. Increased or decreased appetite. Steroid-induced diabetes.	Premedicate with antiemetic. Assess vital signs every 4 hr. Check intake and output. Check weight and edema daily. Check for bleeding. Support during psychological stress. Protect bone from infection and fractures. Check for muscle weakness; may need antacids for heartburn.
MOPP Mechlorethamine Nitrogen mustard (Mustargen)	Bone marrow depression. Nausea and vomiting.	Premedicate with antiemetic. Nausea more severe during administration. Check urine and stools for blood. Increase fluids to 2000 cc daily. Patient may need wig. Avoid extravasation.
Vincristine (Oncovin)	Paralytic ileus. Bone marrow depression. Constipation. Headache. Paresthesias.	Premedicate with antiemetic. Assess for sensory loss and decreased peristalsis, give stool softener. Protect from infection. Avoid extravasation.
Procarbazine (Matulane)	Bone marrow depression. Nausea, vomiting. Skin reaction. Dizziness, headache, paresthesins, ataxia.	Assess for skin and neurologic changes. Premedicate with antiemetic. Instruct patient to avoid food for 2 hr after treatment; and to entirely avoid eating cheese and ripe bananas. Avoid rapid IV injection. Oral hygiene is important.

(continued)

Table 9-3. (*Continued*)

Malignant lymphoma*

Drug	Effect/response in the elderly	Nursing implications
Prednisone		Protect from infection. (Patrick et al 1986)
MVPP (Nitrogen mustard)		
Vinblastine (Velban)	Bone marrow depression. Nausea, vomiting. Stomatitis. Headache. Alopecia.	Premedicate with antiemetic. Check for bleeding and infection. Patient should use wig for hair loss. Assess for sensory loss and decreased peristalsis. Give stool softener or laxative. Encourage oral hygiene. Avoid extravasation.
COPP (Cytoxan)		Premedicate with antiemetic. Protect from infection. Patient may experience nausea. Check urine and stool for blood. Give fluids to 2000 cc daily. Patient may need wig. Check lab work. (Patrick 1986; Stahl 1985).

Chronic lymphocytic leukemia

Corticosteroid prednisone	Fluid retention, GI ulceration and bleeding, mood changes, osteoporosis, hypertension, hypocalemia. Increased or decreased appetite. Cushinoid appearance. Immunosuppression.	Assess vital signs every 4 hr. Check intake and output, weight and edema daily. Check for bleeding. Support during psychological stress, protect from bone fractures, watch for cardiac arrhythmias, dyspnea, or edema. Check for muscle weakness.

(*continued*)

Table 9-3. (Continued)

Chronic lymphocytic leukemia

Drug	Effect/response in the elderly	Nursing implications
Antineoplastic agents		
Chlorambucil (Leukeran)	Bleeding. Bladder irritation. Hair loss. Nausea and vomiting. Bone marrow depression.	Check urine and stools for blood. Increase fluid intake. Check labwork for marrow depression. Patient may need wig. In addition to the above, the patient needs 2–3 liters of fluid before administration.
Cyclophosphamide (Cytoxan)	See above.	See above.

Multiple myeloma

Drug	Effect/response in the elderly	Nursing implications
Antineoplastic agents Melphalan (Alkeran: L-PAM)	Bone marrow depression, nausea, and vomiting.	Premedicate with antiemetic as needed. Protect from infection. Check urine and stools for blood. Check labwork for marrow depression. Check intake and output.
Cyclophosphamide (Cytoxan)	Bone marrow depression. Nausea and vomiting. Bleeding.	See above.
Antibiotic adriamycin	Nausea and vomiting. Bone marrow depression. Decrease in platelets. Calcium elevation. Liver toxicity. Possible cardiac toxicity. Complete alopecia. Stomatitis and esophagitis.	Premedicate with antiemetic. Watch for bleeding, bruising, ulceration. Check liver function studies. Check intake and output. Do baseline cardiac studies. Limit total dose to 550 mg/m^2. Maintain oral hygiene. Avoid drug infiltration at injection site.

(continued)

Table 9-3. *(Continued)*

Giant cell arteritis and polymyalgia

Drug	Effect/response in the elderly	Nursing implications
Corticosteroid prednisone	Fluid retention. Steroid-induced diabetes, hypertension, impaired immune response. Mood changes. Osteoporosis. G.I. bleeding.	Assess vital signs every four hours; intake and output. Check weight and edema daily. Check for bleeding. Support for psychological stress, protect from bone fractures.

Hematology/immune system iron deficiency anemia

Oral iron

Ferrous sulfate	Gastric irritant dyspepsia, abdominal discomfort, nausea and diarrhea.	Administer orally following meals or a snack. Give with orange juice to promote absorption (McNally et al, 1985).
Ferrous gluconate	Staining of teeth. Change color of stools; constipation.	Dilute liquid iron preparation and administer through straw (Sheridan, 1984). Iron excreted in stools. Feces have tarry appearance.

Parenteral iron

Iron dextran	Darkening and discoloration around injection site. Headaches, hypotension, nausea, joint and muscle pains, and bronchospasm may occur. Allergic-like reactions occur occasionally.	Give IM injection properly. 1. One needle to withdraw iron dextran. 2. Change needles to administer. 3. Use Z tracking. 4. Inject "deep" into site— 2"-3" with 19 or 20-gauge needle. 5. Make certain needle is not in vein. 6. DO NOT massage site. 7. Encourage patient to ambulate.

(continued)

Table 9-3. (Continued)

Hematology/immune system iron deficiency anemia

Drug	Effect/response in the elderly	Nursing implications
		8. Observe for: pain at injection site, sterile abscess, fever, headache, urticaria.
		9. You may have to give a test dose for IV/IM Therapy.
		10. Monitor response to and effects from iron therapy (Patrick et al., 1986)

* Specific drug doses vary according to patient's physical status; the drug dose changes when used in combination, and drug protocols differ from one institution to another.

Nursing care plans

Medical diagnosis: Iron deficiency anemia

1. Nursing diagnosis: Knowledge deficit of disease, treatment, and risk factors related to lack of instruction

Goal

Patient will verbalize understanding of risk factors and the recommended therapy for iron deficiency anemia.

Nursing interventions

1. Discuss importance of maintaining normal hemoglobin levels as it relates to health (*e.g.,* describe the function that iron serves).
2. Discuss the relationship between nutrients and increased erythrocyte production.
3. Instruct patient in the maintenance of a diet high in iron.
4. Instruct patient in the signs and symptoms of early anemia: pallor, fatigue, shortness of breath, tachycardia on exertion.

continued

Nursing interventions

5. Outline signs and symptoms of anemia of rapid onset: weakness, heart palpitation, chest pain.
6. Emphasize importance of preventing infection.
7. Emphasize compliance with medication regimens.
8. Instruct patient to report promptly signs and symptoms of bleeding or infection, bruising, fever, malaise.

2. Nursing diagnosis: Activity intolerance related to fatigue or dyspnea

Goal

Patient will have sufficient energy to carry out ADL.

Nursing interventions

1. Provide a safe environment.
2. Assist patient with ambulation.
3. Estimate energy for activity levels needed for ADL and have patient prioritize activities.
4. Plan periods of rest and sleep.
5. Have patient do mild exercise for short periods.
6. Have patient shorten periods of work.
7. See Nursing Care Plans, #7, this chapter.

3. Nursing diagnosis: Alteration in oral mucous membrane related to glossitis and stomatitis

Goals

Patient will maintain adequate nutrition level of iron.
Patient will maintain a healthy oral cavity.
Patient will maintain normal mucous membrane, and will be able to eat comfortably.

Nursing interventions

1. Consult dietician to provide diet high in proteins, vitamins, iron, and food supplements.
2. Provide frequent small meals if patient cannot tolerate large meals.
3. Tell patient to avoid hot, spicy, and coarse foods to protect oral mucosa.
4. Feed patient if too weak to feed self.

continued

Nursing interventions

5. Administer oral care. Inspect mouth daily. Arrange for oral hygiene before and after meals, and before bedtime to prevent infection and promote comfort. Schedule frequent oral rinses. Lubricate lips with petroleum jelly to prevent cracking. Remove dentures if necessary between meals, cleanse, and replace.

6. Administer iron supplements as ordered by physician after meals or snack. Give orange juice with iron supplement. Have patient use straw when giving liquid iron supplement. Describe effects of iron supplement with tarry stools (Marcus and Freedman 1985).

7. Initiate dental consultation if needed.

8. Instruct patient to use soft toothbrush with nonabrasive toothpaste.

9. Have patient floss with unwaxed dental floss.

10. Assess oral cavity, and need for prophylactic use of oral antifungal or antibacterial agents. Request physician order if necessary.

11. Discourage smoking.

12. Teach rationale for oral hygiene regimen.

13. Discuss signs and symptoms of oral burning or pain, reddened areas in oral cavity, and open lesions on lips or in mouth (Marcus and Freedman 1985).

14. Provide appropriate fluid and nutritional intake. Instruct patient to avoid acidic fruit juices and spicy foods, extremes in food temperatures, and rough and crusty food. Encourage bland foods and fingerfoods high in proteins (Sheridan 1984).

15. Evaluate for infection (*i.e.*, painful clusters of vesicles or ulcerations, soft white patches [*Candida albicans*] or eruptions of dry, brownish-yellowish patches).

16. Evaluate patient's ability to chew and swallow.

continued

Nursing interventions

17. Do daily evaluations of patient's hydration status, checking turgor.
18. During each shift, monitor intake and output.

4. Nursing diagnosis: Potential for infection related to decreased resistance

Goal

Patient will be free of the risk of infection.

Nursing interventions

1. Monitor vital signs and report elevated temperature.
2. Implement measures to protect patient from infection, including the following: wash hands frequently; use aseptic techniques when performing patient-care activities and treatments; keep staff and visitors with infection away from patient; maintain environmental hygiene for patient; assist with total body and personal hygiene.
3. Report any signs or symptoms of infection to the physician immediately.
4. Teach patient to avoid crowds and people with active infections.
5. Implement measures to maintain skin integrity. See Nursing Care Plans, #7, this chapter.
6. Provide a nutritious diet.
7. Provide mouth care.
8. Promote rest.
9. Maintain ADL and physical safety. See Nursing Care Plans, #11, this chapter.

5. Nursing diagnosis: Potential impairment of skin integrity related to dry skin and hypothermia

Goal

Patient will have intact integument.

Nursing interventions

1. Inspect skin daily.
2. Avoid drying agents to the skin.
3. Lubricate skin with non-oily agents.
4. Protect skin from injury. Change patient's position frequently. Reinforce role of nutrition.
5. Maintain warm and clean environment. Use light, warm blankets. Provide warm, soft clothing such as exercise suits. Use nonrestrictive clothing.
6. Provide nail care.
7. Wash patient's hair and dry with warm towels.

Medical diagnosis: Chronic lymphocytic leukemia

6. Nursing diagnosis: Knowledge deficit of disease, treatment, prognosis related to lack of instruction

Goal

Patient will discuss factors relating to chronic lymphocytic leukemia and will verbalize an understanding of the nature of treatment.

Nursing interventions

1. Explain about and answer questions about diagnostic studies, (*e.g.,* bone marrow aspiration).
2. Instruct patient to observe self for chronic exhaustion, anorexia, and swollen lymph nodes.
3. Advise patient to avoid situations in which he or she is likely to contract infection (crowds and inclement weather).
4. Teach patient to observe and report signs and symptoms of infections: fever, sore throat, tenderness, redness, nonhealing wound.
5. Discuss with patient the need for seeing a physician regularly and keeping appointments.

continued

Nursing interventions

6. Instruct patient in signs and symptoms of early anemia: pallor, fatigue, shortness of breath.
7. Teach patient to maintain a well-balanced diet in protein, fiber, and fluids. Arrange for a dietary consultation if needed.
8. Instruct patient to maintain a clean body and a clean environment.
9. Teach patient to avoid smoking and oral stimulants.
10. Instruct the patient to drink large volumes of fluids especially urine-alkalizing juices.
11. Teach the patient to observe urine for change in color or amount.

7. Nursing diagnosis: Activity intolerance related to fatigue and weakness

Goal

Patient will be able to balance rest with periods of activity.

Nursing interventions

1. Instruct patient to avoid overexertion by maintaining a schedule of periods of activity and rest.
2. Assess sleep patterns (present and past) regarding arising time, bedtime, staying asleep, awakening, nap patterns. Determine if this is usual pattern or a new one that has developed.
3. Provide measures to assist with sleep (*e.g.,* quiet atmosphere, back rub, warm milk) if appropriate.
4. Assess ADL patterns at work and leisure, and assist in setting up a less-fatiguing schedule.
   - Minimize environmental activity. Schedule treatments and diagnostic procedures allowing for periods of uninterrupted rest.
   - Limit number of visitors if patient appears stressed by their presence.
   - Assist with self-care activities.
   - Keep personal objects in easy access to patient.

continued

Nursing interventions

5. Discuss activities patient desires to perform and cannot. Allow time for listening.
6. Assist patient to engage in diversional activities, checking with occupational therapist.
7. Encourage independence in ADL according to patient's current capabilities.

8. Clinical nursing problem: Alteration in oral mucous membrane: stomatitis related to poor nutrition or cytotoxic agents.

Goal

Patient will maintain a healthy oral cavity.

Nursing interventions

1. Observe for any changes in the mouth (*e.g.*, ulcerated areas).
2. Report changes to physician and obtain cultures.
3. Rinse patient's mouth with dilute solution of hydrogen peroxide or baking soda and water.
4. Inform patient to avoid alcohol, lemon-glycerin swabs, and commercial mouthwashes with alcohol, which will dry out the mouth.
5. Encourage use of oral saliva agents to ease dryness and lubricate mucous membranes.
6. Encourage fluid intake of 2500 cc/day unless contraindicated.
7. Encourage client to not smoke.
8. Instruct patient to avoid hot, spicy, or acidic foods.
9. Refer to Nursing Care Plans, #3, this chapter, for further suggestions.

9. Nursing Diagnosis: Alteration in nutrition (less than body requirements) related to anorexia, nausea, vomiting, stomatis.

Goals

Patient will initiate measures to ensure adequate nutritional status.

Patient or significant other will be informed about nutritional necessities for health.

Nursing Interventions

1. Discuss potential causes of nausea and vomiting.
2. Obtain a dietary consult to provide a balanced diet.
3. Monitor laboratory values: HCT, WBC, BUN, serum albumin.
4. Monitor calorie intake daily.
5. Monitor intake and output each shift.
6. Give small frequent feedings of soft, bland, cold snacks.
7. Pay particular attention to oral care.
8. Encourage patient to select diet.
9. Provide hard candy before meals to promote salivation.
10. Balance rest with exercise.
11. Instruct patient to avoid spices and greasy foods, or adding extra sweeteners to foods.
12. Encourage fluid intake.
13. Measure body weight weekly and document.
14. Administer antiemetic before meals.
15. Provide restful environment.
16. Encourage family to bring foods from home.
17. Instruct family to avoid coaxing, threatening, or bribing in relation to dietary intake (Marcus and Freedman 1985).

10. Nursing diagnosis: Alteration in sensory perception related to 8th cranial nerve damage from cytoloxic drugs.

Goal

Patient will be able to communicate appropriately with staff. Patient will report tinnitus if experienced.

Nursing interventions

1. Observe patient cues (*i.e.*, speaking loudly, wandering attention instead of listening, giving inappropriate responses).
2. Instruct patient to report any dizziness.
3. Facilitate communication (*e.g.*, provide light, reduce noise, use simple sentences, face client, and avoid use of an intercom).
4. Teach family measures to promote communication.

11. Nursing diagnosis: Potential for infection related to immunosuppression

Goal

Patient will not develop symptoms of infection.

Nursing interventions

1. Monitor baseline vital signs, reporting any changes, increased pulse, adventitious breath sounds.
2. Observe patient for restlessness, temperature, elevation, sore throat, sniffles, skin lesions, chills.
3. Check blood studies, CBC, WBC.
4. Observe for change in urine—color, output, odor. Instruct patient to keep perineal area clean.
5. Examine lymph nodes for enlargement and tenderness.
6. Encourage good nutritional intake of foods high in protein and fluids.
7. Wash hands frequently and consistently.
8. Teach patient and family good handwashing techniques.
9. Screen visitors with infections.
10. Encourage rest and limited activity.
11. Maintain warm, clean environment.
12. Use sterile supplies and aseptic technique.
13. Provide oral hygiene after meals and *prn.*

continued

Nursing interventions

14. Use sterile precautions for IV therapy and invasive procedures.
15. Provide good skin care and hygiene for patients on a daily basis.
16. Teach patient to observe signs and symptoms of infection by self when discharged.

12. Nursing diagnosis: Self-care deficit related to inability to perform ADL

Goals

Patient will verbalize knowledge of resources for assistance in the community to assist with ADL.
Patient will demonstrate the ability to perform the necessary self-care practices before discharge.

Nursing interventions

1. Teach maximum use of present self-care abilities.
2. Discuss cause and duration of potential disability (particularly short-term effects of radiation and chemotherapy).
3. Assess preferred patterns of self-care. What is it that the patient does best for himself or herself?
4. Discuss planned therapy and its duration.
5. Determine patient's understanding of disease, treatment, and potential loss of self-care by asking for feedback.
6. Assess availability and nature of support systems in community (*e.g.,* local chapter of American Cancer Society/Leukemia Society).
7. Evaluate effect of illness and potential self-deficits on: patient's self-concept, family function, perception of patient by family.
8. Explore environmental conditions and possible alternatives that will assist at home.

13. Nursing diagnosis: Potential for injury related to weakness from complications of treatment

Goal

Patient will not have accidental falls.

Nursing interventions

1. Observe patient for paresthesia, fatigue, and generalized weakness.
2. Assess environment for hazards (*i.e.,* clutter, scatter rugs, poor lighting, improperly fitting shoes).
3. Remove hazards from environment, instructing patient and family in necessary safety measures (*e.g.,* keeping needed items within reach, using ambulatory aids [canes, walker]).

Medical diagnosis: *Multiple myeloma*

14. Nursing diagnosis: Knowledge deficit of disease and treatment related to lack of instruction

Goal

Patient will verbalize understanding of disease process and recommended therapy.

Nursing interventions

1. Ascertain from the patient how much he or she knows about the disease, filling in with appropriate information.
2. Listen actively to pick up cues associated with fear and anxiety possibly from misinterpretation.
3. Discuss the plans for therapy.
4. Teach methods of pain control: pain-reducing measures and medications.
5. Explain the need for mobility with good body mechanics, balance, and use of mechanical support.
6. Encourage regular exercise, as tolerated.
7. Instruct patient about the medications used in pain control, and then side-effects.
8. Discuss chemotherapy treatment with effects on myeloma and the treatment's side-effects.
9. Discuss the need for a well-balanced diet,

continued

Nursing interventions

> encouraging foods that are high in calcium, protein, and vitamins.
> 10. Teach the patient the importance of adequate fluids (Habin 1983; Steffl 1984).

15. Nursing diagnosis: Alteration in mobility related to impaired physical condition and activity intolerance

Goal

Patient will maintain a level of activity within limitations of disease

Nursing interventions

1. Assess for factors impairing mobility (*e.g.*, chemotherapy treatment, radiation treatment, disease progression or metastasis to bone, lung, liver, brain) and consult with physician about course of action.
2. Determine activity level.
3. Observe gait, coordination, and stability.
4. Evaluate for tenderness or pain with movement.
5. Eliminate environmental barriers (*e.g.*, chairs, tables, rugs).
6. Explain problems related to immobility and possibility of muscle degeneration from disuse.
7. Arrange for consultation from physician for physical therapy for evaluation and baseline data.
8. Note problems and alteration in nutritional status (*e.g.*, any recent weight loss, food likes).
9. At each shift, assess skin, elimination, respiratory, and cardiac states.
10. Evaluate psychosocial status, noting any reactive depression (See Chapter 15, Nursing Care Plans, #1 and 2.)
11. Refer patient to social worker, therapist, or mental health nurse for counseling and long-range planning if appropriate.
12. Document care plan goals for progression toward maintaining maximum mobility (Steffl 1984).

16. Nursing diagnosis: Potential for injury related to impaired mobility secondary to pathologic fractures

Goal	Nursing interventions
Patient will not experience additional fractures.	1. Handle patient gently. 2. Change patient's position frequently and slowly. When patient is on bed rest, set up a schedule. 3. Maintain patient's body alignment. 4. Log-roll the patient. 5. Avoid jarring the bed. 6. Assess body alignment and complaints of pain every time position is changed. 7. Support patient's spine with brace, traction, or pillows at all times. 8. Assess motor function, sensation, and reflexes; report abnormalities to physician.

Medical diagnosis: *Giant cell arteritis*

17. Nursing diagnosis: Knowledge deficit of disease process and treatment related to lack of instruction

Goal	Nursing interventions
The patient will verbalize treatment regimen and signs and symptoms of disease.	1. Instruct patient about side-effects of steroid therapy (*e.g.*, hunger, euphoria) and encourage patient to discuss these with physician if distressed. 2. Teach patient the importance of compliance with therapy and that medication is not to be self-adjusted. 3. Teach patient to report headache pain. 4. Teach patient to report any visual disturbances immediately. 5. Teach patient the importance of compliance with laboratory tests for erythrocyte sedimentation rate.

Medical diagnosis: Polymyalgia

18. Nursing diagnosis: Knowledge deficit of disease, treatment, and risk factors related to lack of instruction

Goals

Patient will monitor self for complications. Patients will verbalize understanding of the disease process, risk factors and recommended therapy.

Nursing interventions

1. Teach patient the importance of and side-effects of prednisone therapy.
2. Explain that giant cell arteritis may be a complication.
3. Teach patient to monitor temporal scalp treatment plan, (*e.g.,* tenderness, headaches, and visual disturbances).
4. Encourage a program of balanced rest and activities.
5. Counsel patient that this disorder responds well to corticosteroid therapy.
6. See Nursing Care Plans, #17, this chapter.

19. Nursing diagnosis: Anxiety related to fear of disease progression

Goal

Patient will exhibit positive coping strategies.

Nursing interventions

1. Counsel patient that disorder responds well to corticosteroid therapy.
2. Use direct and open-ended questions in short, simple sentences.
3. Clarify and validate useful information as needed.
4. Describe signs and symptoms associated with disease process.
5. Support patient's search for information.
6. Use active listening skills.
7. Offer reassurance through touch, quiet physical presence.
8. Encourage ventilation of feelings and tensions.
9. Discuss anxiety. Mood swings, difficulty concentrating, anorexia, and insomnia are responses related to uncertainties of disease.

continued

Nursing Interventions

10. Instruct patient in stress-reduction techniques and guided imagery.
11. Draw on patient's motivation as a measure of active coping.
12. Assist patient to recognize stressors, events, and potential resolutions.
13. Reinforce positive self-care measures.
14. Note importance of hobbies and physical activities for a sense of accomplishment.

Medical diagnosis: Malignant lymphoma

20. Nursing diagnosis: Knowledge deficit of disease treatment and risk factors related to lack of instruction

Goal

Patient will relate knowledge of risk factors, disease, and treatment.

Nursing interventions

1. Instruct patient to observe for changes in activity level.
2. Teach patient to observe and feel lymph nodes in neck area and report any unusual swelling and tenderness.
3. Teach patient to observe for and report pain, any unusual pressures in abdomen, weight loss, and malaise.
4. Observe and report signs and symptoms of infection: fever, sore throat, tenderness, sweating.
5. Inspect the skin for any unusual lesions.
6. Discuss with patient how to maintain a well-balanced diet high in protein, fiber, and fluids.
7. Explain to patient the reasons for all tests and procedures.
8. Discuss with patient the side-effects of chemotherapy.
9. Provide psychological support to patient and family.

21. Nursing diagnosis: Potential for injury related to alteration in body temperature

Goal

Patient will maintain temperature within normal limits.

Nursing interventions

1. Monitor oral temperature level and pattern each shift.
2. Increase fluid intake as needed.
3. Encourage rest mixed with judicious activity.
4. Maintain room temperature appropriate to the patient's need.
5. Cover patient with light-weight blankets or clothing.
6. Bathe patient in cool water or alcohol sponge bath if febrile.
7. Apply cool, damp cloth to patient's face.
8. Observe increases in temperature, pulse, and respirations (McNally 1985).

Medical diagnosis: *Carcinoma of the larynx*

22. Nursing diagnosis: Anxiety related to fear of pain and mutilation

Goals

Patient will be able to verbalize fears about the laryngectomy.
Patient will be able to look at the stoma, and will begin to participate in self-care.

Nursing interventions

1. Encourage communication preoperatively, giving patient time to ventilate fears.
2. Listen attentively.
3. Plan for an alternative method of communication.
4. Arrange for visits pre- and postoperatively from laryngectomy associations.
5. Provide patient with a mirror to allow viewing of the stoma.
6. Gently encourage patient to participate by coughing secretion into a tissue and changing gauze pads as necessary.
7. Work together with social service department to plan now for discharge, including patient and family in all preparations.

23. Nursing diagnosis: Knowledge deficit of postoperative expectations and outcomes

Goal

Patient will discuss post-operative routines and demonstrate some of the anticipated postoperative self-care activities.

Nursing interventions

1. Provide information regarding specific expectations postoperatively regarding: purpose and care of tracheostomy tube, tube feedings, no smoking, humidifier and nebulizer.
2. Discuss postoperative phase.
3. Inform patient of self-care activities anticipated postoperatively; demonstrate oral hygiene techniques that will be used postoperatively, (*i.e.,* power spray, irrigations with saline or hydrogen peroxide and water).
4. Demonstrate exercise to prevent shoulder and neck dysfunction on the affected side.
5. Allow time for clarification, return demonstration, and questions.

24. Nursing diagnosis: Potential for ineffective airway clearance related to tracheal compression, excessive secretions and possible obstruction from tracheal tube

Goal

Patient will maintain a clear and patent airway.

Nursing interventions

1. Suction *prn* to remove pooled secretions.
2. Monitor respiratory function. Monitor VS q hour for the first 12–24 hr, then q 4 hr.
3. Liquify secretions by administering O_2 by nebulizer and placing humidifier in room.
4. Position to promote breathing. Turn q 2 hr and discourage coughing.
5. Assess thorax for adventitious sounds.
6. Provide oral care q 4 hr.
7. Have sterile extra tracheostomy tube at bedside.

25. Nursing diagnosis: Impaired verbal communication related to laryngectomy

Goals

Patient will initially learn alternative methods of communication with staff and family. Patient will be introduced to an esophageal or electronic verbal communication before discharge.

Nursing interventions

1. Establish a system of communication before surgery (*e.g.,* pad, magic slate, chart, flashcards).
2. Keep call button in easy reach at all times.
3. Alert staff to the created system to promote continuity and diminish frustrations.
4. Establish social source referral to obtain communication device.
5. Demonstrate use of the device before discharge.

26. Nursing diagnosis: Ineffective individual coping related to depending on others, loss of ability to cry audibly

Goal

Patient will demonstrate elective coping through use of available support systems.

Nursing interventions

1. Monitor patient for ineffective coping (*i.e.,* uncooperative, sleeping disturbances, increased pain, and discomfort).
2. Sit, after care and comfort measures have been performed, and speak quietly to your patient about the future, the role or roles available, and of your understanding
3. Assist patient to identify support systems and community resources, securing social worker intervention.
4. If needed, ask physician for a psychiatric consultation if the wish of patient is to arrange for spiritual support.

References

Aiken LH, Gortner SR: Nursing in the 1980's: Crises, Opportunities and Challenges. Philadelphia, JB Lippincott, 1983

Billings JA: Outpatient Management of Advanced Cancer. Philadelphia, JB Lippincott, 1985

Calloway NO: The Basic Laws of Biological Senenscense. J Amer Geriatr Soc 17:638, 1969

Carnevali D, Patrick M: Nursing Management for the Elderly. Philadelphia, JB Lippincott, 1986

Cohen HJ: Multiple myeloma in the elderly. In Freedman ML (ed): Clinics in Geriatric Medicine, pp 827–855. Philadelphia, WB Saunders, 1985

Eisek MT: The Adult Leukemia Patient in the Intensive Care Unit. Heart and Lung 13:183–192, 1984

Finkelstein MS: Aging immunocytes and immunity. In Freedman ML (ed): Clinics in Geriatric Medicine, pp 899–911. Philadelphia, WB Saunders, 1985

Freedman ML (ed): Clinics in Geriatric Medicine. Philadelphia, WB Saunders, 1985

Gallucci BB, Rokosky JS: Immune response. In Patrick ML, Woods SL, Craven RF et al (eds): Medical-Surgical Nursing: Pathophysiological Concepts, p 186. Philadelphia, JB Lippincott, 1986

Gioiella EC, Bevil CW: Nursing Care of the Aging Client: Promoting Healthy Adaptation. Norwalk, Connecticut, Appleton-Century-Crofts, 1985

Gluckman RA, Eposito AL: Fever of unknown origin in the elderly: Diagnosis and treatment. Geriatrics 41:45–52, 1986

Habin BH: Arthritis, connective tissue disorder and extracellular rheumatism. In Steinberg FU (ed): Care of the Geriatric Patient. St. Louis, CV Mosby, 1983

Luckman J, Sorensen KC: Medical–Surgical Nursing: A Psychosocial Approach, 2nd ed. Philadelphia, WB Saunders, 1980

Marcus DL, Freedman ML: Clinical disorders of iron metabolism in the elderly. In Freedman ML (ed): Clinics in Geriatric Medicine, pp 729–745. Philadelphia, WB Saunders, 1985

McIntire S, Ciappa A: Cancer Nursing: A Development Approach. New York, J Wiley and Sons, 1976

McNally JC, Stair JC, Somerville ET: Guidelines for Cancer Nursing Practice. New York, Grune and Stratton, 1985

Mezey M, Rauckhorst LH, Stoker SA et al: Health Assessment of the Older Individual. New York, Springer Publishing, 1980

Patrick ML, Woods SL, Craven RF, et al: Medical–Surgical Nursing: Pathophysiological Concepts. Philadelphia, JB Lippincott, 1986

Rossman I: Clinical Geriatrics, 2nd ed. Philadelphia, JB Lippincott, 1979

Schoulen J: Important Factors in the Examination and Care of Old Patients. J Am Geriatr Soc 23:180–183, 1975

Sheridan ES: Drugs in the elderly. In Steffl BM (ed): Handbook of Gerontological Nursing. New York, Van Nostrand Reinhold, 1984

Spitzer WO, Dobson AJ, Hall J et al: Measuring the quality of life of cancer patients. J Chron Dis 16:585–597, 1981

Stahl RL, Silber R: Chronic lymphocytic leukemia. In Freedman ML (ed): Clinics in Geriatric Medicine, pp 857–867. Philadelphia, WB Saunders, 1985

Steffl BM: Handbook of Gerontological Nursing. New York, Van Nostrand Reinhold, 1984

Steinberg FU (ed): Care of the Geriatric Patient, 6th ed. St. Louis, CV Mosby, 1983

Stromberg MF: Early detection of cancer in the elderly: Problems and solutions. Int J Nurs Stud 19:3, 139–152, 1982

Thompson JM, McFarland GK, Hirsch JE, et al: Clinical Nursing. St. Louis, CV Mosby, 1986

Tyan ML: Marrow stem cell during development and aging. In Makinodan T (ed): CRC Handbook of Immunology in Aging. Boca Raton, Florida, CRC Press, 1981

Walsh JR: Hematological disorders of the elderly. In Steinberg FU (ed): Care of the Geriatric Patient, pp 182–198. St. Louis, CV Mosby, 1983

Wexsler ME: The senescence of the immune system. Hosp Pract 16:53–64, 1981

Wobin EM: Cancer in the geriatric patient. In Steinberg FU (ed): Care of the Geriatric Patient, pp 74–91. St. Louis, CV Mosby, 1983

Ulrich S, Canale S, Wendell S: Nursing Care Planning Guides. Philadelphia, WB Saunders, 1986

Yurick AG, Spier BE, Robb SS, Ebert SS: The Aged Person and the Nursing Process. Norwalk, Connecticut, Appleton-Century-Crofts, 1984

Suggested readings

Baranovsky A, Myers MM: Cancer incidence and survival in patients 65 years of age and older. Can J Clin 36:27–31, 1986

Samel J, Hunt WC, Key C: Choice of cancer therapy varies with age of patient. JAMA 255:3385–3390, 1986

Snyder RE: Detection of breast cancer in the elderly woman. In Yancik R, Carbone RR, Peterson WB (eds): Perspectives on Prevention and Treatment of Cancer in the Elderly, p 467. New York, Raven Press, 1983

Stromberg M: Early detection of cancer in the elderly: Problems and solutions. Int J Nurs Stud 16:139–156, 1982

Sherlock P, Winawer S: Cancer and diagnosis of colorectal cancer in older persons. In Yancik R, Carbone RR, Peterson WB et al (eds): Perspective in Prevention and Treatment of Cancer in the Elderly, pp 113–120. New York, Raven Press, 1983

Serpick AA: Cancer in the elderly. Hosp Prac 13:101–112, 1978

Adrianne Linton

Gastrointestinal system *10*

Although much has been written on the physical changes of aging, comparatively little material is available concerning age-related changes of the gastrointestinal tract. Brocklehurst (1985) attributes this situation to the fact that gastrointestinal problems may be worrisome but are rarely a direct cause of death. For many practitioners, mention of the aged gastrointestinal tract conjures images of constipation, laxative abuse, and bowel fixations. Even though the frequency of actual dysfunction is under debate, nurses find that their elderly patients often express digestive and elimination concerns. When such complaints are presented, the health-care worker must assess each situation on an individual basis. Knowledge of normal versus pathological changes is essential, as well as the ability to determine what constitutes "normal" for each elderly patient.

Age-related changes

Oral cavity

The changes that occur in the oral cavity can have significant impact on the elderly person's general well-being. The most obvious change in the mouth is loss of teeth. More than 50% of all Americans aged 65 and older are edentulous (Ebersole 1981). Storer (1985) notes that the two main causes of the loss of natural teeth are caries and periodontal disease. Even in the absence of periodontal disease, the teeth are mechanically worn down so that their height is reduced. Secondary dentin, a hard fibrotic material, gradually replaces the normal dental pulp. The teeth may become somewhat transparent or darker.

Gingival tissues recede, exposing the cement-covered roots of the teeth. The vascularity and elasticity of gum tissues decline. New layers of cement are deposited in the apical region, which elongates the root and helps to maintain the stability of the teeth (Storer 1985). The recession of gingival tissues permits the accumulation of debris, plaque, and calculus on and between the teeth. This process can result in an inflammatory condition, *periodontal disease,* and is characterized by progressive destruction of the periodontal ligament and resorption of surrounding alveolar bone. As a result, there is a loss of support and the affected teeth become more mobile (Fig. 10-1). When one tooth is lost, those nearby experience a reduction in support; and there can be a domino effect, with additional subsequent tooth losses. Factors other than plaque that contribute to the development of periodontal disease include overhanging margins on restorations, food impaction, unilateral mastication, mouth breathing, decreased saliva, and trauma. Periodontal disease increases in frequency and severity with age. When it occurs, decisions must be made regarding the advisability of extraction. Storer (1985) notes that moderately mobile teeth in the elderly respond well to periodontal management and occlusal adjustment so that extraction may be delayed for up to several years. The removal of plaque and calculus is the most important single measure to reduce periodontitis (Kamen 1983).

The advantages of healthy, natural teeth to the elderly are readily apparent to anyone who works with this patient population. Appearance, communication, and nutrition are enhanced by a healthy mouth and teeth. Nevertheless, nurses often find that elderly patients wear only one plate or none at all. Many of these patients report that their plates no longer fit properly, and slip or rub the gums painfully. This maladjustment of the fit occurs over years as the edentulous gums shrink and change shape. Nursing personnel need to assess problems that occur with dentures and arrange for modifications to be made. At the other end of the spectrum are those patients who continue to wear dentures that do not fit properly and thus constantly irritate oral tissues. This is a bad practice because these fragile tissues are susceptible to the development of malignant lesions and need to be protected and inspected on a routine basis.

The tastebud receptors may decrease in number with age, resulting in a loss of ability to discriminate between flavors. This change, compounded with diminished olfactory sensitivity and reduced saliva production, may contribute to a lack

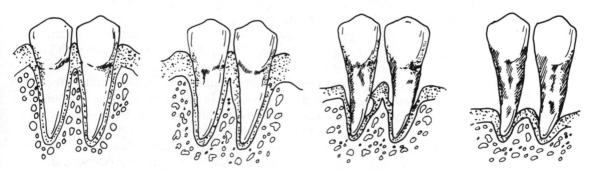

Figure 10-1. Periodontal disease: progressive gum recession and destruction of alveolar bone.

of enjoyment of food, resulting in the development of poor eating habits. Many menopausal women report abnormal taste and burning sensations in the tongue, a phenomenon that may be caused by hormonal factors or vitamin deficiencies (Ebersole 1981).

It is generally thought that, with aging, saliva decreases in volume and acidity. The resulting decrease in ptyalin theoretically affects the initial breakdown of starches, but this change has not been shown to have detrimental effects on food digestion. Baum (1985) has questioned the generalization that saliva production decreases significantly and cites research to support his contention that dry mouth is not a normal part of aging. Regardless of the origin of the complaint, it is not unusual for the elderly person to report discomfort related to dryness of the mouth. Changes in salivary flow among the elderly often have their origin with medication administration, particularly antidepressants, anticholinergics and antihypertensives. Dry mouth (*xerostomia*) can be burdensome to the patient. Some simple interventions such as sugar-free gum or lozenges, artificial saliva, oral hygiene, and maintenance of adequate hydration can relieve the feeling, as well as prevent development of caries (Ofstehage and Magilvy 1986).

A common myth is that tooth loss is normal with aging; however, lack of dental care or follow-up care can cause severe caries that often go untreated. Visits to the dentist become a low priority in situations of chronic health problems, loss of income, and lack of insurance. Normal age-related changes are attrition; the wearing away of a tooth as the result of tooth-to-tooth contact, as in chewing; abrasion from friction over the years; and erosion or the loss of dental tissue from chemical processes.

Esophagus

The walls of the esophagus in the elderly person become thinner and more sensitive as the secretion rate of protective mucin decreases (Forbes 1981). Dilation of the lower esophagus with abnormal contractions and alterations in the pressure of the lower esophageal sphincter may lead to feelings of fullness, dysphagia, and even substernal pain (Heitkemper and Bartol 1986).

Hiatal hernia develops in 40% to 60% of people over 60 years of age. Reflux flow of gastric juices into the esophagus is common and is thought to be a contributing factor in the development of the hernia (Almy 1985a). Although most hiatal hernias are asymptomatic, they may produce varying degrees of heartburn, dysphagia, belching, and pain (Knudsen 1984). The pain that occurs with esophageal reflux resembles, and must be differentiated from, angina. It is helpful to remember that anginal pain usually occurs during exertion and is often accompanied by changes in pulse and blood pressure. Esophageal pain, on the other hand, is usually associated with eating and recumbency and is not associated with changes in vital signs (Heitkemper and Bartol 1986).

Factors that may contribute to the occurrence of hiatal hernia include weakness of the diaphragmatic muscles around the esophagogastric opening, advanced age, and activities and conditions that increase intra-abdominal pressure.

Conservative management usually consists of antacid treatment of heartburn and measures to reduce intra-abdominal pressure. Other drug therapy might include bethanecol chloride to increase gastroesophageal sphincter pressure, and alginic acid with sodium bicarbonate, which forms a protective coating against gastric secretions (Elrod 1983). For severe esophagitis with ulceration, Dymock (1985) notes that cimetidine or ranitidine with metoclopramide can be prescribed. Additional information about drugs used for hiatal hernias is provided in Table 10-1.

The primary dietary alterations recommended are the scheduling of smaller, more frequent meals, and the restriction of some foods. Substances that decrease sphincter tone such as caffeine, nicotine, fats, and chocolate should be avoided. Gradual dilatation of the esophagus is sometimes indicated after esophagitis has subsided. Mild irradiation of the gastric fundus is also used to decrease acid output from the stomach in patients who are poor surgical risks (Berman 1983).

If conservative management fails to control symptoms or the patient develops stenosis, chronic esophagitis, or bleeding, surgical interventions may be necessary. Fundoplication is the procedure used to reinforce the esophagogastric sphincter. Either the abdominal or thoracic approach may be used. A risk of respiratory complications with either approach requires frequent assessment and measures to encourage full lung expansion. Postoperatively the patient will be restricted to intravenous fluids until peristalsis returns. Then the diet is progressed from liquids to small feedings (Elrod 1983).

Stomach

Changes in the stomach include thinning of the gastric mucosa and decreased secretion of acids and digestive enzymes. Generally these alterations are not severe enough to significantly impair the digestive processes. There is also a decrease in motor activity, which accounts for reduced hunger contractions and delayed gastric emptying. Heitkemper and Bartol (1986) make the point that because age-related changes in the stomach are so minor, any gastric complaint should be thoroughly investigated to rule out pathology.

Diseases of the stomach associated with aging include chronic atrophic gastritis, ulcers, gastric malignancies, and pernicious anemia.

Pernicious anemia

When the production of intrinsic factor by the gastric parietal cells ceases, the absorption of vitamin B_{12} also ceases. Without vitamin B_{12} the production of red blood cells is impaired, resulting in large, oval, fragile cells. These abnormal cells have a lifespan of only several weeks (Porth 1986). This condition is known as *pernicious anemia* and is most often seen in the elderly. Because of the loss of parietal cells it always occurs after total gastrectomy or resection of the ileum, but may also occur in persons who do not have this history. Various theories have

Text continues on p 223

Table 10-1. Gastrointestinal drugs

Antacid

General nursing implications

1. Antacids are used to treat ulcers and heartburn because of their ability to neutralize gastric acid.
2. Even though antacids are nonprescription drugs, they do have side-effects and can be abused.
3. Patients with impaired renal function are especially susceptible to the effects of accumulated calcium, aluminum, and magnesium.
4. In general, calcium and aluminum salts tend to be constipating and magnesium salts tend to cause diarrhea. Combinations are often used to counteract these effects (Rodman 1985).
5. Antacid tablets should be chewed before swallowing.
6. Liquid antacids must be followed with enough water to transport the medication to the stomach.
7. Antacids can interfere with the absorption of many other drugs; the patient who has been prescribed other medications should not use antacids without discussing it with his or her physician (Clark et al 1986)

Drugs	Effect/response in the elderly	Nursing implications
Aluminum Hydroxide Gel (Amphogel)	Large daily doses are needed for acid neutralizing. Prevents phosphate absorption, which causes bone demineralization. Elevates blood and urine calcium, increasing risk of renal stones. Aluminum accumulation is possible at high doses, which can produce neurotoxicity and encephalopathy (Rodman 1985)	Encourage 2000 ml/day fluid intake unless contraindicated. Monitor urine output, stools for constipation. Alert to neurological changes such as dementia. Do not give with tetracycline or anticholinergics because it interferes with their absorption (Rodman 1985).
Calcium Carbonate (Tums)	Causes rebound hypersecretion of acid 1–2 hr after intake. Some calcium is absorbed, making it an inexpensive calcium source. In the presence of renal impairment, hypercalcemia could occur. Excessive use may cause alkalosis. It can also cause constipation (Rodman 1985).	Caution patients with renal impairment against self-medication with Tums. Monitor for signs and symptoms of alkalosis—anorexia, nausea and vomiting, muscle pain, irritability, and headache (Rodman 1985). Teach patients that drug is safe for occasional use but should not be used long term. Monitor for signs and symptoms of hypercalcemia: anorexia, lethargy, confusion, depressed reflexes, increased urine (Adams and Lewis 1983).
Magnesium hydroxide (Milk of Magnesia)	In small doses, is used as antacid; larger doses have laxative effect. Dosage required for acute ulcer patient may cause diarrhea.	Monitor for diarrhea. Monitor renal-impaired patient for excess magnesium: lethargy, drowsiness, central nervous system depression (Rodman 1985) Give laxative dose at bedtime.

		Use with caution in the patient with renal impairment because magnesium excess may occur (Rodman 1985) Laxative effect takes 6–8 hr.
Aluminum and magnesium compounds (Aludrox, Maalox)	These compounds are intended to neutralize the diarrhea/constipation effect of aluminum or magnesium given alone.	Monitor for signs and symptoms of aluminum and magnesium excess in the patient who has renal impairment.
Sodium bicarbonate (Baking soda)	Has excellent acid neutralizing effect but action is brief and systemic absorption does occur. This can lead to fluid retention and alkalosis if used frequently, in large amounts, or in the presence of renal impairment. On ingestion, carbon dioxide is released, causing belching and abdominal distention, which could be dangerous if there is potential for perforation (Rodman 1985).	Monitor for signs and symptoms of alkalosis if used in large amounts or over long time. Monitor patient for fluid retention: edema, decreased urine, dyspnea, and increased blood pressure. Monitor for alkalosis: anorexia, nausea and vomiting, irritability. Teach patient that this cooking ingredient is a drug and can be harmful if abused.

Histamine (H₂) receptor antagonist

Drugs	Effect/response in the elderly	Nursing implications
Cimetidine (Tagamet)	Acts by reducing gastric acid secretion. Side-effects of mild diarrhea, dizziness, rash, or headache usually diminish over time. Confusion has occurred in the elderly, as well as slurred speech, delirium, and hallucinations (Berman and Kirsner 1983). Cimetidine reduces metabolism of warfarin, phenytoin, beta adrenergic receptor blockers, lidocaine, and theophylline. It prolongs the halflife of diazepam and increases the effect of morphine. High intravenous bolus doses have caused bradycardia and hypotension (Rodman 1985). This could be especially dangerous for the elderly patient with poor cardiovascular adaptability.	Recent studies have shown that one 800-mg dose at bedtime is as equally effective as multiple doses throughout the day (Tagamet Once A Day 1986). If the patient's dosage schedule is changed to this routine, be able to explain the reason. If dizziness occurs in the elderly patient, take measures to ensure safety. When given intravenously, dilute in 100-ml diluent and administer at a rate of 1 mg to 4 mg/kg/hr (Hahn 1982).

continued

Table 10-1. (Continued)

Histamine (H₂) receptor antagonist

Drugs	Effect/response in the elderly	Nursing implications
Ranitidine (Zantac)	Reduces gastric acid secretion. More potent than cimetidine, and may have fewer side-effects. Adverse effects include headache, malaise, and nausea. Serum enzyme elevations suggest that hepatotoxicity may occur (Rodman 1985). Some cases of persistent headaches have required discontinuing the drug (Nurses Drug Alert 1986). Reduced dosages should be used with renal impairment.	Inform patient that side-effects usually diminish over time, but notify physician if effects persist or are severe.

Antidiarrheals

Drugs	Effect/response in the elderly	Nursing implications
Kaolin mixture with pectin (Kaopectate)	Absorbs irritants and protects the intestinal mucosa. It is relatively safe for the elderly patient, but if used too often might endanger nutritional status by absorbing nutrients and enzymes, as well as irritants (Bergerson 1979).	Discourage chronic use. Chronic diarrhea requires evaluation and specific treatment. The relatively large dosage (45–90 ml) needed for effective treatment may make it unappealing to the elderly patient (Hahn 1982).
Diphenoxylate HCl and atropine (Lomotil)	Acts by decreasing intestinal motility. Useful for chronic functional and inflammatory intestinal conditions. Does not cause dependency if taken in the recommended dosages. There is some disagreement about the use of antiperistaltic drugs for acute diarrhea; critics claim it delays the elimination of irritants from the intestine. Occasional drowsiness and constipation occur at normal doses. It should not be used in patients with liver disease (Rodman 1985).	Monitor continuing need for this drug; take only as long as needed. Record and describe all stools. If drug therapy is not recommended for a diarrhea episode, explain the reason to the patient. If drowsiness occurs, take measures to assure patient safety. Advise patient not to drive until drug effect has been determined.

Laxatives, cathartics, and fecal softeners

General nursing implications

1. Laxatives are used appropriately for temporary treatment of constipation and emptying the gastrointestinal tract for diagnostic procedures.
2. Laxatives are contraindicated with undiagnosed abdominal pain or acute appendicitis, enteritis, diverticulitis, and ulcerative colitis (Rodman 1985).
3. Habitual use can result in physical and psychological dependence.
4. The type used depends on the situation: cathartics act in 6–8 hr, most suppositories within an hour.
5. Repeated use can produce diarrhea with resulting alterations in fluid balance.
6. The hospitalized elderly patient may have a temporary need for laxative therapy as a result of changes in medications, environment, and activity level.
7. Recognize that long-standing laxative dependence in elderly patients may not be correctable.

Drugs	Effect/response in the elderly	Nursing implications
Bisacodyl (Dulcolax)	Can be administered orally or rectally to stimulate colon peristalsis. Frequent rectal administration can cause a mild proctitis. Suppositories should not be used with anal fissures or ulcerated hemorrhoids (Rodman 1985).	Do not give the oral form within 1 hr of milk or antacid ingestion (Clarke et al 1986).
Cascara sagrada extract	One of the mildest cathartics; not for rapid, complete evacuation. A soft stool is usually produced within 6–8 hr. Recommended for bedridden and cardiac patients (Rodman 1985)	Bedtime administration usually provides morning bowel movement. Explain to patient that the drug does not produce immediate results. Inform patient that urine may turn red or brown (Rodman 1985).
Docusate sodium (Colace) Docusate calcium (Surfak)	Relieves constipation by softening the fecal mass. It may be several days before effects can be seen. Docusate facilitates the passage of mineral oil through the intestinal mucosa (Rodman 1985).	This drug must be used regularly to get desired results. Do not administer with mineral oil. Explain drug action to patient so he or she does not expect immediate results. Take other measures to relieve existing constipation.

continued

Table 10-1. *(Continued)*

Laxatives, cathartics, and fecal softeners

Drugs	Effect/response in the elderly	Nursing implications
Hydrophilic colloids (Metamucil)	One of the most natural and least irritating of all laxatives. A natural substance that absorbs fluids to produce a gelatinous mass to facilitate the passage of soft stool. The powder form is mixed in water or juice and will "set" if not consumed quickly (Rodman 1985).	Patients receiving this type of laxative must consume adequate fluids to prevent hardening of the mass and subsequent obstruction (Rodman 1985).

Cholinergic

Drugs	Effect/response in the elderly	Nursing implications
Bethanechol (Urecholine)	Used to reduce gastric reflux with hiatal hernia. As a smooth muscle stimulant, it is contraindicated with asthma, COPD, bladder-neck obstruction, coronary artery disease, severe bradycardia, hypotension or hypertension, and Parkinsonism. Causes detrusor muscle of bladder to contract, and urinary urgency. Antagonized by procainamide and quinidine. Enhanced by other cholinergic drugs.	Monitor voiding. Assess for toxicity: salivation, sweating, flushing, nausea, abdominal cramps. Have atropine sulfate as antidote. Give on empty stomach to prevent nausea and vomiting (Govoni and Hayes 1978).

proposed genetic and autoimmune explanations for the lack of intrinsic factor production (Jennings 1983).

The onset usually takes several months. Fatigue, palpitations, irritability, and exertional dyspnea are common symptoms, related to tissue hypoxia. Manifestations involving the gastric mucosa include sore tongue, anorexia, nausea and vomiting, and abdominal pain. The tongue may have a glazed, smooth appearance. Neurological effects may also develop such as paresthesias of the feet and hands, reduced vibratory and position senses, and impaired thought processes. Unfortunately, many of these signs and symptoms may be attributed to the aging process and thus neglected until they have become severe. Without treatment, patients with pernicious anemia die within one to three years (Jennings 1983).

The only successful treatment at this time is the administration of regular vitamin B_{12} injections. This therapy corrects the faulty production of red blood cells, but may be less successful in reversing neurological deficits (Shank 1985). For this reason, early detection and treatment is especially important. It is critical that the patient understand the need for lifelong therapy in the management of this condition. It must also be stressed that oral vitamin B_{12} cannot be absorbed and therefore cannot be substituted for the injections.

Small intestine

The small intestine undergoes some structural changes with age but these are not thought to cause significant impairment of digestive processes in most people. Some sources claim that absorption of calcium and B vitamins is diminished in the elderly. Others believe that nutritional inadequacies are more likely the result of pathology of the gastrointestinal tract or poor diet rather than the aging process. Although inflammatory conditions are generally associated with young adults, they do occur in elderly persons and may be very debilitating (Heitkemper and Bartol 1986).

Large intestine

The age-related changes in the large intestine are similar to those in other body structures: atrophy of the muscle layer and the mucosa, decreased tone of intestinal smooth muscle, increased connective tissue, and arteriolar sclerosis (Brocklehurst 1985; Jessup 1984; Resnik 1985). The significant findings from numerous studies on the large intestines of elderly people are as follows:

- Elderly people tolerate a higher volume of rectal distention without discomfort.
- The incidence of diverticula increases with age.
- The elderly person may be less able to distinguish between feces, fluid, and flatus in the rectum, a factor that might contribute to incontinence.

- Bowel patterns of people over 60 are basically the same as those of younger people, but 30% of those over 60 who were surveyed used a laxative more than once a week (Brocklehurst 1985).

Despite these identified changes, Jessup (1984, 201) states, "there is no good evidence of major changes in the motor or secretory activity of the colon or rectum." In other words, age-related structural changes alone do not cause significant changes in the function of the large intestine. Why then do people believe that constipation and aging are almost synonymous? One obvious reason is that elderly people often complain of constipation. When the current elderly population were young, it was commonly believed that a daily bowel movement was essential to good health. Periodic laxatives were taken to rid the body of *toxic* substances. Considering this orientation, it is not so surprising that an elderly person may report constipation if he or she goes a day or two without a bowel movement. Since frequent use of laxatives and enemas through the years impairs spontaneous, natural bowel movements, many may have constipation related to laxative abuse. Also, health-care providers most often encounter the ill elderly person who often has multiple risk factors for constipation. Such risks include hypothyroidism, drug use, depression, decreased mobility, diet low in fiber, and poor fluid intake. Complications, which are most common in debilitated and bedridden patients, include fecal impaction, necrosis of the colon wall, anal ulcers, anal mucosa prolapse, internal and external hemorrhoids, varices in the legs, pulmonary embolism, and volvulus of the colon (Almy 1985b).

The usual management of constipation in the elderly patient stresses dietary fiber, adequate fluids, and regular exercise. Changes in fiber or fluid intake or activity level must be instituted slowly. The addition of large amounts of natural fiber or bulk may be impractical if the patient has chewing or swallowing difficulties. Raw fruits or vegetables served to the edentulous patient are usually wasted. Fruit juices, coarse grain cereals, stewed fruit, and bran muffins might be more acceptable. Bran has proved to be very effective in increasing bulk in the gastrointestinal tract. Recommended amounts vary considerably. Because the sudden addition of bran to the diet sometimes produces nausea and distention, it should be increased gradually. Try adding one teaspoonful to a semisolid food at each meal. This amount can be gradually increased until regular elimination is established. Bran is a very light, powdery substance that cannot be consumed without being mixed in some medium (Almy 1985b).

The elderly person's diminished cardiac reserve makes him or her less able to adapt to sudden increases in blood volume. Therefore increasing fluid intake requires that the nurse consider the patient's cardiac and renal status and monitor for fluid excess as fluid intake is increased. When these measures cannot be instituted or are unsuccessful, it may be necessary to use stool softeners, laxatives, suppositories, or enemas to induce bowel evacuation. Beside teaching the elderly patient healthy measures to promote elimination, the hazards of frequent laxative or enema use should be described. If the patient has used mild laxatives or stool softeners without problems for a prolonged period, however, the nurse must question the wisdom of trying to discontinue the medications. The benefits may exceed the risks in such cases. The actions and nursing implications of specific laxatives, cathartics, and stool softeners are outlined in Table 10-1.

Also, the patient with idiopathic megacolon will generally require frequent and regular enemas to achieve bowel evacuation. This condition is characterized by a chronic grossly distended tympanitic abdomen and chronic constipation that does not respond to conservative management (Brocklehurst 1985).

Because bowel elimination is patterned, patients should be advised to select a regular time for bowel elimination and adhere to that schedule closely. This routine can be established even with the confused patient if he or she consistently is taken to the toilet at the same time each day. Physiologically, the best time is within one hour after breakfast. Advise the patient to always heed the defecation reflex as promptly as possible. Other considerations in trying to control constipation include provision for privacy and management of actual or anticipated pain.

Despite conservative measures, fecal impactions develop in some patients. The immobilized or cognitively impaired elderly patient must be monitored closely to detect the presence of impactions. Impaction should be suspected if the patient complains of an inability to pass stool despite feelings of pressure in the rectum, or the occurrence of watery diarrhea in the patient who has not had a normal bowel movement for several days. A digital examination of the rectum will often reveal a firm mass of feces, although sometimes it will be located too high to be palpated. If fecal impaction is confirmed, measures should be taken promptly to remove it. Many long-term-care facilities have protocols for removal of the mass. In other agencies, policies may necessitate obtaining specific orders from the physician. Almy (1985a) suggests the following process: instill into the rectum 150 ml of mineral oil or 5 ml dioctyl sodium sulfosuccinate 1% solution diluted in 100 ml of water; follow this with a hypertonic phosphate enema. If necessary, gently break up and remove the impacted stool. Severe impactions may require that this process be repeated over several days.

Diverticular disease is especially common among the elderly. Diverticuli are sac-like herniations of mucous membranes through the muscularis layer (Fig. 10-2) that are usually multiple and most often found in the sigmoid colon (Porth 1986). Because the occurrence is generally confined to people in developed countries, lack of dietary residue is suspected as a major contributing factor. Brocklehurst (1985) cites studies from 1937 when data from 700 autopsies revealed diverticuli in 17% of white men, 15% of white women, 2% of black men, and 3% of black women. Studies conducted in 1967 found frequencies between 42% and 47%. Porth (1986) reports 1978 figures that diverticular disease was present in about 50% of all people over 60 years of age. Nondietary factors that are thought to contribute to the development of diverticuli include constipation, obesity, and emotional tension (Knudsen 1984). Although most people with diverticuli are asymptomatic (Porth 1986), symptoms often include a change in bowel habits. Constipation occurred in about 35%, diarrhea in 19%, and alternating diarrhea and constipation in 9% of diverticular patients studied by Parks (cited in Brockle-

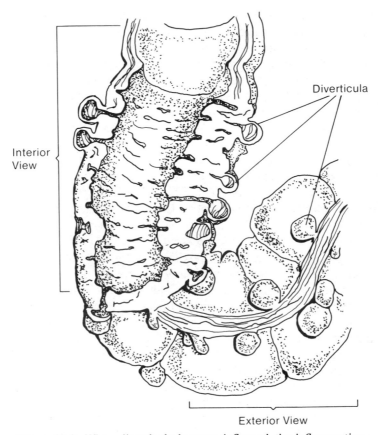

Diverticula

Interior View

Exterior View

Figure 10-2. When diverticula become inflamed, the inflammation may spread to other areas.

hurst 1985). Various patients also experienced rectal bleeding, abdominal pain, flatulence and heartburn, nausea and vomiting, and urinary problems. Pain in the left lower quadrant often occurs after meals and is usually relieved by having a bowel movement (Knudsen 1984). Inflammation may be precipitated by irritating foods, alcohol, straining at defecation, and coughing. The recognition of diverticulitis in the elderly patient may be difficult because it is more likely to manifest less-dramatic fever, leukocytosis, or pain than in a younger patient (Almy 1985b).

Potential complications include perforation with peritonitis, severe bleeding, obstruction, abscess formation, and fistula formation to the bladder or vagina (Brocklehurst 1985; Porth 1986; and Knudsen 1984). Some bleeding occurs in 10% to 25% of all diverticular patients, but severe bleeding develops in only 3% to 5% (Almy 1985b). Current management consists of a high-residue, nonspicy diet, and control of constipation without harsh laxatives. For acute pain, meperidine is the analgesic of choice. Opiates are contraindicated because they increase sigmoid intra-luminal pressure (Almy 1985b). Some experimental studies have reported that pain relief of 24-hour to 48-hour duration has been obtained with the intravenous injection of glucagon (Almy 1985b).

Surgical treatment may be necessary if complications occur. With medical treatment, 43% of patients studied had persistent or recurrent symptoms compared with 33% of those patients who were treated surgically (Brocklehurst 1985). The decision to intervene surgically may be influenced by the fact that the fatality rate for emergency surgery is 15% to 25%, whereas elective surgery carries only a 2% to 3% risk (Smith 1983).

Diarrhea receives less attention than constipation in the geriatric literature, presumably because it is less common, tends to be self-limiting, and is usually marked by complete recovery. To the frail elderly person, however, diarrhea may pose a serious threat. Baillie and Stoltis (1985) cite several studies documenting the increasing incidence of ulcerative colitis and Crohn's disease in the population over 60 years of age.

Diarrhea is characterized by the passage of frequent watery stools. It may be caused by many factors including foods, low serum albumin, diverticulosis, infection, malabsorption, neoplasms, zinc deficiency, diabetic neuropathy, chronic stress, and fecal impaction (White 1983; Anderson 1986). Drugs that may cause diarrhea include antibiotics, antiarrhythmics, aminophylline, digitalis, and potassium supplements. Severe diarrhea may result in fluid and electrolyte imbalance (hypovolemia, hyponatremia, hypokalemia), loss of nutrients, and anal excoriation. Assessment of fluid balance includes monitoring intake and output, vital signs, mental status, neuromuscular function, and tissue turgor. Since the loss of subcutaneous tissue of the extremities makes the forearm a poor place to assess turgor, it is better to check for tenting over the scapula, the abdomen, or the bridge of the nose. In the elderly patient, diarrhea that is especially severe or persists more than 24 hours warrants medical intervention.

Treatment is directed toward resting the gastrointestinal tract by serving only clear liquids or withholding oral feedings while providing intravenous fluids. Generally, antibiotics are not used. A variety of antidiarrheal drugs may be ordered but the use of drugs that decrease intestinal motility is somewhat controversial. Some experts believe that diarrhea represents an attempt to rid the the body of an irritating substance and that drugs that decrease peristalsis simply prolong infectious diarrhea by keeping the irritants in the system longer (Smith 1983). Some antidiarrheal drugs are described in the gastrointestinal drug table (Table 10-1).

Because elderly patients are often taking one or more medications routinely, the possibility of drug-induced diarrhea must be considered. This form of diarrhea is usually mild and is generally not accompanied by abdominal pain or cramps (Heitkemper and Bartol 1986). Food poisoning is not an uncommon cause of diarrhea in the elderly, who may not store or cook food safely.

The management of diarrhea encompasses efforts to determine the cause, measures to prevent dehydration and electrolyte imbalances, skin-care measures, and emotional support for the elderly patient who may have difficulty controlling unpredictable episodes of diarrhea.

Because intestinal complaints are relatively common among the elderly, health-care workers may not take them seriously. The need to investigate intestinal symptoms, especially change in bowel habits, is emphasized by the fact that colorectal cancer is the most common visceral cancer in elderly Americans. Most deaths from colorectal cancer are in people who are 50 to 75 years old. It may be reassuring to patients who are experiencing suspicious changes in bowel function to know that with early treatment the 15-year survival rate is 95% (Messner and Gardner 1985).

In summary, the age-related changes in the gastrointestinal tract do not generally pose threats to survival. However, the impact that dysfunction can have on the quality of life of the elderly person cannot be denied. The nurse plays a significant role in preventing, detecting, and managing gastrointestinal problems to enhance the health and well-being of the elderly patient.

Assessment parameters

A thorough assessment of gastrointestinal function includes data obtained through the nursing history and the physical examination findings. Ideally, the health-history interview should be conducted in an unhurried private setting. A full description of the chief complaint should be elicited. When the complaint is concerned with upper or lower gastrointestinal function, relevant past medical history includes information about all known illnesses and any current treatment regimens. A number of drugs such as antacids, laxatives, diuretics, anticholinergics, and antidepressants can significantly alter gastrointestinal function. A family history of ulcers, gastrointestinal malignancies, or pernicious anemia may be significant in the diagnostic process. The personal and social history provide information about the patient's daily habits. Activity level, diet, fluid intake, stressors, or recent travels may give clues as to the cause of the patient's problems. Any signs or symptoms of gastrointestinal dysfunction need to be fully described.

The basic format for the physical examination of the elderly patient is essentially the same as for any adult, although it is more important to allow adequate time because they may respond more slowly to numerous requests. Also, because elderly people tend to chill easily, adequate draping and environmental warmth must be provided. The examiner needs to be sensitive to the potential for discomfort when a thin, elderly patient is placed on a hard examination table for a prolonged time.

Assessment of the gastrointestinal system includes physical examination of the mouth, abdomen, and anus. As part of the head and neck examination, the nurse assesses the patient's oral cavity (Fig. 10-3). The lips should be inspected for color, lesions, and crusts. Loss of elasticity and blurring of the vermilion borders of the lips are typical in the elderly person (Fig. 10-4). The edentulous patient who is not wearing dentures will have a typical sunken appearance of the lips and cheeks. The number, location, and condition of the teeth are noted. Because of the changes that have been described, the teeth often appear somewhat

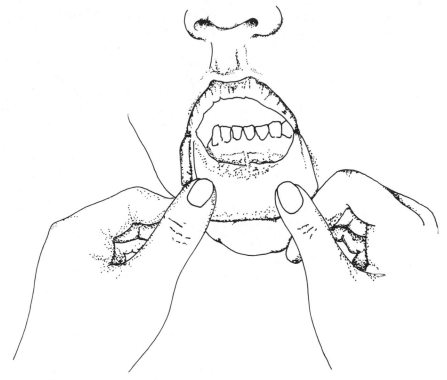

Figure 10-3. Assessment of the oral cavity.

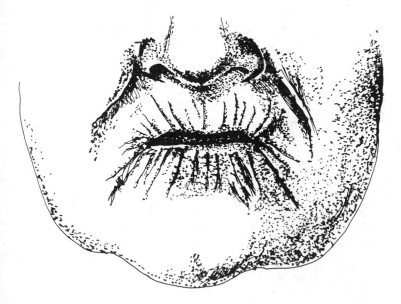

Figure 10-4. "Purse string" appearance of the lips of the elderly person.

transparent and elongated. The chewing surfaces will show varying degrees of wear (attrition) (Fig. 10-5). Exposed dentin on these surfaces may appear yellowish or dark and is usually somewhat depressed. The oral membranes tend to be pale, with the gums becoming waxlike and glossy in appearance. The oral cavity may look drier than does that of a younger person (Gioiella and Bevil 1985). Figure 10-6 shows various oral conditions that may be observed. If the patient wears dentures, they should be removed in order to inspect the gums and palate for irritations or lesions. The dentures and partial plates should be inspected for defects and calculus deposition (Fig. 10-7).

The tongue should be inspected for symmetry and lesions. Atrophy of papillae at the lateral edges is commonly observed in the elderly patient (Spollett 1984). Progressive defoliation of the papillae will give a smoother appearance of the dorsal surface (Kamen 1983). Varicosities on the ventral surface of the tongue and the floor of the mouth may appear as small grapelike clusters and are not cause for concern. Because oral malignancies are more common in the elderly population, the examiner should be especially alert for ulcers or nodules on the base or edge of the tongue. When taste sensation is evaluated, the elderly person often has difficulty differentiating flavors unless stronger-than-usual solutions are used.

For the abdominal examination some elderly persons will not be able to tolerate the supine position and will prefer a semi-Fowler's position. After draping for privacy and warmth, begin by inspecting the abdominal skin for scars, venous patterns, lesions, and striae (Potter and Perry 1985). The shape of the elderly person's abdomen is often protuberant as a result of weight gain and loss of muscle tone. Weight usually declines in men after age 55. Women tend to gain weight up to the fifth decade and do not experience significant weight loss until the mid-seventies (Gioiella and Bevil 1985). The thinning of the abdominal musculature may permit easier visualization of peristalsis (Spollett 1984). The umbilicus should be inspected for position, color, shape, masses, or discharge. Findings should not differ from those in a younger person.

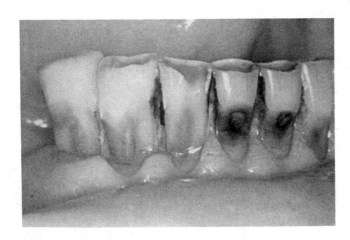

Figure 10-5. Aging dentition. The illustration shows attrition of chewing surfaces, abrasion of lateral surfaces, gingival recession, and cervical caries.

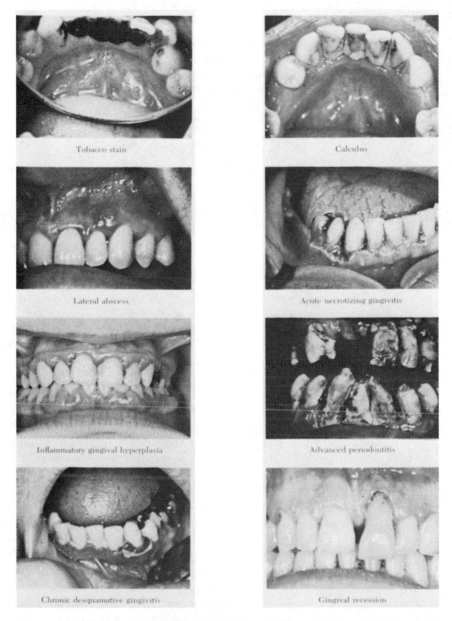

Figure 10-6. *Oral conditions. (Shafer WG, Hine MK, Levy BM: Oral Pathology, 4th ed. Philadelphia, WB Saunders, 1983)*

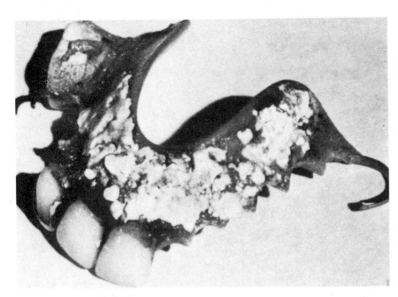

Figure 10-7. Calculus deposited on ill-fitting removable partial denture. (Shafer WG, Hine MK, Levy BM: Oral Pathology, 4th ed. Philadelphia, WB Saunders, 1983)

All four quadrants of the abdomen should be auscultated using the diaphragm of the stethoscope for bowel sounds and the bell for vascular sounds. It may be necessary to listen for as long as five minutes before deciding that bowel sounds are absent (Potter and Perry 1985). Spollett (1984) reports that with decreased esophageal motility, a "popping" sound may be heard in the stomach area.

Percussion enables the examiner to locate organs and masses in the abdomen. Dull sounds are heard over solid organs, whereas air-filled structures elicit tympany. In the elderly patient with kyphosis or emphysema, the liver may be displaced downward, making it detectable below the rib cage margin (Gioiella and Bevit 1985). Otherwise, findings in the elderly patient should be similar to those in a younger adult.

The final step of the abdominal examination is palpation for tenderness and abnormalities. Light palpation provides information about muscle tone and may detect masses or painful areas. Typically, the abdomen of the elderly person feels soft because of loss of muscle tone. While it is easier to palpate some abdominal organs, the kidneys are usually more difficult to feel because they diminish in size with age. It is important to be aware that the elderly person has diminished abdominal sensitivity to pain and may not demonstrate abdominal rigidity in the presence of peritoneal irritation (Jessup 1984). Deep palpation should not be done in the presence of tenderness, incisions, or masses (Potter and Perry 1985). When masses are palpated in the elderly patient, the examiner needs to assess the likelihood that he or she is palpating a full bladder, a constipated colon, or an aortic aneurysm (Gioiella and Bevil 1985). The anal and rectal examinations can be done with the patient in a side-lying position. On inspection, hemorrhoids are commonly found in the elderly patient. When the patient is asked to bear down, decreased sphincter tone and relaxed perineal musculature may be evident (Spollett 1984).

Nursing care plans

Medical diagnosis: Constipation

1. Clinical nursing problem: Alteration in bowel elimination: constipation

Goal	Nursing interventions
Patient will have normal bowel elimination as evidenced by passage of formed stools at regular intervals without cramping, pain, or straining.	*1.* Assess • Usual pattern of bowel elimination • Current pattern (any changes) • Aids to elimination: type and frequency of use • Diet, especially fiber and bulk intake • Activity level: usual, current • Fluid intake • Drug therapy • Characteristics of stools: amount, frequency, color, abnormal constituents. *2.* Note signs and symptoms of constipation • Infrequent passage of dry stool • Anorexia • Bloating • Belching • Flatus • Headache • Weakness • Faintness *3.* Assess indications of fecal impaction • Inability to defecate • Rectal pressure sensation • Watery diarrhea • Firm rectal mass

continued

Nursing interventions

4. Remove fecal impaction according to protocol or physician's orders.
5. If fecal impaction is not present but patient is constipated, consult with the physician or check standing orders to determine the best treatment.
6. When laxatives or suppositories have been administered, alert staff to respond quickly to patient's call for help with toileting.
7. Once immediate bowel elimination needs have been met, institute measures to reduce frequency of constipation.
8. Determine patient's perception of normal bowel elimination.
9. Emphasize that it is not necessary to have a daily bowel movement and that normal, healthy people range from three stools a day to three stools a week.
10. Force fluids, 2000–3000 ml/day, if not contraindicated by renal or cardiovascular impairment. If patient's fluid intake has been poor, gradually increase and monitor for increased pulse and blood pressure, edema, and weight gain.
11. Discourage use of fluid with diuretic effects (coffee, tea).
12. Discuss with patient and dietician the need for increased bulk and fiber in the diet.
13. Add bran to semisolid foods, one teaspoon with each meal. Gradually increase until softer, regular stools occur.
14. If bran is not tolerated, consult with physician regarding the use of fecal softeners.
15. Encourage exercise within the capabilities of patient.
16. Promote adherence to regular schedule for bowel elimination, best within 1 hr after breakfast.
17. Encourage prompt response to defecation reflex.
18. Provide privacy for elimination.
19. Instruct patient to flex the hips if possible to create a modified squatting position.

continued

Nursing interventions

20. Suggest taking a book or crossword puzzle to the toilet to help relax for bowel evacuation.
21. Explain the Valsalva maneuver and why it should be avoided.

2. Nursing diagnosis: Alteration in bowel elimination related to side-effects of drug therapy

Goals

Patient will have regular bowel movements without straining or discomfort.
Patient will state measures to counteract constipating effects of drug therapy.

Nursing interventions

1. Assess patient use of drugs that tend to cause constipation: aspirin, anticholinergics, aluminum hydroxide or calcium carbonate antacids, opiates, tranquilizers, antidepressants.
2. Encourage patient to take at least 2000 ml of fluid daily unless contraindicated.
3. Encourage exercise and activity as permitted.
4. Provide prompt assistance with toileting if needed.
5. Consult with dietician regarding increased bulk in the diet.
6. Teach patient the importance of
   - Heeding urge to defecate promptly
   - Adequate fluid intake
   - Adequate bulk in the diet
   - Regular exercise
7. Discuss alternatives to constipating drugs with physician.

3. Nursing diagnosis: Alteration in bowel elimination related to habitual laxative use

Goals

Patient will have normal stools on a regular basis without straining or pain.
Patient will reduce use of laxatives to no more than once a month.
Patient will verbalize measures to improve bowel elimination.

Nursing interventions

1. Assess the frequency and characteristics of all stools.
2. Assess patient's definition of constipation.
3. Assess patient's understanding of bowel function.

continued

Nursing interventions

4. Identify aids to elimination used by patient: type and frequency of use of laxatives, suppositories, and enemas.
5. Assess patient's diet for adequacy of bulk and fluids.
6. Relieve immediate constipation with laxatives, suppositories, or enemas as ordered.
7. Teach measures to promote normal bowel elimination
   • Minimum of 2000 ml of fluids daily unless contraindicated
   • Inclusion of additional bulk in the diet: whole grains, bran
   • Daily exercise consistent with patient abilities
8. Teach effects of chronic use of laxatives and enemas.
9. Recognize that well-established laxative or enema dependency is not always correctable. Consult with physician for least irritating regimen that will maintain adequate bowel evacuation.

4. Nursing diagnosis: Alteration in bowel elimination related to actual or anticipated pain

Goal

Patient will report painless defecation.

Nursing interventions

1. Assess the cause of patient's pain: hemorrhoids, constipation, anal or rectal lesions.
2. Assist patient to take sitz baths.
3. Teach patient the importance of responding to the defecation urge promptly.
4. Wash and dry the anorectal area thoroughly after each bowel movement.
5. Apply topical creams, ointments, and hemorrhoidal medications as ordered.
6. If hemorrhoids are present instruct patient to avoid straining and prolonged standing.

5. Nursing diagnosis: Alteration in bowel elimination related to lack of privacy

Goal

Patient will have normal bowel movements without unnecessary disruptions or exposure.

Nursing interventions

1. Assess patient-toileting arrangement and its acceptability to patient.
2. If patient is able to use the bathroom, close the door and be sure patient is able to call for assistance.
3. If patient cannot be left alone in the bathroom, stand out of his or her line of vision and remain quiet. The sound of running water may be relaxing.
4. Draw curtains for visual privacy, leave radio or television on for auditory privacy.
5. If safe, step out of the room, first providing patient with a call bell or instructions to obtain assistance.
6. If assistance with perianal cleaning is needed, drape patient appropriately and complete the procedure in a matter-of-fact manner.
7. Remove bedpan or commode chair from patient area. Deodorize the room if necessary.
8. When assisting patient with toileting, be pleasant and businesslike.

Medical diagnosis: Diarrhea

6. Clinical nursing problem: Alteration in bowel elimination: diarrhea secondary to tube feeding

Goal

Patient will pass formed stools.

Nursing interventions

1. Record and describe the characteristics of all stools. Formula stools are usually pasty, but watery stools occurring more than twice daily should be considered diarrhea (Anderson 1986).
2. Inquire about known lactose intolerance.
3. Check the osmolarity of the feeding solution; those exceeding 280 mOsm/liter may be too concentrated (Deters 1983).

continued

Nursing interventions

4. Monitor for signs and symptoms of dumping syndrome after feedings: cold sweat, distention, dizziness, weakness, tachycardia, nausea, and diarrhea (Deters 1983).
5. Administer the feeding slowly, allowing the solution to flow by gravity.
6. If a pump is used, decrease the solution flow rate (25 ml/hr) (Anderson 1986).
7. Gradually increase the strength of the formula, progressing from a quarter to one-half strength.
8. Notify physician for antidiarrheal order.
9. Investigate possible cause of diarrhea other than feedings.
10. Consult with dietician and physician for possible change in formula if other measures are ineffective.

7. Nursing diagnosis: Alteration in comfort related to abdominal cramps and anal irritation

Goals

Patient will verbalize relief of discomfort.
Patient will exhibit relaxed posture and facial expression.
Patient's perianal area will remain free of excoriation.

Nursing interventions

1. Assess the severity, duration, and location of the discomfort and associated signs and symptoms.
2. Record the characteristics of each stool passed.
3. Assess the perianal area for redness, skin breakdown, and maceration.
4. Notify physician to obtain orders for antidiarrheal medications.
5. Administer antidiarrheal medications as ordered, being careful to assess when they are no longer needed.
6. Respond immediately to calls for assistance with toileting from the frail elderly patient.
7. If patient is unable to call for help, check frequently to detect the presence of diarrhea stools.

continued

Nursing interventions

8. Cleanse the perianal area throughly after each stool using warm water and mild soap. Pat dry with a soft towel.
9. Apply protective cream, lotion, or spray to perianal area.
10. Assist patient to take a sitz bath to relieve burning and itching.

8. Clinical nursing problem: Potential alteration in fluid balance: dehydration and electrolyte deficits

Goal

Patient will maintain normal fluid and electrolyte status as evidenced by:
- Normal skin turgor
- Blood pressure and pulse consistent with patient norms
- Normal serum electrolyte values.

Nursing interventions

1. Record number and description of all stools, noting color, amount, frequency, abnormal constituents, and associated symptoms.
2. Record and compare intake and output.
3. Assess for saline deficit: decreased skin turgor, hypotension, thirst, and lethargy.
4. Assess for hypokalemia: weakness, cardiac arrhythmias, abdominal distention.
5. Check vital signs every 4 hr.
6. Check current medications to identify those that may induce diarrhea.
7. Consult with physician regarding laboratory assessment of serum electrolytes and medical treatment. Inquire about withholding diuretics while acute diarrhea is present.
8. Identify and eliminate irritating foods from the diet. Milk products and high-residue foods are usually withheld.
9. Institute physician's orders for NPO and intravenous fluids.
10. Monitor rate of intravenous fluids to prevent circulatory overload.
11. When foods are permitted orally, encourage those high in potassium such as citrus fruits and bananas
12. If oral fluid replacement is used, encourage fluid intake of 2000–3000 ml/day un-

continued

Nursing interventions

less contraindicated by cardiovascular or renal disturbances.

13. Teach patient and family the importance of: prompt treatment of diarrhea, fluid replacement, and home management of occasional mild diarrhea if appropriate.

14. When diarrhea is resolved, provide fermented foods such as yogurt or buttermilk to restore bowel flora.

Medical diagnosis: *Diverticulosis*

9. Clinical nursing problem: Alteration in comfort: abdominal pain, flatulence, and heartburn

Goal

Patient will report decreased frequency and severity of symptoms of diverticular disease.

Nursing interventions

1. Elicit and record complete description of patient's complaints.
2. Teach patient how to reduce the discomfort of diverticulosis:
   - Use high-residue diet, avoiding spicy foods
   - Avoid harsh laxatives
   - Take bulk laxatives as ordered by physicians
   - Take anticholinergic drugs as ordered to reduce bowel contractions
3. Evaluate the need for medication and administer analgesics as ordered. Opiates are contraindicated (Almy 1985b).
4. Teach patient to manage constipation associated with diverticuli:
   - Sprinkle one teaspoonful of bran on semi-solid food at each meal, gradually increasing the amount until constipation is resolved (Almy 1985b).
   - Use whole wheat breads, fresh fruits, and vegetables to increase natural fiber in the diet.
   - Refer to Nursing Care Plans, #1, this chapter, for other measures.

10. Nursing diagnosis: Knowledge deficit of disease risk factors related to lack of instruction

Goals

Patient will identify factors that increase the risk of diverticula formation and measures to reduce personal risk.

Patient will verbalize knowledge of complications of diverticulosis that warrant medical attention.

Nursing interventions

1. Assess the following risk factors that contribute to or aggravate diverticular disease (Steffl 1984):
   - Low-residue diet
   - Constipation
   - Obesity
   - Emotional tension
2. Discuss with patient ways to reduce the risk factors:
   - Increase residue in diet
   - Constipation management
   - Weight reduction, if needed
   - Coping strategies
3. Explain diverticulosis and the potential for inflammation to patient.
4. Identify the signs and symptoms of diverticulitis (Almy 1985b):
   - Increasingly severe pain in the lower left abdomen that may be aggravated by movement
   - Nausea with or without vomiting
   - Bowel change, usually constipation but sometimes diarrhea
   - Fever and chills
   - Urinary frequency or painful urination
5. Explain the possibility of bleeding associated with diverticuli. Severe bleeding is rare but can occur.
6. Instruct patient to seek medical care if he or she passes red, maroon, or black stools. Often this is preceded by sudden mild lower abdominal distress and the urge to defecate (Almy 1985b).
7. Teach measures to control diverticular disease as outlined in Nursing Care Plans, #9, this chapter.

Medical diagnosis: *Hiatal hernia*

11. Nursing diagnosis: Alteration in comfort related to epigastric distress and esophageal reflux of gastric contents

Goals

Patient will state measures to reduce esophageal reflux.

Patient will report decreasing frequency and severity of epigastric distress.

Nursing interventions

1. Assess pain—location, severity, relationship to meals and position.
2. Teach patient relationship between food, position, and intra-abdominal pressure and symptoms of epigastric distress and heartburn.
3. Teach measures to reduce esophageal reflux:
   • Eat slowly, preferably small frequent meals rather than few large meals (Knudsen 1984).
   • If liquids alone are hard to swallow, try soaking bread, cookies, or crackers in them (Knudsen 1984).
   • Omit foods that lower esophageal sphincter tone: fat, coffee, tea, alcohol, chocolate, orange juice, and cola (Knudsen 1984).
   • Do not eat or drink for 2–3 hr before bedtime (Almy 1985a).
   • Elevate the head of the bed on 4–6-in blocks (Knudsen 1984).
4. Administer antacids as ordered or give patient instructions for self-administration if appropriate.
5. Avoid anticholinergics, which enhance esophageal reflux (Berman and Kirsner 1983).
6. Inform patient of measures to reduce intra-abdominal pressure (Knudsen 1984).
   • Avoid bending forward, lifting, and straining
   • Avoid tight clothing
   • Reduce weight if obese
7. Discuss the relationship between emotional stress and symptoms.
8. Explore patient stressors and ways to cope.

12. Nursing diagnosis: Knowledge deficit of disease risk factors and of nutrition related to lack of instruction

Goals

Patient will state symptoms of complications of hiatal hernia that require medical attention.
Patient will identify measures to take to reduce the risk of complications related to hiatal hernia.

Nursing Interventions

1. Explain hiatal hernia to patient and describe how complications may occur.
2. Identify signs and symptoms of complications (Almy 1985a):
   • Esophagitis—substernal pain (heartburn), precipitated by straining, often occurs while lying down and is relieved by sitting up, often relieved by ingestion of food, fluid, or antacids.
   • Erosion with hemorrhage—that is uncommon, but patient should know to report any obvious bleeding to the physician.
   • Aspiration—of particular concern with the immobile elderly patient. Be alert for chest pain, dyspnea, fever.
   • Strictures—characterized by progressive dysphagia, often without pain.
3. Teach patient measures to control discomforts of hiatal hernia (refer to Nursing Care Plan 11, this chapter, on altered comfort with hiatal hernia).
4. Teach patient and family, if appropriate, about drug therapy. See Table 10-1 on gastrointestinal drugs: antacids, bethanechol, and H_2-receptor blockers (cimetidine and ranitidine).

Medical diagnosis: Periodontal disease

13. Clinical nursing problem: Alteration in oral tissue: periodontal disease

Goals

Patient will verbalize measures to maintain or achieve healthy gums and teeth.
Patient will demonstrate correct techniques of brushing and flossing.
Patient's teeth will be free of plaque and caries.

Nursing interventions

1. Assess gums as part of mouth care for signs of gingival inflammation: redness and swelling, fragility with easy bleeding, halitosis, calculus (Hirschel 1985).
2. Advise patient to brush teeth at least twice a day and floss daily (Hirschel 1985).

continued

Goal	Nursing interventions
Patient's gums will be uniformly pale pink and firm without recession.	3. Assess patient's ability to perform oral care. Difficulty with grip, strength, and coordination may create problems. Provide assistance as needed. 4. Provide equipment and help as needed for the ill or immobilized patient. 5. Refer for dental evaluation if signs of gingival inflammation appear. 6. Recommend annual dental checkups to detect problems early. 7. Teach the elderly patient that loss of teeth is not a consequence of old age but of oral disease. Dental problems should be treated aggressively whether a person is seven or seventy.

Medical diagnosis: *Pernicious anemia*

14. Nursing diagnosis: Potential alterations of sensorimotor function related to degenerative changes in the peripheral nerves and spinal column

Goals	Nursing interventions

Patient will retain normal peripheral neural function as evidenced by:
• Intact tactile sensation
• Intact perception of vibration
• Normal balance
Patient will remain free of injury related to neurologic changes of pernicious anemia.
	1. Participate in early detection of pernicious anemia. Screen family members of patients for pernicious anemia.
	2. Assess for: sore tongue, pallor, nausea and vomiting, tachycardia, irritability, weight loss, impaired thought processes, and sensitivity to cold (Jennings 1983).
	3. Once pernicious anemia has been confirmed, explain the condition and treatment to patient and family.
	4. Emphasize the importance of lifelong therapy with vitamin B_{12} injections to correct the anemia and reduce neurological complications.
	5. If neurological deficits are present
	  • Protect extremities from injury
	    a. Use blankets and socks for warmth (Jennings 1983)

continued

Nursing interventions

    b. Never use hot water bottles or heating pads (Jennings 1983)

    c. Assess the feet regularly for signs of irritation or pressure

    d. Make sure shoes fit properly

• Assist with ambulation as needed if balance is poor.

---

15. Nursing diagnosis: Anxiety related to loss of ability to carry out ADL

Goal

Patient will feel less anxious as evidenced by:
- Verbalization of lessened anxiety
- Relaxed posture and facial expression

Nursing interventions

1. Provide opportunities for patient to share concerns about his or her condition.
2. Acknowledge signs of anxiety.
3. Assist patient to focus specific problems of major concern.
4. Help patient prioritize problematic activities.
5. Work together to reach alternative ways of carrying out difficult activities. For example, if fatigue is a problem, look for ways to arrange the daily schedule so that it is less demanding.
6. Emphasize that adherence to drug therapy is critical and it reduces the risk of (further) neurologic symptoms.

---

16. Nursing diagnosis: Knowledge deficit of disease, treatment, and risk factors related to lack of instruction

Goals

Patient will verbalize understanding of pernicious anemia and its treatment.

Patient will describe measures to be taken to protect extremities.

Nursing interventions

1. Assess patient learning needs: what patient knows, wants to know, and needs to know.
2. Respond to patient's immediate questions and concerns.
3. Teach patient that key to management is lifelong use of vitamin B_{12} injections.
4. Emphasize that oral B_{12} is not absorbed and therefore is useless.

continued

Nursing interventions

5. Teach patient to protect extremities that have poor sensation—never apply external heat, assess feet daily, wear properly fitting shoes.
6. Provide written material to supplement verbal information.
7. For illiterate patients, offer to tape-record teaching session.
8. Reinforce key points frequently.

References

Adams NR, Lewis SM: Fluid and electrolyte imbalances. In Lewis SM, Collier IC (eds): Medical–Surgical Nursing: Assessment and Management of Clinical Problems, p 243. New York, McGraw-Hill, 1983

Almy TP: Alterations in gastrointestinal function in old age. In Andres R, Biereman EL, Hazzard WR (eds): Principles of Geriatric Medicine, p 297. New York, McGraw-Hill, 1985a

Almy TP: Some disorders of the alimentary tract. In Andres R, Bierman EL, Hazzard WR (eds): Principles of Geriatric Medicine, p 662. New York, McGraw-Hill, 1985b

Anderson BJ: Tube feeding: Is diarrhea inevitable? Am J Nurs 6:706, 1986

Baillie J, Stoltis R: Systemic complications of inflammatory bowel disease. Geriatrics 2:53, 1985

Baum BJ: Alterations in oral function. In Andres R, Bierman EL, Hazzard WR (eds): Principles of Geriatric Medicine, p 288. New York, McGraw-Hill, 1985

Berman PM, Kirsner JB: Gastrointestinal problems. In Steinberg FU (ed): Care of the Geriatric Patient, 6th ed, p 118. St Louis, CV Mosby, 1983

Bergersen BS, Goth A: Pharmacology in Nursing, 14th ed. St Louis, CV Mosby, 1979

Brocklehurst JC: The gastrointestinal system—the large bowel. In Brocklehurst JC (ed): Textbook of Geriatric Medicine and Gerontology, 3rd ed, p 534. Edinburgh, Churchill Livingstone, 1985

Clark JB, Queener SF, Karb VB: Pharmacological Basis of Nursing Practice, 2nd ed. St Louis, CV Mosby, 1986

Deters G: Problems of nutrition and digestion. In Lewis SM, Collier IC (eds): Medical–Surgical Nursing: Assessment and Management of Clinical Problems, p 907. New York, McGraw-Hill, 1983

Dymock IW: The gastrointestinal system—the upper gastrointestinal tract. In Brocklehurst JC (ed): Textbook of Geriatric Medicine and Gerontology, 3rd ed, p 508. Edinburgh, Churchill Livingstone, 1985

Ebersole P, Hess P: Toward Healthy Aging: Human Needs and Nursing Response. St Louis, CV Mosby, 1981

Elrod RE: Problems of ingestion. In Lewis SM, Collier IC (eds): Medical–Surgical Nursing: Assessment and Management of Clinical Problems, p 885. New York, McGraw-Hill, 1983

Forbes EJ, Fitzsimmons VM: The Older Adult: A Process for Wellness. St Louis, CV Mosby, 1981

Gioiella EC, Bevil CW: Nursing Care of the Aged Client. Norwalk, Connecticut, Appleton-Century-Crofts, 1985

Govoni LE, Hayes JE: Drugs and Nursing Implications, 3rd ed. New York, Appleton-Century-Crofts, 1978

Hahn AB, Barkin RL, Oestreich SJ: Pharmacology in Nursing, 15th ed, p 284. St. Louis, CV Mosby, 1982

Heitkemper M, Bartol MA: Gastrointestinal problems. In Carnevali DL, Patrick M (eds): Nursing Management for the Elderly, 2nd ed, p 423. Philadelphia, JB Lippincott, 1986

Hirschel LA: Is Gum Disease Stealing Your Teeth? Knoxville, Tennessee Dental Health Advisor Information Center, 1985

Jennings BM: Hematologic problems. In Lewis SM, Collier IC (eds): Medical–Surgical Nursing: Assessment and Management of Clinical Problems, p 595. New York, McGraw-Hill, 1983

Jessup LE: The chest, abdomen, and genitourinary system. In Steffl BM (ed): Handbook of Gerontological Nursing, p 193. New York, Van Nostrand Reinhold, 1984

Jones DA, Lepley MK, Baker BA: Health Assessment Across the Life Span. New York, McGraw-Hill, 1984

Kamen S: Oral care of the geriatric patient. In Steinberg FU (ed): Care of the Geriatric Patient, p 388. St Louis, CV Mosby, 1983

Kerr DA, Ash MM Jr, Millard HD: Oral Diagnosis, 6th ed. St Louis, CV Mosby, 1983

Knudsen FS: Gastrointestinal and metabolic problems in older adults. In Steffl BM (ed): Handbook of Gerontological Nursing, p 234. New York, Van Nostrand Reinhold, 1984

Messner RL, Gardner SS: Stop a killer with early detection. J Gerontr Nurs 11:8, 1985

Nurse's Drug Alert: Am J Nurs 6:711, 1986

Ofstehage J, Magilvy K: Oral health and aging. Geriatr Nurs 7:238–241, 1986

Parks TG: Natural history of diverticular disease of the colon: A review of 521 cases. Br Med J IV: 639–645, 1969

Porth CM: Pathophysiology, 2nd ed. Philadelphia, JB Lippincott, 1986

Potter PA, Perry AG: Fundamentals of Nursing. St Louis, CV Mosby, 1985

Resnik B: Constipation: Common but preventable. Geriatr Nurs 6:213, 1985

Rodman MJ, Karch AM, Boyd EH, Smith DW: Pharmacology and Drug Therapy in Nursing, 3rd ed. Philadelphia, JB Lippincott, 1985

Shank RE: Nutrition principles. In Andres R, Bierman EL, Hazzard WR (eds): Principles of Geriatric Medicine, p 444. New York, McGraw-Hill, 1985

Smith IM: Infections in the elderly. In Steinberg FU (ed): Care of the Geriatric Patient, 6th ed, p 231. St Louis, CV Mosby, 1983

Spollett G: Physical assessment. In Jones DA, Lepley MK, Baker BA: Health Assessment Across the Life Span, p 780. New York, McGraw-Hill, 1984

Storer R: The gastrointestinal system—the oral tissues. In Brocklehurst JC (ed): Textbook of Geriatric Medicine and Gerontology, 3rd ed, p 500. Edinburgh, Churchill Livingstone, 1985

Tagamet once a day. Am J Nurs 5:524, 1986

White EH: Problems of absorption and elimination. In Lewis SM, Collier IC (eds): Medical–Surgical Nursing: Assessment and Management of Clinical Problems, p 971. New York, McGraw-Hill, 1983

Yurik AG, Spier BE, Robb SS, Ebert NJ: The Aged Person and the Nursing Process, 2nd ed. Norwalk, Connecticut, Appleton-Century-Crofts, 1984

Barbara K. Penn

Diabetes mellitus *11*

The physiological aspects of aging and the changes in the endocrine system have been linked repeatedly, but the exact relationship remains speculative. Aging has been cited as responsible for changes in the endocrine system, and conversely, the endocrine system has been proposed as the facilitator of the aging process (Cryer 1983; Eckel and Hofeldt 1982; Gioiella and Bevil 1985). Certainly similarities do exist between the often subtle signs and symptoms of various endocrine disorders and those of aging itself; and advancing age can alter the presentation, diagnosis, and treatment of endocrine diseases (Cryer 1983; Eckel and Hofeldt 1982; Gioiella and Bevil 1985; Nasr 1983). This chapter focuses on perhaps the most common age-related endocrine disorder: diabetes mellitus.

Age-related changes

Although diabetes mellitus occurs throughout the human lifespan, prevalence of the disease increases dramatically with age. Over 80% of all diabetic patients are past the age of 45 years, with incidence estimated at less than 2 per 1000 children, 1 in 6 at age 65, and 1 in 4 by age 85 (Bennett 1985; Nasr 1983). The predominant type of diabetes changes with age. Insulin-dependent diabetics, primarily diagnosed at young ages, are living to an advanced age as a result of general improvements in longevity. But in the elderly new cases of diabetes are usually not the more-severe insulin-dependent type (Levin 1983). According to the current internationally recognized classification system, this insulin-dependent diabetes (primarily of young people) is called *Type I diabetes* (Bennett 1985). About 10% of older diabetics have Type I diabetes (Shuman 1984). After the age of 40 new-onset diabetes is almost always noninsulin-dependent, ketosis-resistant, and controllable by diet, exercise, and possibly oral hypoglycemic agents (Gioiella and

Bevil 1985; Laakso and Pyorala 1985; Nasr 1983; Williams 1981). This form of the disease is commonly referred to as *Type II diabetes* (Bennett 1985). Generally, it is associated with lower mortality and greater longevity than Type I diabetes, presumably because the condition is milder (Goodkin 1975). Four of five diabetics have noninsulin-dependent diabetes mellitus (NIDDM) and this type of diabetes is much more common in women than in men (Skillman and Tzagournis 1983). The terms "juvenile-onset" and "maturity-onset," that have been used traditionally to describe diabetes are imprecise, and are no longer used (Bennett 1985; Laakso and Pyorala 1985).

Professional literature confirms overwhelmingly a gradual and continuous age-related decline in glucose tolerance, but findings are inconsistent and controversial, and the relationship between impaired glucose tolerance of aging and diabetes mellitus is unclear (Eckel and Hofeldt 1982; Levin 1983). It must be mentioned that not *all* elderly people have impaired glucose tolerance (Levin 1983). Generally in the NIDDM person, insulin availability and secretion appear normal but blood-glucose levels become progressively higher with age (Gioiella and Bevil 1985; Williams 1981). This appears to be a normal response to aging, resulting from numerous interrelated phenomena, none of which can be considered to be solely responsible for the glucose intolerance. The phenomena that link aging and elevated blood glucose include

- Possibly delayed insulin secretion in response to a glucose load (Gioiella and Bevil 1985; Levin 1983; Williams 1981).
- Decreased sensitivity of beta cells to glucose (Eckel and Hofeldt 1982).
- A higher blood-glucose level required to stimulate insulin release (Levin 1983).
- Decreased cellular sensitivity or tissue responsiveness to insulin (Eckel and Hofeldt 1982; Gioiella and Bevil 1985; Goldberg et al 1985; Levin 1983; Nasr 1983; Williams 1981).
- Increased adipose tissue and decreased lean body mass with a resulting decrease in muscle tissue available for glucose uptake (Eckel and Hofeldt 1982; Goldberg et al 1985; Levin 1983; Nasr 1983; Williams 1981).
- Alimentary hyperlipemia, common in the elderly, which acts as an insulin antagonist or inhibitor (Gioiella and Bevil 1985; Levin 1983).
- Decreased tendency for hyperglycemia to suppress glucagon secretion (Goldberg et al 1985; Levin 1983).
- Increased pancreatic secretion of proinsulin, which is less active biologically than insulin (Gioiella and Bevil 1985; Levin 1983; Nasr 1983).
- Increased secretion of insulin antagonists (Gioiella and Bevil 1985).
- Decreased exercise and its insulin-potentiating effect (Gioiella and Bevil 1985; Goldberg et al 1985; Nasr 1983).

In addition to the changes in carbohydrate metabolism, diabetes is characterized by premature development of nervous and vascular degenerative changes that mimic aging (Eckel and Hofeldt 1982). In fact, the diabetic patient is considered to be ten or more years older than actual chronological age because of the effects of accelerated aging (Levin 1983). Diabetes has been considered a model of aging because of the similarities in physiology between the disease state and aging itself (Eckel and Hofeldt 1982). Phenomena that occur in normal aging and are accelerated in diabetes include the development of atherosclerosis, increased capillary membrane thickness, increased stiffness of collagen, and abnormalities of skin fibroblasts (Eckel and Hofeldt 1982; Levin 1983; Williams 1981). Additional parallels between diabetes and aging have been proposed, including early development of cataracts, macular degeneration, decrease in bone mass, osteoporosis, and antibody formation against the islet cells (Lawrence and Abraira 1980). By far the most clinically significant of these changes is the premature development of atherosclerotic cardiovascular disease (ASCVD), which results in a dramatically higher death rate for diabetics than for nondiabetics (Eckel and Hofeldt 1982; Goodkin 1975; Levin 1983, Williams 1981).

Assessment variables

Medical diagnosis

The phenomenon of elevated blood-glucose levels in elderly patients presents a diagnostic dilemma: when is hyperglycemia a normal response to aging, and when does it indicate pathology that requires treatment? This dilemma has become the source of much controversy. Fasting blood-glucose levels and glucose-tolerance test results are used in the diagnosis of diabetes in the elderly, as well as in younger patients, but in the elderly population clear distinction between normal and abnormal blood-glucose results is not always evident (Goldberg et al 1985).

The fasting blood-glucose test seems to be a useful diagnostic tool for diabetes in the elderly when confirmed by a second test (Gioiella and Bevil 1985; Goldberg et al 1985; Levin 1983; Williams 1981). It is considered reliable because fasting plasma-glucose concentration is relatively unaffected by age and the several variables that can significantly alter glucose-tolerance test results (Eckel and Hofeldt 1982; Gioiella and Bevil 1985, Goldberg et al 1985; Nasr 1983). A test result of fasting plasma-glucose levels above 140 mg/dl (or blood glucose above 120 mg/dl) on more than one occasion is considered diagnostic for diabetes mellitus, and glucose-tolerance testing is considered unnecessary or undesirable (Eckel and Hofeldt 1982; Goldberg et al 1985; Levin 1983; Williams 1981).

Beyond the fasting glucose, glucose-tolerance testing is used widely in the determination of diabetes. Unfortunately, no clear standard exists for evaluating glucose tolerance in the elderly, a fact that makes diagnosis extremely difficult (Levin 1983). A reported 50% of people over the age of 60 have abnormal glucose-tolerance tests when measured by standards taken from a young population (Goldberg et al 1985; Nasr 1983). When the results are age-adjusted, however, the incidence of diabetes drops to about 17% of the population over age 60 (Gioiella and Bevil 1985; Goldberg et al 1985). Glucose-tolerance test results can be affected adversely by acute illness, stress of hospitalization, alterations in diet, physical inactivity, and numerous medications—all potentially characteristic of hospitalized elderly patients. For these reasons, the test should be done only on healthy outpatients (Gioiella and Bevil 1985; Goldberg et al 1985; Levin 1983; Williams 1981). Because of the equivocal nature of diagnosing diabetes among the elderly, it is best to use age-adjusted norms when interpreting glucose-tolerance test results (Gioiella and Bevil 1985). Two such methods are presented below, with a third that is useful although not specifically age-adjusted:

- A nomogram developed by Andres compares plasma-glucose levels of the patient with others of similar age. Although this nomogram is useful in that it is age-adjusted, the diagnosis still remains arbitrary (Gioiella and Bevil 1985; Levin 1983; Nasr 1983).
- The National Commission on Diabetes (1976) graphically represents glucose-tolerance test results on normal, borderline, probable, and confirmed diabetes based on age-adjusted norms (Gioiella and Bevil 1985; Williams 1981).
- The National Institutes of Health developed definitive diagnostic guidelines that consider classic symptoms, fasting-glucose concentrations, and glucose-tolerance test results. Although not adjusted for age, the standards are considered appropriate for diagnosing diabetes in the elderly (Goldberg et al 1985; Nasr 1983; Williams 1981).

Presentation

Typically, the onset of diabetes in youth is abrupt and clearly identifiable by classic signs and symptoms. Presentation in the elderly, however, is very different, and requires astute nursing observation skills both during initial diagnosis and periods of poor control when signs and symptoms might be expected to recur. The typical signs and symptoms of diabetes in young people are contrasted with those of elderly diabetes in Table 11-1.

Additional signs and symptoms of diabetes in the elderly may include fatigue, loss of energy, lethargy, or weakness (Goldberg et al 1985; Guthrie et al 1984; Williams 1981); recurrent infections (Goldberg et al 1985); nonspecific instability of balance or shuffling gait (Williams 1981); skin pruritis or pimples (Burggraf and Donlon 1985; Levin 1983); nocturia (Guthrie et al 1984); or vulvovaginitis (Goldberg et al 1985; Guthrie et al 1984). The first manifestation of diabetes in the elderly patient may be peripheral or autonomic neuropathy, renal dysfunction, or eye disorders (Hayter 1981a; Williams 1981).

Table 11-1. *Signs and symptoms of diabetes in young and elderly patients*

Onset in children	Onset in the elderly
Sudden, obvious onset of symptoms	Gradual, mild, subtle onset. Usually there are no overt clinical symptoms. The disease is discovered during routine examination or during workup for another health problem (Gioiella and Bevil 1985; Goldberg et al 1985; Nasr 1983; Williams 1981).
Clearly elevated blood glucose	Blood-glucose elevation marginal or absent (Gioiella and Bevil 1985; Goldberg et al 1985). As described in text, delineation between normal and abnormal blood glucose is difficult in the elderly.
Glycosuria	Glycosuria may not appear until the blood glucose reaches 200–300 mg/dl (Gioiella and Bevil 1985; Goldberg et al 1985; Hayter 1981a; Spenser 1973; Williams 1981). Glycosuria normally occurs when tubular reabsorption of glucose in the kidneys reaches its maximum. In aging, however, the renal threshold for glucose increases.
Polyuria	Polyuria is uncommon. Hyperglycemia and glycosuria normally exert osmotic influences and result in cellular dehydration and diuresis (Spenser 1973; Stock-Barkman 1983). With neither hyperglycemia nor glycosuria present as a classic sign in the elderly diabetic, polyuria does not commonly follow. The normal urinary frequency of the elderly that results from decreased bladder capacity and tone should not be mistaken for polyuria of diabetes (Burggraf and Donlon 1985).
Polydipsia	Polydipsia is not present. Without the dehydrating effects of hyperglycemia, glycosuria, and polyuria, there is no physiological need to replace fluids (Gioiella and Bevil 1985; Hayter 1981a; Spenser 1973). Also, the elderly in general have a reduced sensation of thirst even when their physical variables indicate dehydration (Lancet 1984).
Polyphagia	Polyphagia is uncommon. This normal response to insufficient insulin may not occur in the elderly patient because most aged diabetics continue to produce some insulin (Gioiella and Bevil 1985; Hayter 1981a; Skillman and Tzagournis 1983). In addition, normal aging results in a decreased sense of smell and taste sensation with a resulting decrease in appetite (Burggraf and Donlon 1985; Gioiella and Bevil 1985; Hayter 1981a).
Weight loss	There will be no weight loss. An estimated 80% or more of elderly diabetics are obese, and many can be treated with diet therapy and exercise alone (Gioiella and Bevil 1985; Levin 1983; Nasr 1983; Williams 1981). NIDDM is so closely linked to obesity that each 20-pound weight gain doubles the risk of diabetes developing (Skillman and Tzagournis 1983). The vast majority of obese elderly diabetics are women. Obese men as a group do not survive to old age (Nasr 1983).
Diabetic ketoacidosis	DKA is uncommon. As described in the text, elderly diabetics are not generally ketosis-prone. Although DKA can and does occur in the elderly, the more common acute complication is HHNK (Gioiella and Bevil 1985; Nasr 1983; Williams 1981). A diabetic emergency, HHNK is most common in the elderly, it has an average age of presentation of 60 years, and the fatality rate is 40–70% (Goldberg et al 1985; Nasr 1983).

Nursing assessment

As is the case with a younger patient, the health history and physical assessment of an elderly diabetic encompasses almost every body system and aspect of the patient's lifestyle. Nurses must be proficient at posing questions that will elicit information about the patient's knowledge of the disease and its management, as well as his or her ability to accomplish self-care measures independently (see boxed material, below). In addition, the many physiological and lifestyle changes common to elderly persons in general must be considered when interviewing and examining the elderly diabetic.

Questions for use in assessing diabetic status

Diet

What kind of dietary program has been recommended to you? By whom?

Do you use the exchange system? How do you figure exchanges? Do you have charts or other literature to help you?

Are your calories restricted? Other restrictions?

Where do you eat most of your meals? (home, dining room, restaurant)

Do you eat your meals at the same time every day?

Who cooks for you? Has that person been instructed about your prescribed diet? By whom?

Do you have any problems with eating, such as appetite, taste, dentures, allergies?

Describe your daily diet for the past three days (foods and beverages consumed, amounts, and times).

Exercise

What has your doctor said about exercise for you?

Do you exercise regularly? If not, why not? If so, what do you do? How much or how long? How often?

Describe a typical day of rest and activity.

Describe a very active day and a very quiet day.

How often do these types of days occur?

Insulin

How long have you been taking insulin?

What kind? How much? When? Do you mix insulin?

Can you describe what insulin does?

What areas of the body do you use for injection?

Do you have a plan for rotating sites?

continued

Questions for use in assessing diabetic status (Continued)

Insulin

Do you have hard, lumpy, or irritated injection areas?

Do you inject yourself? If not, who helps you? What do they do to help?

Do you ever change your insulin dose on your own? Under what circumstances?

Oral agents

How long have you been taking oral agents? What kind? How much? When?

Can you describe what oral agents do?

Have you noticed any side-effects?

Do you ever change your dosage? When?

Metabolic control

What are the signs and symptoms of hypoglycemia?

How often does it happen to you? Under what circumstances?

What do you do?

Have you ever been in the hospital with complications of diabetes? If so, when? What was wrong?

Do you test your urine or blood?

What test(s) do you use? Do you know what each measures?

What results do you usually get? How do you record them? When do you share results with your doctor?

General

Do you have medical conditions other than diabetes?

Do you take medication for these conditions? If so, please list.

How often do you see your doctor for diabetes? For other conditions?

When was your last dental examination? Eye examination?

Do you routinely examine your own legs and feet? How often? Do you know why this is important? What do you look for? Do you have any physical problems with doing this?

Do you do much traveling? How do you adapt your routine when you're away?

Do you live with someone or have frequent visitors?

Does a friend or family member know about your diabetes and its treatment?

Do you need help caring for yourself at home?

Do you have difficulty affording your special diet, testing equipment, or medication?

What is the most difficult aspect of managing your diabetes?

(Data from Bille DA: Tailoring your diabetic patient's care plan to fit his lifestyle. Nurse 86, 16:55–57, 1986; Crigler-Meringola ED: Making life sweet again for the elderly diabetic. Nurse 84, 14:60–64, 1984; Gioiella EC, Bevil CW: Nursing Care of the Aging Client: Promoting Healthy Adaptation. Norwalk, Connecticut, Appleton-Century-Crofts, 1985; Guthrie D, Guthrie R, Walters J: Dealing with diabetes mellitus. In Nurse's Clinical Library—Endocrine Disorders. Springhouse, Pennsylvania, Springhouse Corp, 1984; Miller BK, White N: Diabetes assessment guide. Am J Nurs 80:1314–1316, 1980)

Nursing history

The nursing history offers an opportunity to identify signs and symptoms that may aid in the diagnosis of diabetes and to assess the status and self-care abilities of the known diabetic. Age and circumstances surrounding onset of diabetes need to be established (Miller and White 1980). As previously discussed, the Type I diabetic is more likely to report an abrupt and recent onset of classic signs and symptoms, whereas the Type II diabetic may relate the gradual onset of vague, diffuse symptoms that can involve any part of the body. A discussion of the general course of the disease is useful to assess the patient's understanding of diabetes, the problems that have been encountered, and the degree of success in management (Guthrie et al 1984). Determining the patient's degree of comfort with the fact of the disease can serve as a valuable point of departure for further discussion, instruction, and support (Bille 1986). Specific aspects of diabetes management need to be assessed. Representative questions are presented in the boxed material on pages 254–255.

Physical assessment

The physical assessment should include each body system, and can be guided by the elements discussed below.

Mouth

The diabetic is particularly prone to periodontal diseases, which can result in destruction of bone and loss of teeth. The patient may report or exhibit poor dental hygiene that can facilitate dental problems (Schumann 1981).

Vision

Blurred vision is a common finding in uncontrolled hyperglycemia (Bille 1986; Hayter 1981a; Laakso and Pyorala 1985). Decreased peripheral vision, halos around lights, and photophobia may result from glaucoma or cataracts, both of which are more common in elderly Type II diabetics (Schumann 1981; Carter Center of Emory University 1985). The patient may require a nightlight when getting up during the night to help vision or improve his or her sense of security (Bille 1986).

Cardiovascular

Because atherosclerosis, blood pressure, heart sounds, bruits, and episodes of chest discomfort are more likely to develop in the diabetic, dyspnea or shortness of breath should be evaluated (Gioiella and Bevil 1985; Schumann 1981). Postural hypotension may occur as the result of autonomic neuropathy or either hyperosmolar hyperglycemic nonketotic (HHNK) or diabetic ketoacidosis (DKA) (Gioiella and Bevil 1985; Grace 1985; Stock-Barkman 1983).

Extremities

The extremities are particularly prone to neurovascular compromise and should be examined carefully for color, temperature, peripheral pulses, skin integrity, edema, diminished sensation, and decreased reflexes (Gioiella and Bevil 1985). Skin lesions can occur on the soles of the feet and between the toes, so these areas should not be overlooked (Schumann 1981; Sibbald and Schachter 1984). The patient should be asked about decreased sensation to hands or feet, leg cramps, the occurrence of ulcers or sores on lower extremities, injuries to the hands or fingers, and pain or burning of legs or feet, particularly at night (Gioiella and Bevil 1985; Schumann 1981). Musculoskeletal changes also occur in conjunction with neuropathy, causing irregular alignment of toes, flattened arches, altered gait, and ulcers at new pressure points (Schumann 1981; Sibbald and Schachter 1984).

Gastrointestinal

Autonomic neuropathy can cause loud borborygmi, diarrhea, fecal incontinence, nausea, vomiting, and gastric distention (Gioiella and Bevil 1985).

Genitourinary

Urinary elimination patterns can be informative with regard to the diabetic patient's condition. Polyuria may result from hyperglycemia; urgency, frequency, or straining may indicate a urinary tract infection; and nocturia may indicate both. Infrequent voiding, perhaps only twice a day, may be a sign of hypotonic distended bladder, a condition that occurs frequently in diabetics over the age of 60 (Gioiella and Bevil 1985; Schumann 1981). Proteinuria and edema can indicate nephropathy (Gioiella and Bevil 1985). Although the elderly diabetic may be reticent to discuss sexual dysfunction, the problem occurs, particularly among men, frequently enough to be worth mentioning. Because of neuropathy, men may be impotent or achieve orgasm without ejaculation (retrograde ejaculation), and women may have difficulty achieving orgasm (Bille 1986; Schumann 1981).

Central nervous system (CNS)

Syncope resulting from autonomic neuropathy can cause falls, and poses a particular danger to elderly diabetics (Gioiella and Bevil 1985). Nocturnal hypoglycemia can cause restlessness at night (Hayter 1981a). Headache, drowsiness, lethargy, or weakness may be the only signs and symptoms of impending acute complications (Guthrie et al 1984). A history of seizures may help identify a previous episode of HHNK (Stock-Barkman 1983).

Integument

Shin spots, or diabetic dermopathy, is one of the most-common skin lesions in diabetics, and is more common in elderly diabetics and patients who have had the disease for a long time. Look on the shins for atrophic, scarred brown spots, which are the end stage of small red papules—some of which may still be visible (Sibbald and Schachter 1984). The fragile skin characteristic of the elderly is particularly problematic for the diabetic, who is prone to bacterial, yeast, and fungal infections because of glucose deposits in the skin (Crigler-Meringola 1984; Gioiella and Bevil 1985; Schumann 1981). These infections are especially prevalent in the groin, axillae, and under a pendulous abdomen or breasts, and can result in chafing, generalized itching, or pruritis vulvae in women (Gioiella and Bevil 1985). Dehydration, rather than being attributed solely to aging, must be evaluated carefully as a potential manifestation of DKA or HHNK (Stock-Barkman 1983). Insulin-injection sites may show localized inflammation or surface irregularities as the result of repeated injections, and the patient's site rotation pattern should be discussed in detail (Schumann 1981; Thatcher 1985). Photosensitivity, as evidenced by skin eruptions in patterns of sun exposure or other skin reactions, may occur as a result of sulfonylurea therapy, even as late as 6 months to 24 months after the beginning of therapy (Steffl 1984; Walther and Harber 1984).

General

The patient's weight should be recorded, and the patient questioned about any noticeable, recent gain or loss. The therapeutic diet that the patient describes may appear inconsistent with current weight, and may require additional discussion (Miller and White 1980). Self-care abilities can be assessed indirectly by evaluating the patient's manual dexterity, vision, mobility, mental status, and energy (Gioiella and Bevil 1985).

Management of diabetes in the elderly

Methods of medical treatment and types of chronic complications of diabetes do not significantly differ between the young and the elderly; and the elderly diabetic deserves treatment that is just as aggressive and skillful as that rendered to a younger patient (Goldberg et al 1985; Nasr 1983). However, some ways in which the elderly diabetic responds to the disease or its management differ from those of younger patients, and require particularly attentive nursing care.

Diet and exercise

Diet therapy is an essential component of treatment in diabetes, and dietary goals differ very little between young and elderly diabetics. Diabetes in the elderly often can be controlled by diet therapy and exercise alone (Gioiella and Bevil 1985;

Goldberg et al 1985; Levin 1983; Williams 1981). A common focus of diet therapy for the elderly diabetic is reduction of obesity, but calories may also need to be restricted for the patient with normal weight to compensate for the age-related decreases in activity level, and decline in calories needed to maintain weight (Bierman 1985; Gioiella and Bevil 1985; Hayter 1981a; Levin 1983; Williams 1981). Socioeconomic factors may play a more prominent role in diet therapy for the elderly diabetic and may present unique challenges to health-care professionals. The elderly may have limited funds, a situation that results in an inability to purchase appropriate foods (Levin 1983; Nasr 1983). They may have poor understanding of diet instructions; they may live alone and have a reduced incentive to prepare or eat proper meals; they may eat out at restaurants, or in an institutional setting and have little control over food selection or preparation; and they may have poor dentition (Levin 1983). The role of fiber in the diabetic diet is receiving increasing attention, and may play a part in reducing blood sugar (Bierman 1985; Levin 1983; Williams 1981).

Whatever dietary restrictions are prescribed for the elderly diabetic, diet teaching must be realistic and individualized. If diet instructions are too complex, if restrictions are too severe, or if the diet is radically different from lifelong habits, compliance by the elderly patient will be jeopardized (Gioiella and Bevil 1985; Hayter 1981a). Food preferences need to be determined at the outset, with subsequent teaching and supplementary written materials individualized to these preferences. The elderly patient should not be overwhelmed with rigid written instructions or lists that do not allow flexibility and personal preferences (Bille 1986; Crigler-Meringola 1984; Gioiella and Bevil 1985).

Specific teaching points should be developed in response to the dietary assessment. If the prescribed diet is new or has not been followed, it may be helpful to identify the risk factors that are associated with the patient's current eating habits. Then specific reasons for the new diet must be stressed, and the patient convinced that the therapeutic diet is essential to good health. Most important, the elderly adult must consider the planned change to be valuable in order for it to be successful (Gioiella and Bevil 1985). The elderly diabetic may need to be encouraged to decrease the amount of food eaten rather than to change the types of foods. This may be particularly true for the patient who eats in an institutional setting or restaurant where the plate is prepared for the patron by someone else (Bille 1986). Some patients may be helped by a list of specific foods to avoid (Crigler-Meringola 1984). As with younger patients, general dietary guidelines should be emphasized such as eating meals and snacks at the same time every day, eating about the same amount from day to day, including foods from each exchange group every day, and including occasional sweets and alcohol in the total caloric plan for the day.

Exercise in conjunction with diet is an integral aspects of diet therapy, particularly for the overweight diabetic, and it becomes even more important with age. The beneficial effect of increased peripheral use of glucose with activity decreases with the reduced activity levels that are characteristic of aging. In addition, adipose tissue increases with age, but this tissue uses only a small amount of glucose. The reduction of lean body mass with advancing years means a concurrent decrease in the tissue that is most capable of using glucose (Levin 1983). Unfortunately, the elderly patient may believe that he or she does not have the physical capability to exercise regularly, and the adoption of a sedentary lifestyle further contributes to diminished physical abilities and a decreased sense of well-being (Cryer 1983; Fitzgerald 1985). Although there are physical limitations associated with aging, the healthy elderly person is able to achieve aerobic benefits of conditioning over time that are similar to those created in younger persons. Even the healthy elderly person, however, must have a thorough medical evaluation before starting an exercise program to preclude adverse medication interactions, musculoskeletal abnormalities, cardiovascular disease, or sensory deficits that could endanger him or her (Fitzgerald 1985). This is particularly important for elderly diabetics, whose response to exercise may be variable. The Type I diabetic whose condition is poorly controlled may make his or her hyperglycemia worse with exercise, whereas the patient with well-controlled diabetes may achieve a lowered blood-glucose level. Too, insulin absorption may be enhanced from subcutaneous injection sites that are exercised. Exercise-induced hypoglycemia can occur from this phenomenon, as well as from exercising at the time of peak insulin action. For these reasons, individual treatment patterns need to be assessed (Bergman and Auerhahn 1985; Thatcher 1985). For the Type II diabetic, weight loss and a consistent exercise program may result in increased insulin receptor sites and enhanced insulin sensitivity, but effects of exercise on glucose regulation are not clear (Bergman and Auerhahn 1985; Essig 1983).

Walking is considered one of the best forms of exercise available (Crigler-Meringola 1984). If nothing else in the routine is changed, an extra 2 miles or 30 minutes to 40 minutes of walking a day can result in a 20-pound weight loss over a year (Williams 1981). Although a new program of brisk walking, swimming, or other forms of unaccustomed aerobic activity will require medical approval, the patient can be encouraged and assisted to engage in more daily activity. For example, the institutionalized, inactive patient may be able to assume more self-care activities, be out of bed longer, or be encouraged to walk farther, longer, or more frequently. For the more active elderly patient, group stretching, chair exercises, or dancing improve flexibility and muscle tone while encouraging socialization (Fitzgerald 1985). As with diet therapy, a planned and regular exercise program is essential for all diabetics, but should be tailored to fit the needs and capabilities of each individual patient (Bergman and Auerhahn 1985; Fitzgerald 1985).

Drug therapy

Insulin therapy is required for 20% to 30% of elderly diabetics. It is used routinely for Type I diabetics, occasionally as a treatment for Type II diabetics who do not achieve control by diet or oral agents, and frequently for elderly, diet-controlled Type II diabetics whose conditions need close control during illness, infection, or surgery (Eckel and Hofeldt 1982; Essig 1983; Levin 1983; Shuman 1984; Skillman and Tzagournis 1983; Williams 1981). Insulin is not recommended to treat the hyperglycemia of obese diabetics because insulin actually can aggravate hyperglycemia in these cases (Shuman 1984; Skillman and Tzagournis 1983). Although insulin therapy is the same as with younger diabetics, management goals should be modified. Hyperglycemia should be reduced, but not to the point of hypoglycemia, a danger to which the elderly diabetic is especially vulnerable (Gioiella and Bevil 1985; Goldberg et al 1985; Levin 1983; Shuman 1984). For elderly patients, the diet plan should be established first, within American Dietetic Association (ADA) guidelines, and normal living patterns identified, with insulin therapy prescribed to accommodate the patient's lifestyle (Gioiella and Bevil 1985; Shuman 1984). As with younger diabetics, formal insulin site rotation is important to prevent lipohypertrophy or lipodystrophy, and to allow for differing absorption rates in different parts of the body (Thatcher 1985). The success of insulin therapy may be jeopardized, however, by the elderly diabetic's decreased visual acuity, mobility, memory, or coordination. The nurse must carefully assess the elderly patient's ability to independently self-administer insulin if it is prescribed, and consider alternatives as necessary. These may include teaching a friend or family member to administer the injections; having a visiting nurse draw up, label, and refrigerate a week's supply of single-type (unmixed) insulin; or helping the patient identify useful devices such as a syringe scale magnifier or measuring guides to draw up the correct dose, or an injection device to help with the injection itself (Crigler-Meringola 1984; Gioiella and Bevil 1985).

Oral hypoglycemic agents are considered safe and effective for use with symptomatic, older Type II diabetics when dietary management alone fails (Eckel and Hofeldt 1982; Skillman and Tzagournis 1983). These medications should be used as an adjunct to diet therapy and an exercise program, never as a substitute for them (Essig 1983; Williams 1981). All oral agents approved for use in this country are sulfonylureas (Govoni and Hayes 1985):

First Generation

    Acetohexamide (Dimelor, Dymelor)

    Chlorpropamide (Apo-Chlorpropamide, Chloronase, Diabinese, Novopropamide, Stabinol)

    Tolazamide (Tolinase)

    Tolbutamide (Mobenol, Novobutamide, Orinase, Rastinon, Sk-Tolbutamide)

Second Generation

    Glipizide (Glucotrol)

    Glyburide (DiaBeta, Euglucon, Micronase)

Phenformin, a biguanide agent, was withdrawn from the market in 1978 because of the increased incidence of lactic acidosis associated with its use (Essig 1983; Gioiella and Bevil 1985).

It is thought by some researchers that oral hypoglycemic agents are misused or used to excess in the elderly (Levin 1983; Skillman and Tzagournis 1983). There is much controversy regarding the use of oral agents in the presence of cardiovascular disease because these medications may increase mortality (Campbell 1984; Hayter 1981a; Levin 1983; Williams 1981). In addition, oral agents must be used with extreme caution in patients who have renal or hepatic disease. Since most oral agents reach the kidneys in active form, impairment of renal function can result in accumulation of the drug and prolonged hypoglycemia. In the case of impaired hepatic function, the drug is not metabolized (Levin 1983).

Chlorpropamide (Diabinese), in particular, causes an unpleasant Antabuse-like reaction when even a small amount of alcohol is ingested (Campbell 1984; Essig 1983; Skillman and Tzagournis 1983). In addition, it can cause fluid retention by enhancing the secretion and effect of antidiuretic hormone (ADH), so must be used with caution in patients with cardiovascular disease, and may not be recommended at all for use with elderly patients (Eckel and Hofeldt 1982; Essig 1983; Gioiella and Bevil 1985; Levin 1983). It is the oral agent with the longest halflife and duration of action is most likely to cause prolonged hypoglycemia (Eckel and Hofeldt 1982; Essig 1983; Hudson 1984; Steffl 1984). It is, however, the oral agent recommended for patients with hepatic disease (Eckel and Hofeldt 1982). Of all the sulfonylureas, tolbutamide (Orinase) is the one recommended for use with diabetics having concurrent renal disease (Eckel and Hofeldt 1982). Because it is converted by the liver into inactive metabolites, however, it may accumulate in patients with impaired liver function (Hudson 1984).

The second-generation sulfonylureas, glipizide and glyburide, are able to be prescribed in lower effective doses than the first-generation drugs. The type and incidence of side-effects are similar to those attributed to the original agents, but they may be less frequent (Campbell 1984; Essig 1983; Prendergast 1984; Skillman and Tzagournis 1983). The second-generation drugs do not appear to be superior therapeutically to other sulfonylureas, and they are contraindicated in patients with renal or hepatic impairment (Prendergast 1984). Adverse interactions with alcohol are extremely rare with second-generation agents (Campbell 1984; Prendergast 1984).

Less than 5% of patients taking oral hypoglycemic agents experience adverse effects, the primary ones being gastrointestinal distress and allergic skin reactions (Campbell 1984; Essig 1983; Levin 1983). The risk of severe hypoglycemia is as real with oral agent therapy as with insulin, a fact that requires vigilance on the part of patients, families, and health-care professionals (Campbell 1984; Eckel and Hofeldt 1982; Goldberg et al 1985; Levin 1983; Steffl 1984; Williams 1981). Use of oral agents is the primary cause of hypoglycemia in diabetics over 60 years of age (Gioiella and Bevil 1985).

Information concerning many of the antidiabetic drugs used with the elderly is presented in Table 11-2. In addition, numerous medications have an effect on blood sugar when used in conjunction with insulin or oral hypoglycemic agents. Examples are presented in the boxed material on page 267.

Text continues on p 266

*Table 11-2. **Anti-diabetic drugs***

Oral anti-diabetic agents

Drug	Effect/response in the elderly	Implications
Acetohexamide (Dymelor)	Exhibits hypoglycemic actions; has a plasma half-life of 5 hr. Has a rapid onset of 1 hr and duration of effect is 14–24 hr. Useful in the management of mild to moderately stable, nonketotic type II diabetes mellitus.	Instruct patient to test urine and acetone at least 3 times daily and report to physician if acetone is detected. GI symptoms such as nausea, vomiting, diarrhea, heartburn, and headache may be dose-related. Inform patient that alcohol intolerance disulfuram-life reaction (*i.e.*, facial flushing, pounding headache, sweating, abdominal cramps, nausea, tachycardia) may occur within minutes and last for 1–4 hr. Advise patient to maintain body weight, control exercise, and practice good hygiene and infection-control measures. Avoid using propranolol to prevent masking hypoglycemia responses such as sweating and palpitations.
Chlorpropamide (Diabinese)	Exhibits longterm hypoglycemic effect. Has a rapid onset of 1 hr and duration of action of 65–72 hr. May be given by once daily regimen. Needs at least 7 days to reach a steady state. Thus, dosage adjustment requires 1 wk or more. Has antidiuretic activity, preventing free water clearance. May be used for the treatment of neurogenic diabetic insipidus.	Geriatric patients may be more sensitive to the hypoglycemic effect of chlorpropamide and a dosage reduction is suggested. A transition period from other sulfonureas may be unnecessary. Advise patient about facial flushing when drug is used together with alcohol. Caution patient on the enhanced effect when sulfonylureas are administered with thiazide diuretics. Monitor adverse reaction from enhanced effect of anticoagulant phenytoin salicylates, nonsteroidal anti-inflammatory drugs (NSAID), and sulfonamides, as a result of protein-bending site displacement.
Glipizide (Glucotrol)	Effective hypoglycemic agent. One of the most potent sulfonylureas. Glipizide 5 mg is similar in effect to acetohexamide 500 mg, chlorpropamide 250 mg, tolbutamide 1 g, or glyburide 5 mg. Has rapid onset and long duration of effect (24 hr). Can be given on a once-a-day schedule.	The protein-binding glipizide is non-ionic and is less likely to be displaced by other highly protein-bound drugs. Appears to have displacement action when administered with salicylates, NSAIDs, or warfarin. Advise patient to take glipizide before a meal. Has a low incidence of disulfiram-like reaction when taken with alcohol. Hypoglycemic effect may be the result of inhibition of hepatic metabolism. Caution patient to check increased urine glucose level when thiazide diuretic is added to the regimen.

continued

Table 11-2. (Continued)

Oral anti-diabetic agents

Drug	Effect/response in the elderly	Implications
		Avoid concomitant use of beta-adrenergic blocking agents and sulfonylurea when possible. If necessary, beta-1 selective adrenergic-blocking agent (*e.g.,* metoprolol may be preferred).
Glyburide (DiaBeta, Micronase)	Exhibits potent hypoglycemic effect. Structurally similar to actohexamide and glipizide. Oral absorption is incomplete (only 24%). Completely metabolized by the liver to nonactive derivatives. Minimally dialyzable by hemodialysis. Has a long duration of action (24 hr).	Appears to be the agent of choice in patients with renal disease. Disulfiram-like reaction is rarely seen when given with alcohol. Ineffective as sole therapy in patients with diabetes mellitus complicated by acidosis, ketosis, or coma. Caution patient on the potency of glyburide (*i.e.,* a hypoglycemic reaction may occur with as little as 2.5 mg daily). Elderly are particularly susceptible to glyburide-induced hypoglycemia. Can be given once daily. Caution patient on dose-related GI effects such as nausea and heartburn. Avoid using beta-adrenergic-blocking agents.
Tolbutamide (Orinase)	A rapid-onset hypoglycemia agent with 6 hr to 12 hr duration. Totally metabolized to an inactive form and excreted by way of the kidney. Especially useful in patients with kidney disease.	Caution patient not to take the drug at bedtime, to avoid nocturnal hypoglycemia. Elderly are more sensitive to oral hypoglycemic agents. The starting dose should be low and given before breakfast. Patient should abstain from alcohol to avoid a disulfiram-like reaction. Advise patient to report signs of hepatic dysfunction (pruritis, jaundice) or renal impairment (dysuria, anuria) to prevent hypoglycemic reactions.
Tolazamide (Tolinase)	Slow onset (4–6 hr) and moderate duration of 10–16 hr. May be effective in patients with history of ketoacidosis or coma.	Side-effect profile is similar to tolbutamide and patient will need close observation and monitoring. Patient should be told of the hazards of a disulfiram-like reaction when taken with alcohol. To control diabetes during stress (fever, infection, or surgery) temporary use of insulin, alone or in combination with tolazamide may be needed. Not recommended for patient with concurrent liver, renal, or endocrine disease.

continued

Table 11-2. (Continued)

Insulin (rapid-acting)

Drug	Effect/response in the elderly	Implications
Animal source (pork, beef, or mixture)		
Actrapid Simitard Velosulin Regular Iletin II Purified Regular Regular Semilente Regular Iletin I Semilente Iletin	Rapid onset: immediate to 0.5 hr. Peak effect achieved in 2–4 hr. Duration of effect 6–8 hr.	Educate the patient about insulin shock. Can be administered IV or subcutaneously (SC). However, by IV infusion 20%–30% of potency is lost by interaction with plastic bag and tubing. Caution patient about substituting brands without first checking with the physician. Can be stored at room temperature. However, after opening vial, store in refrigerator to minimize bacterial growth.
Human source		
Novolin R. Humulin R.	Same as animal-source insulins.	Produced by semisynthetic or DNA-recombinant technology. Less antigenic than animal-source insulin. May require dosage reduction in selective patient population when converting from an animal to a human source of insulin.

Insulins (intermediate-acting)

Drug	Effect/response in the elderly	Implications
Animal source (pork, beef, or mixture)		
Protaphane Mixtard Monotard Lentard Insulatard NPH NPH Iletin II Purified Isophane NPH Lente Iletin II Purified Lente Isophane NPH Lente NPH Iletin I Lente Iletin I	Onset of effect 1–2 hr. Duration of effect is 18–26 hr. Peak effect is achieved in 6–12 hr. Mixtard is a mixture of 70% isophane insulin and 30% regular insulin that provides rapid onset with a duration of 24 hr.	Content of vial is cloudy. Administer subcutaneously. May be used with regular insulin to achieve rapid onset. *Never* give an intermediate-acting insulin by *IV* route.

continued

Table 11-2. (Continued)

Insulins (intermediate-acting)

Drug	Effect/response in the elderly	Implications
Human source		
Humulin N Novolin N	Same as animal source.	Should be administered subcutaneously. Instruct patient to use same type of syringe to avoid dosage errors. Rotate injection sites to prevent lipodystrophy. Educate patient about insulin-requirement changes in the event of unpredicted stressors. Any dosage change should be only on the advice of a physician. Caution patient that alcohol and salicylates may potentiate the hypoglycemic effect of insulin.

Insulin (long-acting)

Drug	Effect/response in the elderly	Implications
Animal source (pork, beef, or mixture)		
Ultratard PZI Iletin II Ultralente PZI Ultralente Iletin I PZI Iletin I	Onset of effect 4–6 hr. Duration of effect 26–36 hr. Peak effect achieved in 14–24 hr.	Thiazide diuretics elevate blood glucose level and may antagonize insulin's hypoglycemic effect. Avoid concomitant use of beta adrenergic blocking agent, which may delay recovery from a hypoglycemic episode and may mask signs and symptoms of hypoglycemia.

Compensating for decreased visual acuity

The normal decline in visual acuity and accommodation of the elderly may adversely affect the diabetic patient's ability to perform self-care (Gioiella and Bevil 1985; Goldberg et al 1985; Yurick et al 1984). In addition, continued hyperglycemia of diabetes may change the shape and clarity of the lens as a result of sorbitol deposits, causing myopia. Normal vision returns, however, when glucose control becomes regulated; patients should not be fitted for glasses until this occurs (Hayter 1981a; Skillman and Tzagournis 1983). Because vision can deteriorate so profoundly in diabetic patients, regular eye examinations are recommended at

Drug interactions with insulin and sulfonylureas

Drugs that potentiate hyperglycemia (or decrease hypoglycemia effect)

Alcohol (chronic, heavy use)
Bulk laxatives
Chlorpromazine
Diazoxide
Digitalis
Epinephrine (sympathomimetics)
Estrogens
Ethacrynic acid
Furosemide
Indomethacin
Isoniazid
Levodopa
Lithium
Nicotinic acid
Phenytoin
Rifampin
Thiazides
Thyroid hormone

Drugs that potentiate hypoglycemia

Alcohol
Antithyroid drugs
Aspirin (salicylates)
Chloramphenicol
Chlorpropamide
Clofibrate
Guanethidine
MAO inhibitors
Oxyphenbutazone
Phenylbutazone
Probenecid
Propranolol (beta blockers)
Sulfonamides
Warfarin

(Data from Essig M: Update your knowledge of oral antidiabetic agents. Nurs 83, 13:58–63, 1983; Gioiella EC, Bevil CW: Nursing Care of the Aging Client: Promoting Health Adaptation. Norwalk, Connecticut, Appleton-Century-Crofts, 1985; Hayter J: Why response to medication changes with age. Geriatr Nurs 2:411–416, 1981b; Hudson M: Drugs and the older adult—take special care. Nursing 84, 14:46–51, 1984; Levin MD: Diabetes Mellitus. In Steinberg F (ed): Care of the Geriatric Patient, 6th ed, pp 154–181. St. Louis, CV Mosby, 1983; Nasr H: Endocrine disorders in the elderly. Med Clin N Amer 67:481–495, 1983; Podolsky S, Krall L, Bradley RF: Treatment of diabetes with oral hypoglycemic agents. In Podolsky S (ed): Clinical Diabetes: Modern Management, pp 149, 154–158. New York, Appleton-Century-Crofts, 1980; Skillman TG, Tzagournis M: Diabetes Mellitus. Kalamazoo, Michigan, Upjohn Co, 1983; Steffl BM: Handbook of Gerontological Nursing, pp 417–418. New York, Van Nostrand Reinhold, 1984)

three to six month intervals for the elderly diabetic (Gioiella and Bevil 1985). Decreased vision may require the use of premeasured insulin or special appliances for the visually impaired, increased assistance from family or home-care agencies, and modification of the many self-care measures that require clear sight.

The deterioration of color perception with age also has potentially serious effects on self-care abilities of elderly diabetics who test urine or blood glucose with a color scale. The ability to discriminate among blues, greens, and violets decreases with normal aging, and these colors are used frequently with commercial testing products (Burggraf and Donlon 1985; Gioiella and Bevil 1985; Hayter 1981a; Yurick et al 1984). In addition to the normal changes of aging, color vision has been shown to deteriorate further with increasing severity of diabetic retinopathy (Green et al 1985).

Metabolic control

Although there is disagreement among researchers, maintenance of good metabolic control is thought to be an important measure for the prevention or reduction of chronic complications associated with diabetes (Eckel and Hofeldt 1982; Goodkin 1975; Hayter 1981a; Levin 1983; Nasr 1983; Williams 1981). Even for the elderly diabetic whose therapeutic regimen often is more flexible than that of a younger person, the goal of treatment remains relief of symptoms and achievement of satisfactory control (Eckel and Hofeldt 1982; Gioiella and Bevil 1985; Goldberg et al 1985; Hanuschak and Duncan 1985; Hayter 1981a; Nasr 1983). Because of the particular hazards of hypoglycemia in elderly diabetics, these patients may be allowed to maintain a higher blood glucose level and demonstrate a small amount of glycosuria as their norm (Gioiella and Bevil 1985; Levin 1983).

The mechanism for monitoring the degree of control among elderly diabetics is controversial. Routine urine testing is often recommended for both Type I and Type II diabetics (Eckel and Hofeldt 1982; Williams 1981). Urine testing several times a day, however, is thought to be unnecessary for the elderly patient, except in the event of unstable diabetes (Gioiella and Bevil 1985; Clinical Brief 1984). The routine measurement of urine ketones is considered unnecessary for elderly diabetics except during times of poor glucose control, illness, or major stress, when ketosis is more likely to occur (Eckel and Hofeldt 1982; Shuman 1984; Williams 1981). In addition, the need for routine use of a second-voided specimen for testing is arguable (Eckel and Hofeldt 1982; Gioiella and Bevil 1985; Hayter 1981a; Williams 1981).

There seems to be persuasive evidence that blood-glucose testing is more reliable and appropriate than urine testing for the elderly diabetic, for the following reasons:

- The high renal threshold for glucose in elderly diabetics makes urine testing an inaccurate indicator of control (Crigler-Meringola 1984; Gioiella and Bevil 1985; Goldberg et al 1985; Hanuschak and Duncan 1985; Hayter 1981a; Shuman 1984).
- A poor correlation exists between concurrent urine and blood-glucose levels (Goldberg et al 1985; Hanuschak and Duncan 1985).
- In persons who have a large postvoiding residual volume from neurogenic bladder, or impaired bladder-emptying caused by aging, the urine being tested could be old and give a false impression of current physiological status (Burggraf and Donlon 1985; Eckel and Hofeldt 1982; Gioiella and Bevil 1985; Hayter 1981a; Shuman 1984).
- The aforementioned decline in color discrimination of the elderly patient makes independent testing against a color chart unreliable.
- Urine specimens may be difficult and time-consuming to obtain from the elderly patient for various reasons (Hanuschak and Duncan 1985; Clinical Brief 1985).

· The elderly diabetic may be on numerous prescribed medications that have variable effects on urine test results such as salicylates, pyridium, levodopa, and probenecid (Gioiella and Bevil 1985; Hayter 1981a; Kelly 1979).

If the patient has adequate vision and has been successful in monitoring control with urine tests, there may be no reason to change methods (Crigler-Meringola 1984; Hayter 1981a). In fact, the patient with decreased visual acuity but normal color vision may benefit from extra-large urine dipsticks, which are available (Gioiella and Bevil 1985; Hayter 1981a). Even though urine testing has been prevalent in the past, home blood-glucose monitoring is being recommended as easier and much more accurate for both Type I and Type II diabetes. Blood testing helps the patient see promptly the physiological response to treatment, and encourages more patient responsibility. The patient can associate blood-glucose levels with what has been eaten, how much insulin or oral agent has been taken, and how exercise or stress has affected metabolism (Surr 1983a). The patient who has consistently negative urine sugars cannot use urine tests to interpret the efficacy of treatment and could benefit from blood testing. The elderly patient who repetitively experiences hypoglycemia without warning is also an excellent candidate for blood-glucose monitoring because of its accuracy (Hanuschak and Duncan 1985). Blood testing with a digital display meter is particularly appropriate for the patient who needs monitoring but whose color perception makes urine testing inaccurate (Crigler-Meringola 1984; Hanuschak and Duncan 1985; Clinical Brief 1986). Type I diabetics are urged to test blood as frequently as they formerly tested urine, before meals and at bedtimes, and they should continue to test for urine ketones in response to illness or hyperglycemia (Guthrie et al 1984). The well-controlled Type II diabetic may need to test blood only a few times a week or once a month (Hanuschak and Duncan 1985; Clinical Brief 1986). Depending on the patient's visual acuity and color perception, blood testing can be done either manually, with reagent strips compared against a color chart, or using the expensive but more accurate meters with a dial or digital display (Surr 1983a, 1983b). These tests require adequate vision and manual dexterity, as do urine tests, so a family member may have to help the patient with testing.

Acute complications

Hypoglycemia

Hypoglycemia is precipitated by the same factors in young and elderly diabetics: overmedication with insulin or oral agents, omitting meals, eating less than usual, or unplanned exercise without changes in diet or medication (Gioiella and Bevil 1985; Guthrie 1984). The usual signs and symptoms so common and classic in younger patients, however, may not appear in the elderly. Hypoglycemia manifests itself atypically in elderly patients, is more poorly tolerated, and may be prolonged (Goldberg et al 1985; Nasr 1983). In the elderly diabetic, the release of catecholamines in response to hypoglycemia can precipitate cardiac ischemia, arrhythmia, myocardial infarction, cerebrovascular accident, and death (Gioiella and Bevil 1985; Levin 1983). In addition, cerebral function and level of consciousness may be affected. Changes in the level of consciousness may be slow and insidious and progress through confusion, disorientation, slurred speech, somnolence, bizarre behavior, stupor, convulsions; and coma or unconsciousness may occur without warning (Eckel and Hofeldt 1982; Gioiella and Bevil 1985; Goldberg et al 1985; Levin 1983). At night, the elderly patient who is hypoglycemic may exhibit restlessness, headache, sleep disturbance, unusual positions, or difficulty in being aroused (Gioiella and Bevil 1985; Hayter 1981a).

Emergency treatment of hypoglycemia is the same for elderly diabetics as for the young. A blood specimen should be obtained first to validate the diagnosis and document for future reference the point at which signs and symptoms occurred. A rapid-acting carbohydrate should then be administered—by mouth if the patient is conscious (orange juice, soft drink, sugar), or intravenously if unconscious (50% dextrose) (Guthrie et al 1984; Stock-Barkman 1983). Subcutaneous or intramuscular glucagon is another treatment method for insulin-induced hypoglycemia because it raises blood sugar by mobilizing liver glycogen. In the patient who has been critically hypoglycemic for some time, however, glycogen stores may have been used, and the only helpful treatment will be IV glucose (Luckman and Sorensen 1980). Glucagon is not recommended for treatment of hypoglycemia induced by sulfonylureas (Lawrence and Abraira 1980; Lefebvre and Luyckx 1983). Emergency carbohydrates should be augmented as soon as possible by ingestion of a complex carbohydrate or protein (milk, crackers, cheese, peanut butter) to replace liver glycogen and prevent further hypoglycemia (Guthrie et al 1984; Stock-Barkman 1983). Unlike the prompt reversal of signs and symptoms of hypoglycemia in the young, neurological manifestations in the elderly patient may take several days to resolve completely (Levin 1983).

Diabetic ketoacidosis (DKA)

Although DKA occurs in Type II diabetes, the patient most at risk is the Type I diabetic (Stock-Barkman 1983; Carter Center of Emory University 1985). This acute complication is precipitated most commonly by concurrent illness, particularly infection, to which elderly diabetics are especially susceptible (Goldberg et al 1985; Stock-Barkman 1983). Common infections among diabetics include pulmonary tuberculosis, urinary tract infections, gingivitis, infected foot ulcers, and monilial vulvovaginitis in women (Goldberg et al 1985). Urinary tract infections and pulmonary tuberculosis are the most common precipitators of DKA among the elderly, but this complication also can occur in some elderly diabetics from omission of insulin or in response to physical or emotional stress (Gioiella and Bevil 1985; Guthrie et al 1984; Steiner 1981). Treatment is the same in young and elderly diabetics, but the response of the latter to DKA and its treatment can be very different.

Although there is a smaller incidence of DKA in the elderly, the fatality rate is higher (Goldberg et al 1985). Only 9% of patients hospitalized with DKA die, but most of those deaths occur in elderly diabetics who have concurrent acute, nonmetabolic diseases such as infection, cerebrovascular accident (CVA), myocardial infarction (MI), vascular thrombosis, intestinal obstruction, or pneumonia (Goldberg et al 1985; Carter Center of Emory University 1985). DKA is more likely to be fatal when associated with infection. For this reason, when infection is suspected as the cause of DKA, its source must be found and treated promptly (Goldberg et al 1985).

In addition to infection, arterial thrombosis and hypovolemic shock are responsible for large numbers of deaths among elderly DKA patients (Goldberg et al 1985). The elderly are at high risk for developing arterial occlusion after DKA, and the occlusion may be a direct result of both DKA and its treatment (Gioiella and Bevil 1985; Goldberg et al 1985). Evidence of occlusion typically appears hours or days after treatment for DKA has begun, and patients remain at risk for several days after treatment has been successful. For this reason, heparin therapy may be a part of DKA treatment (Goldberg et al 1985; Stock-Barkman 1983). The risk of thrombosis is heightened in elderly patients who have pre-existing atherosclerosis. Hypovolemic shock also causes a large number of DKA deaths in elderly diabetics, particularly when dehydration is not adequately or promptly reversed (Goldberg et al 1985).

The goals of DKA treatment are the same for all ages:

- Stop endogenous acid production by administration of insulin (Gioiella and Bevil 1985; Guthrie et al 1984; Surr 1983b; Stock-Barkman 1983). The preferred route is by IV bolus and drip, but it must be remembered that insulin may bind to plastic IV bags and tubing. Administration of sodium bicarbonate in DKA is controversial (Skillman and Tzagournis 1983; Stock-Barkman 1983).
- Restore fluid volume and blood pressure by prompt administration of 0.9% sodium chloride as the preferred first IV solution, followed later by 0.45% sodium chloride at a reduced rate when circulatory volume has been restored (Goldberg et al 1985; Skillman and Tzagournis 1983; Stock-Barkman 1983). Typically, 10% of body weight is lost in fluid (Goldberg et al 1985). About 3 liters of IV fluid over 4 hours to 6 hours is average for replacement (Skillman and Tzagournis 1983).
- Observe for and correct electrolyte imbalances: sodium, chloride, potassium, and phosphate. Hypokalemia and hypophosphatemia commonly occur in DKA (except in the presence of renal failure) and potassium phosphate may be given to reverse these deficits once renal function is adequate (Guthrie et al 1984; Skillman and Tzagournis 1983; Stock-Barkman 1983).
- Treat the underlying cause of the DKA (Guthrie et al 1984).

Specific treatment of DKA in the elderly is individualized according to the patient's cardiopulmonary and renal status. The patient with chronic kidney disease may have fewer functioning nephrons and a decreased ability to handle the excess hydrogen ion loads of acidosis (Gioiella and Bevil 1985). Too, as previously mentioned, these patients may have an altered electrolyte status in response to DKA. The patient with cardiac compromise will have a decreased ability to tolerate the cardiac effects of hypokalemia that are almost inevitably induced by DKA (Skillman and Tzagournis 1983; Stock-Barkman 1983). The hypotension from dehydration can critically reduce renal and cerebral blood flow, resulting in oliguria, CVA, and shock. Hydration therapy, however, must restore adequate circulatory volume without overloading the elderly person's cardiopulmonary system (Gioiella and Bevil 1985; Goldberg et al 1985). An elderly diabetic who has had DKA requires longterm insulin therapy (Goldberg et al 1985).

Hyperglycemic hyperosmolar nonketosis (HHNK)

HHNK is a life-threatening acute complication, similar to DKA but without the ketoacidosis. It occurs most often in the elderly, in persons with no previous diagnosis of diabetes, or Type II diabetes thought to be under control, and particularly affects those with underlying renal impairment (Gioiella and Bevil 1985; Grace 1985; Guthrie et al 1984; Hayter 1981a; Levin 1983; Nasr 1983; Stock-Barkman 1983; Williams 1981). Occurring equally in men and women, HHNK may be the initial presentation of previously undiagnosed diabetes, or may occur in controlled diabetes when a new stress is experienced such as an acute or chronic illness other than diabetes (Gioiella and Bevil 1985; Levin 1983; Nasr 1983; Williams 1981). It may occur over 24 hours or 10 days to 12 days (Williams 1981). There are numerous potential precipitating factors, including diuretic therapy, severe illness or infection, surgery, dialysis, hyperalimentation, and a wide variety of medications (Goldberg et al 1985; Grace 1985; Guthrie et al 1984).

The pathophysiology of HHNK is very similar to that of DKA with the exception of ketoacidosis (Guthrie et al 1984; Stock-Barkman 1983); however, approximately 30% of HHNK patients do exhibit metabolic acidosis, either from renal failure or lactic acidosis precipitated by shock (Grace 1985). It is thought that some insulin is available in HHNK—enough to prevent ketosis, but not enough to respond to the increased demands brought about by stress (Gioiella and Bevil 1985; Goldberg et al 1985; Hayter 1981a; Nasr 1983; Williams 1981). The absence of ketonemia and ketonuria are what distinguish HHNK from DKA (Stock-Barkman 1983).

Hyperglycemia is worse in HHNK than in DKA, and may reach or exceed 1000 mg/dl (Gioiella and Bevil 1985; Guthrie et al 1984; Hayter 1981a; Stock-Barkman 1983; Williams 1981). Glycosuria results in osmotic diuresis, severe dehydration, hypotension, and possible renal failure or shock (Gioiella and Bevil 1985; Grace 1985; Guthrie et al 1984; Williams 1981). The dehydration of HHNK is also worse than in DKA, and up to 25% of total body water may be lost (Goldberg et al 1985; Grace 1985; Guthrie et al 1984; Skillman and Tzagournis 1983; Stock-

Barkman 1983). Because fluid is lost in greater amounts than solutes, hyperosmolality results (Goldberg et al 1985; Grace 1985). The dehydration and hyperosmolality further can produce

- Variable neurological signs and symptoms, ranging from confusion to coma (Gioiella and Bevil 1985; Goldberg et al 1985; Grace 1985)
- Hemoconcentration and thromboembolitic episodes (Goldberg et al 1985; Grace 1985; Guthrie et al 1984)
- Decreased insulin release, which further increases hyperglycemia and decreases insulin responsiveness (Gioiella and Bevil 1985; Hayter 1981a; Williams 1981)
- Paradoxical depression of thirst in the presence of severe dehydration that results in further volume depletion (Goldberg et al 1985; Guthrie et al 1984).

HHNK is a life-threatening emergency that usually requires transfer to an intensive care unit and constant monitoring (Hayter 1981a; Stock-Barkman 1983; Williams 1981). Mortality has been reported at 40% to 70% (Goldberg et al 1985; Grace 1985; Skillman and Tzagournis 1983). Treatment is very similar to that for DKA

- Fluid replacement is of primary importance, and more fluid is administered than in DKA (Goldberg et al 1985; Guthrie et al 1984; Stock-Barkman 1983). The average amount of replacement fluid needed is 9 liters given over from 36 hours to 48 hours. Hypotonic 0.45 sodium chloride is recommended unless hypovolemic shock is evident (Goldberg et al 1985; Grace 1985; Williams 1981). Care must be taken to observe the patient's hydration status carefully because of pre-existing cardiovascular or renal compromise typical of elderly patients, or reduced renal function as a result of the HHNK (Grace 1985; Stock-Barkman 1983).
- Electrolyte imbalances must be monitored and corrected as in DKA. Serum sodium may be elevated rather than decreased as in DKA (Gioiella and Bevil 1985; Goldberg et al 1985; Grace 1985; Williams 1981). Generally, potassium replacement should start earlier in HHNK than in DKA, and the amount administered is usually more. As in DKA, potassium supplementation is not started until renal function is adequate (Goldberg et al 1985; Grace 1985).
- Smaller doses of insulin generally are required than in DKA (Goldberg et al 1985; Guthrie et al 1984; Stock-Barkman 1983; Williams 1981).
- Complications must be observed for and treated. Thromboembolitic episodes may be prevented by heparin therapy (Goldberg et al 1985; Grace 1985; Stock-Barkman 1983). Seizures occur in 25% of HHNK patients, and are stopped by reversal of the metabolic disorder itself. Phenytoin (Dilantin) administration is not recommended because it can inhibit

insulin release and potentiate hyperglycemia (Grace 1985; Stock-Barkman 1983).
- The underlying precipitating factor(s) should be identified and corrected (Goldberg et al 1985; Grace 1985). It is estimated that in over half of HHNK episodes, a precipitating factor can be identified (Skillman and Tzagournis 1983).

Slow treatment over about 2 days is believed to be safer than rapid reversal of HHNK. Too-rapid correction can result in convulsions, deepening coma, and death (Williams 1981). After an episode of HHNK, a few diabetic patients become insulin-dependent (Goldberg et al 1985; Grace 1985).

Chronic complications

The most common chronic complications of diabetes mellitus are of three types that will be considered separately—microvascular complications (retinopathy, nephropathy), neuropathy, and macrovascular disease. As previously mentioned, there are positive correlations among the incidence and severity of chronic complications, the duration of diabetes, and the degree of metabolic control. The exception appears to be large-vessel disease (Frazin 1984; Hayter 1981a; Levin 1983).

Microvascular changes

The primary characteristic of microvascular disease in the diabetic patient is capillary basement membrane thickening, and the retina and kidney are primarily affected (Skillman and Tzagournis 1983).

Microangiopathy, while occurring in both Type I and Type II diabetes, is associated with higher morbidity and mortality in Type I diabetes. Although many Type I diabetics have microvascular changes later in life, a surprisingly large number do not (Eckel and Hofeldt 1982). The clinical significance of capillary basement membrane thickening is unclear, but may be associated with the diabetic's decreased resistance to infection by its effect upon the permeability of the capillary walls (Campbell 1984; Gioiella and Bevil 1985; Levin 1983).

Retinopathy

Retinopathy occurs in about 45% of diabetics over 60 years of age (Gioiella and Bevil 1985) and accounts for 10% to 15% of new blindness among the elderly in the United States (Levin 1983). Diabetes is the leading cause of new blindness among Americans (Levin 1983; Skillman and Tzagournis 1983; Carter Center of Emory University 1985). In Type I diabetes, 87% of legal blindness is attributable to retinopathy, as is 33% of blindness in Type II diabetes. Retinopathy includes

- Retinal disease alone: Physical changes are confined to the retina alone and there is little risk from blindness (Skillman and Tzagournis 1983). Over 60% of diabetics with impaired vision have this type of retinopathy (Gioiella and Bevil 1985). In Type II diabetes, visual impairment beyond age 60 is usually caused by vascular insufficiency to the macula (Levin 1983).
- Proliferative retinopathy: New vessel growth from the retina extends into the normally nonvascular vitreous chamber (Gioiella and Bevil 1985; Skillman and Tzagournis 1983). These vessels are fragile and tend to hemorrhage (Levin 1983). This type of retinopathy occurs much more often in Type I diabetes (Eckel and Hofeldt 1982; Carter Center of Emory University 1985). Medical treatment has not been particularly helpful in retinopathy; however, surgical procedures such as photocoagulation, vitrectomy, and scleral buckling have been useful (Eckel and Hofeldt 1982; Levin 1983; Skillman and Tzagournis 1983). Hypertension may be a precipitating factor in retinopathy and should be carefully controlled (Eckel and Hofeldt 1982; Levin 1983).

In the older diabetic, retinopathy often occurs in addition to the other eye changes to which the elderly are vulnerable, including macular degeneration, cataracts, and glaucoma (Levin 1983). In fact, these three conditions are more frequent causes of blindness in Type II diabetes than is diabetic retinopathy. Evidence indicates that all these disorders occur earlier or with greater frequency in diabetes (Eckel and Hofeldt 1982; Levin 1983; Skillman and Tzagournis 1983). The elderly diabetic should undergo an ophthalmologic examination every three to six months, and the patient with retinopathy should avoid heavy lifting or straining (Gioiella and Bevil 1985).

Nephropathy

Renal failure as a result of nephropathy is the leading cause of death in Type I diabetes, but it is fairly uncommon in Type II diabetes (Eckel and Hofeldt 1982; Skillman and Tzagournis 1983). Slowly progressive renal capillary basement membrane thickening occurs, however, in about 90% of Type II diabetics, although it rarely results in renal failure (Eckel and Hofeldt 1982; Gioiella and Bevil 1985). The first indication of nephropathy is proteinuria, but this sign also may be a normal response to aging (Eckel and Hofeldt 1982). According to Levin (1983), it takes a juvenile diabetic about 17 years to exhibit the proteinuria of glomerulosclerosis. Once signs and symptoms of severe renal failure are evident, death usually follows in a very short time. Therefore, patients in whom diabetic nephropathy develops rarely live to old age. This trend may reverse, however, as well-managed juvenile diabetics live long enough for renal failure to develop.

In elderly diabetics, there may be many causes of decreased renal function other than nephropathy. These include nephrosclerosis, pyelonephritis, renal or ureteral calculi, prostate enlargement in men, congestive heart failure, the overuse of diuretics to control hypertension or edema, and urinary tract infections (Eckel and Hofeldt 1982; Levin 1983).

Once renal mass and function are reduced, insulin breakdown and excretion are decreased, and insulin requirements also may decrease (Eckel and Hofeldt 1982; Levin 1983). As previously mentioned, renal impairment affects excretion of oral hypoglycemia agents and can cause accumulation of the medication and profound hypoglycemia. As with retinopathy, good metabolic control is the best means to prevent or minimize nephropathy. Control is not, however, as beneficial in elderly diabetics whose renal disease may be complicated by atherosclerosis of renal arteries (Levin 1983). Control of hypertension and smoking cessation are thought to decrease progression of renal failure (Skillman and Tzagournis 1983). Prevention of fluid overload, low-protein diet, and decrease in insulin dose are palliative measures useful in the presence of symptoms of renal impairment, but hemodialysis or peritoneal dialysis and kidney transplantation are the only major treatments (Gioiella and Bevil 1985; Skillman and Tzagournis 1983). These treatments, however, have drawbacks for the diabetic. Diabetics do not tolerate hemodialysis as well as nondiabetics; this is particularly true of elderly patients who have compromised vascular status and susceptibility to infection. In these patients, vascular access is difficult to maintain (Gioiella and Bevil 1985; Levin 1983). Renal transplant is becoming more common in diabetic end-stage renal disease, but postoperative recovery is much more problematic because of the diabetes (Levin 1983).

Neuropathy

Diabetic neuropathy is one of the most common and debilitating complications of diabetes mellitus, but statistics on its occurrence are rare because of disagreement about definition, classification, and pathophysiology (Carter Center of Emory University 1985). Neuropathy is particularly common in diabetics over 50 years of age and may be the initial presentation of undiagnosed diabetes (Gioiella and Bevil 1985; Levin 1983; Williams 1981). The pathophysiology is unclear, but seems to be related to poor glucose control (Skillman and Tzagournis 1983). It is postulated that persistent hyperglycemia results in the production of sorbitol that deposits in nerve cells, causes dilation, and results in decreased nerve conduction velocity (Campbell 1984). Further, sorbitol contributes to the degeneration of the myelin sheath that is associated with diabetic neuropathy (Levin 1983).

Two very different types of neuropathy affect diabetics: peripheral and autonomic. Peripheral neuropathy, the more common type, generally affects the lower extremities bilaterally and symmetrically. There are losses of vibratory sense, temperature, touch and pain sensation, proprioception, and deep tendon reflexes. The patient may suffer pain (particularly with movement), hyperesthesia, and paresthesias or "burning" feelings in legs or feet, which may be worse at night (Eckel and Hofeldt 1982; Frazin 1984; Gioiella and Bevil 1985). However distressing hyperesthesia or paresthesia may be to the patient, hypoesthesia is particularly problematic. Insensitivity of the legs and feet creates an opening for injury and subsequent infection, gangrene, and amputation; this situation makes patient education about foot care a priority (Gioiella and Bevil 1985; Levin 1983). Diabetic foot lesions that require hospitalization occur more often from neuropathy than from primary vascular disorders (Frazin 1984). Destruction of the weight-bearing foot bones, footdrop, and osteomyelitis can be particularly devastating longterm problems that can dramatically curtail mobility (Skillman and Tzagournis 1983). Amyotrophy, another form of peripheral neuropathy, is serious but usually self-limiting. It is most frequently seen in elderly men and is characterized by asymmetrical wasting of hip and thigh muscles, severe pain, and limited mobility. It is usually seen in newly diagnosed or poorly controlled diabetes and generally resolves over several months of good control (Eckel and Hofeldt 1982; Gioiella and Bevil 1985).

Autonomic neuropathy is particularly disruptive to the lifestyle of the elderly diabetic because of its serious effects on multiple body systems. Cardiovascular signs and symptoms include postural hypotension and syncope, which place the elderly diabetic at risk for falls and injury. Genitourinary problems include neurogenic or hypotonic bladder, a problem particularly prevalent in diabetics over 60 years old, which results in incomplete bladder emptying and can lead to urinary tract infections and kidney dysfunction (Gioiella and Bevil 1985; Schumann 1981). A second genitourinary problem is sexual dysfunction—for both men and women. Although they retain their interest in sexual activity, as many as 50% of diabetic men experience impotence as a result of nerve impairment. Erectile dysfunction may develop slowly, but is irreversible. Retrograde ejaculation occurs in some men who are able to achieve orgasm but who do not ejaculate. Bladder neck incompetence causes semen to flow back into the bladder (Funnell and McNitt 1986; Garofano 1980; Schumann 1981). Information about sexual dysfunction in women is less clear, but orgasmic difficulty has been documented (Funnell and McNitt 1986; Garofano 1980).

Gastrointestinal difficulties include delayed gastric emptying, nausea, vomiting, constipation, severe diarrhea, fecal incontinence, loud borborygmi, nutritional deficiencies, and fluid and electrolyte problems (Eckel and Hofeldt 1982; Funnell and McNitt 1986; Gioiella and Bevil 1985). Autonomic neuropathy is also characterized by abnormal sweating of the trunk or head, which is annoying, and for which no therapy is successful (Skillman and Tzagournis 1983).

Neuropathy is managed the same way in both young and elderly patients (Goldberg et al 1985). Unfortunately, there is no definitive treatment for neuropathy because the pathophysiology is so poorly understood (Eckel and Hofeldt 1982). There are numerous symptomatic treatments available, but the best approach to treatment is good metabolic control to reduce hyperglycemia, which aggravates symptoms (Funnell and McNitt 1986; Garofano 1980; Levin 1983; Skillman and Tzagournis 1983). Unfortunately, even well-controlled diabetics may have signs and symptoms of neuropathy.

Macrovascular disease

Macrovascular complications of diabetes are of three major types: coronary heart disease, cerebrovascular disease, and peripheral vascular disease. The incidence of all three increases dramatically with age in the general population, but even when adjusted for age, hypertension, and other factors, the incidence of each type is at least twice as high among diabetics than among nondiabetics. Atherosclerotic cardiovascular disease occurs in both Type I and Type II diabetes, but it seems to be more severe in Type II diabetics, for whom this complication is the major cause of death (Eckel and Hofeldt 1982; Skillman and Tzagournis 1983; Carter Center of Emory University 1985). The presence and progression of heart, cerebrovascular, and peripheral vascular diseases are not as strongly related to the duration and severity of diabetes as they are to age (Eckel and Hofeldt 1982). Unfortunately, glycemic control does not appear to prevent or reduce the severity of macrovascular complications in diabetes (Eckel and Hofeldt 1982; Frazin 1984; Levin 1983).

The pathology of atherosclerosis in diabetes mellitus is qualitatively similar to that which affects nondiabetics, but in diabetes, it is more common, has an earlier onset and more rapid progression, involves small vessels, and affects women more frequently (Frazin 1984; Levin 1983; Steiner 1981). Macrovascular and microvascular complications may occur simultaneously in the same patient, but progress at different rates (Frazin 1984; Skillman and Tzagournis 1983).

Age alone is a major predisposing factor to transient ischemic attacks (TIA) and CVA, but diabetes in conjunction with advancing age greatly increases the predisposition to stroke. Of all MIs in diabetic patients, silent or painless MIs are more common in elderly patients (Levin 1983). In addition, elderly diabetics have a higher fatality rate after MI than do nondiabetics (Eckel and Hofeldt 1982). Vascular changes leading to gangrene occur 53 times more often in diabetic men and 71 times more often in diabetic women than in nondiabetics, and the incidence of gangrene in the diabetic increases markedly after age 50 years (Levin 1983). Of lower-extremity amputations performed in the United States, 50% are done on diabetics (Carter Center of Emory University 1985).

Management of heart and vascular disease is the same in diabetics and nondiabetics (Eckel and Hofeldt 1982; Frazin 1984; Levin 1983). Because of the potential severity of neurologic and vascular complications in elderly diabetics, however, particular attention must be given to foot care. Specific foot care measures are presented in the boxed material on the opposite page.

Regardless of a patient's age, diabetes mellitus is a serious chronic disease. However, the cumulative effects of aging and other system disorders superimposed upon diabetes can make it a particularly disruptive disease for elderly patients, and a particularly challenging one for health-care providers. Because manifestations of the disease and responses to treatment are so different in the elderly patient than in the young, health-care professionals must be especially vigilant to meet unique needs of the elderly diabetic client. The elderly diabetic must be helped to live a full, comfortable, independent, and productive life.

Foot-care measures

Daily examination

Examine both feet entirely, including between toes. Use a mirror if necessary to see bottoms of feet.

Observe for cuts, scratches, areas of redness, and chafing.

Observe for signs of poor circulation such as pallor or cyanosis, coolness, altered hair growth, and swelling.

Daily care

Exercise feet regularly to increase circulation.

Wash feet with mild soap and warm water every day. Check water temperature with hand or elbow before putting feet into it. Pat or blot feet dry instead of rubbing.

Cut or file nails straight across.

Use lubricating lotion or cream to soften skin, but use sparingly. Don't use between toes.

Use talcum powder if feet have tendency to sweat. If used between toes, be sure to clean and dry toes well every day.

Continuing care

If your vision or mobility is seriously impaired, have someone else examine and care for your feet.

See a podiatrist every two months for care of toenails, corns, calluses, or ingrown toenails. Visit more often for blisters, sores, pain, redness, cracked nails, or swelling.

Guidelines on shoes and socks

Wear clean, unmended socks or hose every day.

Wear well-fitting, comfortable, supportive leather shoes. Don't buy shoes that will have to be "broken in" to be comfortable.

Wear extra layers of socks in cold weather. Keep feet dry in snowy and rainy weather.

Inspect shoes before wearing for foreign objects, exposed nail points, or torn linings that can cause injury.

Do not do the following

Use hot water bottles or heating pads on feet. Instead, wear socks for warmth, even in bed at night.

Wear girdles, garters, or socks and hose with tight elastic.

Go barefooted—even at home.

Use chemical agents to remove corns or calluses.

Continue to smoke.

Cut into or dig out corners of toenails.

(Adapted from Bille DA: Tailoring your diabetic patient's care plan to fit his life-style. Nurse 86, 16:55–57, 1986; Crigler-Meringola ED: Making life sweet again for the elderly diabetic. Nurse 84, 14:60–64, 1984; Frazin R: Preventing diabetic foot problems. Nurse Practitioner 9:40–41, 44–46, 50–52, 1984; Garofane CD: Helping diabetics live with their neuropathies. Nurse 80, 10:42–44, 1980; Guthrie D et al: Dealing with diabetes mellitus. In XXXX (ed): Nurses's Clinical Library—Endocrine Disorders. Springhouse, Pennsylvania, Springhouse Corp, 1984)

Nursing care plans

Medical diagnosis: Diabetes mellitus

1. Nursing diagnosis: Alteration in nutrition (more than body requirements) related to impaired carbohydrate metabolism

Goals

Patient will identify rationale and goals of diabetic diet therapy and exercise in general, and his or her diet and exercise program in particular (*items 1–4*).

Patient will adhere to therapeutic diet (*items 5–9*).

Patient will maintain or lose weight in accordance with medical plan (*items 10 and 11*).

Nursing interventions

1. Determine who is responsible for preparation of patient's meals. Include preparator in planning and teaching.
2. Assess patient's usual diet. Ascertain that it reflects the following elements.
   - Knowledge of and adherence to therapeutic diet
   - Types and amounts of foods consumed
   - Preferred, disliked foods, beverages
   - Regularity and consistency of mealtimes
   - Snacking pattern—foods and times
   - Assistance needed with food selection or preparation
   - Other family members' dietary habits and their impact on patient
   - Any difficulty associated with eating (appetite, chewing, swallowing)
3. Identify patient's usual exercise pattern.
4. Clarify misconceptions and provide instruction as needed regarding diet therapy and exercise program. (Refer to Chapter 3, Patient Education.)
5. Arrange dietary consult as needed to plan an individualized therapeutic diet or to reinforce instruction about the diet.
6. Observe and document patient's appetite and adherence to dietary regimen.
7. Use select menu system if possible to observe patient's ability to select appropriate foods. Assist and reinforce as indicated.

continued

Nursing interventions

8. Consult with dietician regarding significant changes in patient's ability to eat, appetite, activity level, or severity of illness.
9. Consult with other health-care providers as necessary to resolve poor dentition, dysphagia, or other impediments to eating.
10. Weigh the patient at regular intervals and record results.
11. Encourage maintenance of a reasonable exercise program, as possible, during hospitalization, and resumption of regular exercise upon return home.

2. Clinical nursing problem: Potential for acute complications: alterations in glycemic control

Goals

Patient will identify signs and symptoms of acute complications, their causes, and actions to be taken if they occur (*items 1–3*).
Patient will exhibit stable glycemic control (*item 4*).
Patient will demonstrate proficiency with blood and urine testing procedures (*items 5–9*).

Nursing interventions

1. Evaluate patient's ability to differentiate among and respond to acute complications. Advise that only early and mild hypoglycemia should be self-treated and that prolonged hypoglycemia, DKA, and HHNK all require immediate medical attention.
2. Identify the most likely time for a hypoglycemic reaction to occur according to the duration of action of prescribed insulin or oral agent.
3. Ensure that at least one accessible family member, neighbor, or friend is aware of signs, symptoms, and treatment of acute complications.
4. Observe for signs of acute complications and take immediate action. Be particularly alert to subtle neurologic changes that may be the only signs of impending complication.
5. Assess patient's (or family's) knowledge of usual blood and urine testing procedure and proficiency with performing the test(s).

continued

Nursing interventions

6. Identify physical or physiological factors that might interfere with accurate hospital or home testing (*e.g.,* physical limitations, procedural errors, medication interactions) and modify testing as indicated.

7. Encourage patient to continue testing as independently as possible during hospitalization after procedure has been acceptably demonstrated.

8. Ensure that test results are documented consistently and accurately. If urine glucose is tested, identify the specific test used and record results in % rather than + amounts. If patient is not doing the testing, ensure that he or she is aware of each test result, as appropriate.

9. Identify particular risk factors that make urine testing inaccurate and evaluate the need for and patient's ability to do home blood-glucose monitoring. Evaluate products and equipment available, with patient, and teach the use of chosen method.

3. Nursing diagnosis: Potential for impaired skin integrity and infection related to vascular or sensory deterioration

Goal

Patient will describe and demonstrate appropriate skin and foot-care measures and will not have skin breakdown.

Nursing interventions

1. Assess home and hospital environments and patient's habits for potential sources of injury to the skin, particularly the lower extremities (*e.g.,* ill-fitting shoes or clothing, walking barefoot, foreign objects on floor).

2. Inspect patient's skin and lower extremities daily and record findings. Share observations with patient.

3. Review and augment patient's knowledge of specific foot-care measures. Encourage as much independence in foot care as possible.

4. Insist that the patient wear shoes while out of bed.

continued

Nursing interventions

5. Discourage use of artificial heat sources for comfort or therapy (*e.g.*, hot water bottle, heating pad). If medically ordered, supervise closely.
6. Initiate a podiatry consultation as indicated for initial evaluation, treatment, or instruction of patient.

4. Clinical nursing problem: Alteration in comfort: neuropathy

Goals

Patient will verbalize symptoms of peripheral neuropathy (*items 1 and 2*):
  • Decreased touch, pain, and temperature sensation in lower extremities
  • Decreased touch and temperature sensation in hands
  • Pain or burning of legs particularly at night or on movement

Patient will verbalize symptoms or describe episodes of autonomic neuropathy (*item 3*):
  • Postural hypotension, syncope, resting tachycardia
  • Loss of bladder sensation and incomplete bladder emptying (neurogenic or hypotenic bladder) (*second subentry under item 3*)

Nursing interventions

1. Assess patient's presentation and respond symptomatically:
  • Observe daily for injury or skin breakdown that is likely and might otherwise be unnoticed. Reinforce foot-care measures.
  • Evaluate patient's use of cigarettes, matches. Assess impact on ability to perform self-care measures.
  • Elevation of legs, use of bed cradle, and decreased activity during pain may be helpful. Do not use heat as a pain-relief measure. Evaluate quality of rest and sleep.
2. Solve for and evaluate glucose control carefully since this complication is associated with poor control. Advise patient that signs and symptoms may decrease as control is regained and maintained.
3. Assess patient's presentation and respond symptomatically:
  • Protect from injury by use of side-rails, slow and progressive ambulation, assistance with ambulation, placing call bell within patient's reach. Take and record vital signs frequently, particularly during symptomatic episodes. Use elastic stockings to increase venous return if not contraindicated. Use blood glucose monitoring to differentiate hypotensive from hypoglycemic episodes.
  • Teach patient to prevent infection by emptying bladder every few hours in smaller

continued

Nursing interventions

amounts rather than longer intervals with larger amounts. Instruct patient in Credé's maneuver to assist in emptying bladder. Do not rely on urine glucose test results to indicate glycemic control in patient. Teach patient to recognize early signs and symptoms of bladder infection, as well as preventive measures. (Refer to Nursing Care Plans, #12 in Chapter 12, the Genitourinary System.)

5. Clinical nursing problem: Alteration in comfort: neuropathy (continued)

Goal

Patient will not have
  • Sexual dysfunction (*item 1*)
  • Nausea and vomiting, delayed gastric emptying (*item 2*)
  • Constipation (*item 3*)
  • Diarrhea, fecal incontinence (*item 4*)
  • Profuse sweating (*item 5*)

Nursing interventions

1. Refer to Nursing Care Plans, #13, Chapter 12.
2. Evaluate impact on patient's appetite, food, and fluid intake, and ability to maintain glycemic control, prevent ketosis, and maintain fluid and electrolyte balance.
3. Refer to Nursing Care Plans, #1, Chapter 10.
4. Refer to Nursing Care Plans, #7 and #8, Chapter 10.
5. Evaluate site of sweating (legs and feet versus head and trunk) and determine options. Reinforce foot-care and skin-care measures. Evaluate food-induced diaphoresis and eliminate offending foods from diet. Use blood-glucose monitoring as necessary to differentiate this condition from hypoglycemia.

6. Nursing diagnosis: Potential self-care deficit related to visual or physical impairment

Goal

Patient will demonstrate ability to perform self-care measures that require visual acuity and neuromuscular coordination.

Nursing interventions

1. Evaluate patient's ability to
  • Read (labels, instructions, menus)
  • Prepare and administer insulin or oral hypoglycemic agents
  • Perform blood and urine tests
  • Inspect own skin and feet

continued

Nursing interventions

2. Consult with ophthalmologist or optometrist to determine if decreased visual acuity is the temporary result of poor glycemic control or a longterm problem.
3. Identify alternative resources or equipment to help the impaired diabetic patient continue to perform self-care measures, or to assist with activities which he or she can no longer do adequately or safely.

7. Nursing diagnosis: Potential for impaired home-maintenance management related to lack of knowledge or acceptance of disease

Goal

Patient will adequately describe the disease process of diabetes, its treatment, complications, and the lifestyle modifications that are required.

Nursing interventions

1. Encourage and allow patient to describe his or her understanding of the following aspects of diabetes:
   - Pathophysiology
   - Signs and symptoms
   - Therapeutic diet
   - Exercise, including sexual activity
   - Insulin or oral agents—drug name, action, route, use, dose, side-effects, precautions with administration
   - Skin and foot care
   - Acute complications
   - Chronic complications
   - Urine and blood testing measures
   - Limitations imposed by disease, and concerns regarding self-care at home
2. Clarify misconceptions and provide written and verbal information about each above topic as required. (Consult the current professional literature, and Chapter 3, Patient Education.)
3. Evaluate patient's acceptance of the disease, and plan support accordingly. (Refer to Chapter 15, Psychosocial Care.)
4. Encourage patient to assume as much independence and responsibility for self-care as possible during hospitalization.

References

Bennett PH: Basis of the present classification of diabetes. Adv Exp Med Biol 189:17–29, 1985

Bergman M, Auerhahn C: Exercise and diabetes. Am Fam Phys 32:105–111, 1985

Bessman A, Kasim S: Managing foot infections in the older diabetic patient. Geriatrics 40:54–63, 1985

Bierman EL: Diet and diabetes. Am J Clin Nutr 41(suppl 5):1113–1116, 1985

Bille DA: Tailoring your diabetic patient's care plan to fit his life-style. Nurs 86, 16:55–57, 1986

Burggraf V, Donlon B: Assessing the elderly. Am J Nurs 85:974–984, 1985

Campbell K: Treating diabetes in the 1980's and beyond. American Pharmacy NS24:52–65, 1984

Carter Center of Emory University: Closing the gap: The problem of diabetes mellitus in the United States. Diabetes Care 8:391–406, 1985

Clinical Brief: Thirst and osmoregulation in the elderly. Lancet 2:1017, 1984

Clinical Brief: Urine testing: Ritual with no reason? Am J Nurs 85:13–14, 1985

Clinical Brief: Testing blood glucose in type II diabetes. Am J Nurs 86:647, 1986

Crigler-Meringola ED: Making life sweet again for the elderly diabetic. Nurs 84, 14:60–64, 1984

Cryer PE: Endocrinology. In Steinberg F (ed): Care of the Geriatric Patient, 6th ed, p 275. St. Louis, CV Mosby, 1983

Eckel RH, Hofeldt FD: Endocrinology and metabolism in the elderly. In Schrier R (ed): Clinical Internal Medicine in the Aged, pp 225–255. Philadelphia, WB Saunders, 1982

Essig M: Update your knowledge of oral antidiabetic agents. Nurs 83, 13:58–63, 1983

Fitzgerald PL: Exercise for the elderly. Med Clin N Am 69:189–196, 1985

Frazin R: Preventing diabetic foot problems. Nurs Prac 9:40–41, 44–46, 50–52, 1984

Funnell MM, McNitt P: Autonomic neuropathy: Diabetic's hidden foes. Am J Nurs 86:266–270, 1986

Garofano CD: Helping diabetics live with their neuropathies. Nurs 80, 10:42–44, 1980

Gioiella EC, Bevil CW: Nursing Care of the Aging Client: Promoting Healthy Adaptation. Norwalk, Connecticut, Appleton-Century-Crofts, 1985

Goldberg AP, Andes R, Bierman EL: Diabetes mellitus in the elderly. In Andres R, Bierman E, Hazzard W: Principles of Geriatric Medicine, p 750. New York, McGraw-Hill, 1985

Goodkin G: Mortality factors in diabetes. J Occup Med 17:716–721, 1975

Govoni LE, Hayes JE: Drugs and Nursing Implications, 5th ed. Norwalk, Connecticut, Appleton-Century-Crofts, 1985

Grace T: Hyperosmolar nonketotic diabetic coma. Am Fam Phys 32:119–125, 1985

Green FD, Ghafour IM, Allan D et al: Colour vision of diabetics. Br J Ophthalmol 69:533–536, 1985

Guthrie D, Guthrie R, Walters J: Dealing with diabetes mellitus. In XXXX (ed): Nurse's Clinical Library—Endocrine Disorders. Springhouse, Pennsylvania, Springhouse Corp, 1984

Hanuschak LN, Duncan TG: Why having older diabetics self-monitor blood sugar pays off. Geriatrics 40:91–92, 95–96, 98, 1985

Hayter J: Diabetes and the older person. Geriatr Nurs 2:32–36, 1981a

Hayter J: Why response to medication changes with age. Geriatr Nurs 2:411–416, 441, 1981b

Hudson M: Drugs and the older adult—take special care. Nurs 84, 14:46–51, 1984

Kelly B: Methods of glycosuria testing: A reference for nursing personnel. Diabetes Educator 5(2, Summer):7–12, 1979

Laakso M, Pyorala K: Age of onset and type of diabetes. Diabetes Care 8:114–117, 1985

Lawrence AM, Abraira C: Glucagon and diabetes mellitus. In Podolsky S (ed): Clinical Diabetes: Modern Management, p 594. New York, Appleton-Century-Crofts, 1980

Lefebvre P, Luyckx A: Hypoglycemia. In Ellenberg M, Rifkin H (eds): Diabetes Mellitus: Theory and Practice, 3rd ed, p 1001. New Hyde Park, New York, Medical Examination Publishing, 1983

Levin ME: Diabetes mellitus. In Steinberg F (ed): Care of the Geriatric Patient, 6th ed, pp 154–181. St. Louis, CV Mosby, 1983

Luckman J, Sorensen KC: Medical–Surgical Nursing: A Psychophysiologic Approach, 2nd ed, p 1571. Philadelphia, WB Saunders, 1980

Miller BK, White N: Diabetes assessment guide. Am J Nurs 80:1314–1316, 1980

Nasr H: Endocrine disorders in the elderly. Med Clin N Amer 67:481–495, 1983

Podolsky S, Bradley RF: Treatment of diabetes with insulin. In Podolsky S (ed): Clinical Diabetes: Modern Management, p 113. New York, Appleton-Century-Crofts, 1980

Podolsky S, Krall L, Bradley RF: Treatment of diabetes with oral hypoglycemic agents. In Podolsky S (ed): Clinical Diabetes: Modern Management, pp 149, 154–158. New York, Appleton-Century-Crofts, 1980

Prendergast BD: Glyburide and glipizide, second generation oral sulfonylurea hypoglycemia agents. Clin Pharm 3:473–485, 1984

Schumann D: Mastering the art of assessment. In Nursing Skillbook—Managing Diabetes Properly, pp 101–114. Horsham, Pennsylvania, Intermed Communications, 1981

Shuman CR: Optimum insulin use in older diabetics. Geriatrics 39:71–89, 1984

Sibbald RG, Schachter RK: The skin and diabetes mellitus. Int J Dermatol 23:567–584, 1984

Skillman TG, Tzagournis M: Diabetes Mellitus. Kalamazoo, Michigan, Upjohn Co, 1983

Spenser RT: Patient Care in Endocrine Problems, p 141. Philadelphia, WB Saunders, 1973

Steffl BM: Handbook of Gerontological Nursing, pp 417–418. New York, Van Nostrand Reinhold, 1984

Steiner G: Diabetes and atherosclerosis—an overview. Diabetes 30(suppl 2):1–7, 1981

Stock-Barkman P: Confusing concepts—is it diabetic shock or diabetic coma? Nurs 83, 13:33–41, 1983

Surr CW: Part I: Teaching patients to use the new blood-glucose monitoring products. Nurs 83, 13:42–45, 1983a

Surr CW: Part II: Teaching patients to use the new blood-glucose monitoring products. Nurs 83, 13:58–62, 1983b

Thatcher G: Insulin injections—the case against random rotation. Am J Nurs 85:690–692 (as corrected 85:836), 1985

Thirst and osmoregulation in the elderly. Lancet (2) 8410:1017–1018, 1984

Walther RR, Harber LC: Expected skin complaints of the geriatric patient. Geriatrics 39:67–69, 72–74, 79–80, 1984

Williams TF: Diabetes mellitus. Clin Endocrinol Metab 10:179–194, 1981

Yurick AG, Spier BE, Robb SS, Ebert NJ: The Aged Person and the Nursing Process. Norwalk, Connecticut, Appleton-Century-Crofts, 1984

Suggested readings

Cleary M: Aiding the person who is visually impaired from diabetes. Diabetes Educator 11(winter):12–23, 1985

Controlling the insulin balance. Am J Nurs 86:1239–1258, 1986

> Haire-Joshu D, Flavin K, Clutter W: Contrasting type I and type II diabetes, pp 1240–1243

> Flavin K and Haire-Joshu D: The pharmacologic repertoire, pp 1244–1250

> Haire-Joshu D, Flavin K, Santiago J: Intensive conventional insulin therapy, pp 1251–1255

> Bates S, Ahern J: Tight control: What does it mean? pp 1256–1258

Heins J, Wylie-Rosett J, Davis SG: The new look in diabetic diets. Am J Nurs 87:196–198, 1987

Jeffries MR, McIntosh EN: Diabetes education and the older patient. Diabetes Educator 11(summer):27, 34, 1985

Nemchik R: Diabetes today: Facing up to the long-term complications. RN 46:38–44, 1983

Thomas K: Diabetes in the elderly. In VanSon A (ed): Diabetes and Patient Education: A Daily Nursing Challenge, pp 115–128. New York, Appleton-Century-Crofts, 1982

Schumann D: Appraisal of the diabetic patient. The Diabetes Educator: Part I—7(4, Winter):15–21, 34, 1982; Part II—8(1, Spring):24–29, 1982; Part III—8(2, Summer):19–22, 1982

Mary Jackle

Genitourinary system 12

In general, the age-related changes in the genitourinary system of the elderly are similar to those of other body systems. Normal aging is not a deterrent to continence or sexual functioning; however, mental health, physical illness, and cognitive functioning of the elderly person can have a significant impact on his or her renal and genitourinary system. The nurse's attitude and treatment of the subject can spell success or failure in situations such as a bladder-training program or a counselling session for a distorted self-image after a prostatectomy.

Age-related changes

Kidneys

Many studies have been done of the aging process in the kidneys. It is difficult to differentiate changes that result from aging from those caused by disease. The nurse needs to know the age-related changes that are common to the kidneys and genitourinary tract in order to distinguish the normal from the disease-related.

The renal capacity of a healthy young person far exceeds the body's needs for regulating hemostasis. An elderly person's renal function is substantially diminished, but still provides for adequate regulation under ordinary circumstances; however, the ability to respond to physiological stress and challenge is reduced. Therefore, when under the stress of illness, the kidneys take longer to make needed adjustments (Sourander and Rowe 1985).

Nephrons and blood vessels

Aging causes a decrease in the size and weight of all the body organs, including the kidneys. The number and size of the nephrons are reduced and are replaced by interstitial connective tissue.

The glomerular tufts, which make up the filtering surface of the kidneys, become sclerotic with age (Fig. 12-1). From age 30 years to 50 years, 1% to 2% of the nephrons are lost, increasing to a 12% loss after age 70. When a glomerular tuft collapses, the lumen of the preglomerular arteriole is obliterated and blood is shunted from the afferent to efferent arterioles without being filtered.

Sclerotic changes are also common in the walls of the larger renal vessels, decreasing the amount of blood presented to the glomeruli for filtration. Additionally, diseases such as hypertension, diabetes mellitus, and pyelonephritis often cause damage to the smaller renal arteries, further diminishing blood flow (Sourander and Rowe 1985).

Functional results of changes

Clearance.   These sclerotic changes cause the glomerular filtration rate (GFR) to progressively decline in healthy persons by about 5% per decade after the age of 40. By the age of 80 the GFR in many elderly persons may be 50% of former capacity (Sourander and Rowe 1985). This level of function is adequate unless illness or severe environmental stress occurs. Overmedication and illnesses such as shock, severe dehydration, inflammatory processes, and hypertension may damage the remaining glomeruli, quickly resulting in renal failure. The elderly patient

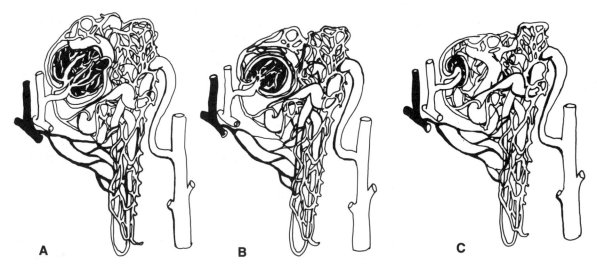

*Figure 12-1. Loss of glomeruli in the aging kidney. **A.** Narrowing of glomerular artery. **B.** Partial degeneration of glomerular tuft. **C.** Loss of glomerulus.*

also excretes drugs more slowly, resulting in higher blood levels and toxicity if the dose is not titrated.

Fluid and electrolyte balance. Aging renal tubules have a decreased ability to concentrate urine, thus their ability to conserve water is also decreased. Concentrating ability is lost at a rate of about 5% per decade after age 40. The healthy elderly person's kidneys, however, are able generally to maintain normal fluid, acid-base, and electrolyte balance (Sourander and Rowe 1985).

In stress conditions, however, the elderly are at much greater risk of dehydration. Along with the impairment of water conservation in the kidney, intake of fluids may be diminished because of immobility, inability to communicate, and a decreased sensation of thirst with age (Lye 1985). A large volume of body water may be lost if the elderly patient is stressed by gastrointestinal disorders, uncontrolled diabetes mellitus, respiratory infection with increased respiration, or conditions that cause fever.

Hypernatremia (serum sodium >145 mEq/L) may occur because of the relative decrease in body water. Sodium depletion is sometimes seen in elderly patients because of excessive loss caused by diuretics (especially the thiazides), vomiting, diarrhea, burns, and pancreatitis (Lye 1985).

Hypokalemia (serum potassium <3 mEq/L) may result from gastrointestinal tract losses through vomiting and diarrhea, and through laxative abuse. Thiazide and loop diuretics also cause loss of potassium, and require use of potassium supplements. If an elderly patient's medication is switched to a potassium-sparing diuretic, but the patient continues to take the potassium supplement, hyperkalemia (serum potassium >5.5 mEq/L) may result. Hyperkalemia may also develop in patients who have large areas of tissue necrosis because potassium is liberated from the injured cells (Lye 1985).

Genitourinary tract

Bladder

Aging also causes changes in the structure and function of the lower urinary tract (Fig. 12-2). The capacity of the bladder is reduced from about 500 ml to 250 ml because of loss of elasticity of smooth muscle and other changes in the bladder wall. Bladder filling may be interrupted by bladder contractions, which cause a desire to void. Loss of muscle tone may impair complete emptying of the bladder. The urinary stream is slower and at lower pressure, and a large residual urine may remain (Gioiella and Bevil 1985).

Because of these changes, elderly patients feel the need to void more frequently and in smaller amounts. Incomplete emptying may predispose the patient to bladder infections, which increases symptoms of urgency and frequency. These changes in voiding patterns, accompanied by decreased mobility, set the stage for the development of incontinence. In addition, nocturia can cause safety problems, when the patient attempts to walk to the bathroom in darkness. If the patient is

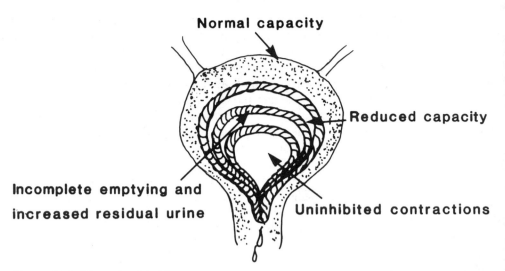

Figure 12-2. The aging bladder.

able to use the bathroom unassisted, leave a nightlight on, the side-rail down and walking aids within reach. If the patient needs assistance, offer the urinal on rounds. How often is an elderly patient labeled "incontinent" when he or she couldn't possibly get out of the bed or call for help for lack of a call button?

Pelvic diaphragm

Women often lose muscle tone in the pelvic floor, with a resulting prolapse of the urethra at the external meatus. Contributing factors include weakened pelvic musculature associated with birth trauma and tissue changes in the vaginal epithelium from estrogen deficiency. These changes also affect the trigone area of the bladder and may cause urinary symptoms such as burning, pain, frequency, and stress incontinence (Gioiella and Bevil 1985).

Prostate

In men, nodular hyperplasia of the prostate begins during the fifth decade. This process is usually not malignant, but still results in a narrowing of the urethra near the neck of the bladder and protrusion into the cavity of the bladder that mechanically obstructs bladder emptying (McNeal 1985).

The patient may complain of difficulty initiating voiding, diminished stream of urine, and frequent voidings of small quantities of urine. If large amounts of urine are retained in the bladder, a feeling of heaviness or dull pain is present, and distension can be palpated. Chronic urinary retention often is complicated by urinary infection, with the classic symptoms of frequency, urgency, and burning on urination.

In the longterm-care setting, it is important to maintain on-going vigilance regarding the adequacy of urinary output in elderly male patients. Assessment should include examination of the lower abdomen to check for bladder distension.

Surgical repair of bladder prolapse in women and prostatic hypertrophy in men requires the usual nursing considerations in caring for elderly surgical patients. Specific potential postoperative problems that must be considered are: urinary retention, dysuria, and re-establishment of urinary continence. The surgical procedure may disrupt nerves and muscles involved in voiding. Usual sensations of bladder fullness and the need to void may be masked by incisional pain and the use of analgesics. In addition, the patient's normal voiding habits will be changed by hospitalization. Anxiety and embarrassment about urinary function, use of urinals and bedpans, and asking others for help with elimination may also cause difficulty in re-establishing normal patterns.

Malignancy

Malignant changes in the lower urinary tract occur in many elderly patients. Carcinoma of the prostate accounts for 18% of malignancies in American men, and the rate of incidence increases rapidly with old age (Karr and Murphy 1984). Bladder cancer is the second-most-common neoplasm of the genitourinary tract. The incidence is three times higher in men than women and the average age of onset is 68 years (Riehle and Vaughan 1984). Depending on location, stage, and type of malignancy, medical treatment may include surgery, radiation, and chemotherapy.

Bladder control problem

Incontinence is estimated to be a problem for about one in ten older people in the community and one in two of the institutionalized elderly population. The incidence increases progressively with age, and most of these patients are also limited in mobility (Brocklehurst 1985). The estimated annual cost of incontinence care in nursing homes is 8 billion dollars, or a third of the total cost of institutional care in the United States (Whitehead et al 1984). This problem is devastating to continued independent living and self-esteem in elderly persons and is a frequent cause for seeking institutional care.

Neurological causes

The ability to control bladder emptying can be impaired by a number of diseases or injuries at various levels within the central nervous system (CNS). Lesions in the cerebral cortex (seen in cerebral vascular accident [CVA], tumor, dementia, Parkinsonism, and normal pressure hydrocephalus) may cause an *uninhibited neurogenic bladder* (Fig. 12-3), in which the sensation of bladder filling is retained but the ability to inhibit bladder emptying is lost (Brocklehurst 1985).

DISORDERS OF NEUROLOGIC CONTROL

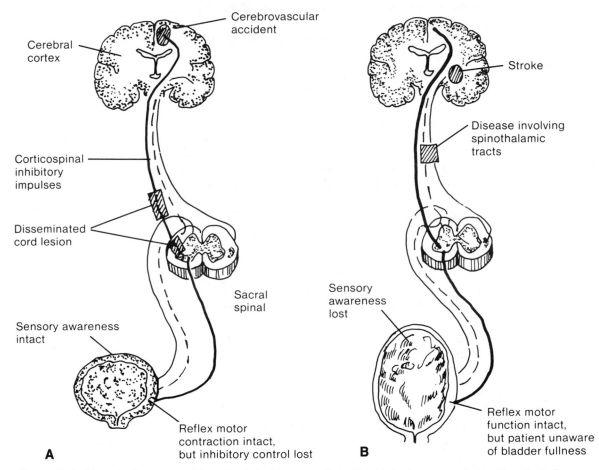

Figure 12-3. Neurologic causes of impaired bladder control. **A.** *Uninhibited neurogenic bladder.* **B.** *Reflex neurogenic bladder.*

Any pathological process that interrupts sensory pathways in the spinal cord (such as tumors, disc prolapse, infarct) can lead to a loss of sensation of bladder fullness, while the reflex motor function remains unimpaired. The result is a *reflex neurogenic bladder* (Fig. 12-3) with overflow incontinence (Brocklehurst 1985).

Diseases such as tabes dorsalis and diabetic neuropathy can cause *atonic bladder,* an impairment of the voiding reflex, resulting in bladder distention, urinary retention, and overflow (Brocklehurst 1985).

Some elderly patients have no evidence of neurologic disease, but still have an *unstable bladder,* which develops uninhibited contractions as a response to filling, or to stimuli such as coughing, laughing, or changing position. These patients may be otherwise asymptomatic, or may also have frequency, nocturia, urgency, and urge incontinence (Brocklehurst 1985).

Transient causes

Sometimes incontinence accompanies other underlying disease, and clears up as the disease is successfully treated. Some examples are

- Acute confusional disorders, resulting from pneumonia, cardiovascular disease, and toxemias
- Acute CVA with cerebral edema that affects bladder control pathways for several days
- Acute urinary tract infection
- Becoming bedfast for any reason and thus unable to maintain usual routines.

Precipitating factors

Incontinence in the elderly may be precipitated by sensory loss and inability to find the lavatory, mobility problems, constipation, use of tranquilizers and night sedation, powerful diuretics, inappropriate fluid intake, clothing that is difficult to manage, and impaired manual dexterity.

Anxiety, fear, grief, and depression from loss of significant others, home, and so forth, may also be associated with incontinence. Because incontinence is a cultural taboo, the elderly person may respond to it with embarrassment, denial, fear, or anxiety. In a recent study, psychological testing implied that emotional disturbances were secondary to voiding dysfunction, rather than its cause (Millard and Oldenberg 1983).

Treatment

The evaluation of an incontinent patient is a collaborative responsibility of both physicians and nurses. The medical diagnosis includes a history, physical examination, and urinalysis with a culture. Causes such as urinary tract infection, constipation, and gynecologic problems such as stress incontinence from cystocele, are found in about 60% of elderly women evaluated. If none of these causes is identified, then invasive tests such as cystoscopy, cystography, and cystometry are undertaken to uncover neurologic causes or bladder-outlet obstruction. Medical treatment may involve surgical removal of obstruction, a trial of antispasmodic drugs for unstable bladder, and treatment of any underlying disease (Stanton 1984). Nursing evaluation includes specific information about the behavioral and environmental influences that affect a patient's voiding profile, and the patient's perception of the problem. On the basis of their evaluations, the health-care team decides whether a behavioral program to control or cure the problem is warranted, or if a consultation is needed on measures and products to manage incontinence (McCormick and Burgio 1984).

A number of behavioral measures to control incontinence are within the scope of nursing practice. *"Kegel exercises"* have been used for many years to treat stress incontinence in women, and are appropriate for patients who have intact cognitive function. The patient is taught to tighten the perineal muscles as though stopping the expulsion of urine, and is also instructed to repeatedly start and stop the flow of urine while voiding. These exercises are done with four repetitions, four times a day, for 2 months to 3 months, to improve bladder control (Gettrust et al 1985).

Biofeedback involves using a manometer attached to a bladder catheter to provide visual, and sometimes auditory, feedback of bladder pressure during filling, the sensation of abdominal pressure and external anal sphincter activity. The patient learns to correlate bladder sensation with actual capacity and pressure. If contractions start, the patient is taught to inhibit them. On average, six one-hour sessions are needed to acquire the skills. Biofeedback may be used in combination with other methods (Millard and Oldenburg 1983).

Habit training, also called bladder training or drill, aims to achieve two-hour to four-hour voiding schedules with no accidents. It is used frequently in nursing homes, and some studies have shown success rates of 75% (Clay 1980). A record is kept for several days of the patient's voiding patterns to identify preventable causes of incontinence and to provide a baseline against which the effects of treatment can be evaluated (Fig. 12-4). Then the patient is taught to void at predetermined times, whether or not a sensation to void is present. The following procedure is used

Day 1	Ask the patient to void every 2 hours. Record all voiding on the bladder record.
Day 2	Toilet the patient at the time he or she was dry and able to void on day 1.
	Toilet the patient one half-hour earlier than the time he or she was wet on day 1.
Day 3 and after	Continue to adjust the schedule until the patient is continent. Then continue this schedule for 5 days. After 5 days of continence, gradually increase the length of the intervals by 1/2 hour until the patient is continent at 3-hour to 4-hour intervals (Clay 1980).

To break the habit of very frequent voiding that may have been established before treatment, patients who are cognitively intact may be taught to use controlled breathing, mental distraction, and perineal pressure to postpone voiding for 5 minutes each time (Millard and Oldenburg 1983).

Date ___March 27___

Instructions:
1. In the 1st column, mark the time every time you void.
2. In the 2nd or 3rd column, mark every time you accidently leak urine.
3. Write "dry" if no accident occurs in the 2-hour interval.

Time interval	Urinated in toilet	Leaking accident	or	Large accident	Reason for accident
6–8 am	✓				
8–10 am	✓	✓			
10–12 am	dry				
12–2 pm	✓				
2–4 pm	dry				
4–6 pm				✓	Drank 3 cups of tea
6–8 pm	✓				
8–10 pm	✓				
10–12 pm	dry				
Overnight				✓	Didn't wake up

Figure 12-4. Record of bladder control.

The use of reinforcers such as tokens for special privileges or treats, snack-foods, verbal praise, and social interaction have been helpful in reducing incontinence, particularly with institutionalized patients.

Rewards for staff members who successfully carry out habit-training with patients are also appropriate. The nurse is the leader of the caregiving team, and must be aware that caring for incontinent patients is a burden for staff members and family caregivers. Incontinence of urine is a stigma; it commonly elicits ostracism and psychological and social discrediting from other persons. Observing genitalia and handling excreta, combined with the heavy and unremitting physical efforts of care, become sources of emotional stress for caregivers. Dehumanization of the patient, anger, and abuse may result unless caregivers are assisted to manage the problem (Wells 1984).

The changes in the genitourinary tract seen in aging can cause a number of symptoms besides incontinence. Most common are:

Nocturnal frequency: Resulting from loss of renal ability to concentrate urine, and decreased bladder capacity, estimated to affect 50% to 70% of the elderly

Difficulty in initiating voiding: A result of benign prostatic hypertrophy or neurological deficit in the voiding reflex, seen in 10% to 20% of the elderly

Urinary infection: Often a chronic condition in the elderly, which may be asymptomatic, although progressive (Brocklehurst 1985).

Altered sexual patterns

So much emphasis is placed on sexual performance that those elderly persons who are not interested in sex can be made to feel that something is wrong with them. As Carnevali and Patrick (1986) point out, "This is not consistent with the beliefs and values of many people born and raised in the 1900s. As in all other areas of aging, there is a wide range of interest and activity in sexual matters."

The material in the box (below) lists the normal sexual changes associated with aging. It can be assumed that normal sexual functioning can take place into the eighth and ninth decades. Once again, professional nursing attitudes play a large part in how elderly patients respond. In actuality, the skills required for sexual-health care are not so very different from the skills needed for comprehensive nursing care. Nurses should be able to provide the following care:

- Use the nursing process of assessment, planning, implementation, and evaluation to promote positive sexual health

---

Age-related sexual changes in men and women

Male	*Female*
An erection takes longer to develop and may not be as full or firm as in younger years.	More time is needed to respond to sexual stimulation.
Ejaculation lasts a shorter time and has a less forceful emission.	Lubrication takes longer and may be less effective.
The erection subsides rapidly after ejaculation.	The vagina has a reduced elasticity.
Semen volume is reduced and testes are decreased in size.	The clitoris is reduced in size but still very responsive.
There is an increased refractory period between erections.	Orgasms are less intense and of shorter duration (Kart et al 1978).

- Provide education and counseling in sexuality
- Make referrals to appropriate sources for sexual problems needing intervention beyond the nurse's ability (Burnside 1981)

History and assessment

Gathering specific subjective and objective information from persons who have renal and genitourinary problems requires sensitivity and tact because the subject is intensely personal to clients, who may find difficulties with elimination to be embarrassing. One study found that 84% of women who were incontinent of urine initially reported no problem on interview (Yarnell et al 1981). Many people consider such problems to be an inevitable and untreatable part of old age. Consistently, the sexual history of elderly patients is omitted in histories, most often because of the embarrassment of the interviewing nurse. The nurse should be concerned with the status of past as well as current significant relationships that involve sexual activity, and the degree to which these relationships satisfied the patient. The interview section concerning sexual information can be handled in a variety of ways, delaying it until after a comfortable rapport has been established, and broaching the subject when discussing family relationships or loss of significant others. These data can also be obtained from female patients during the gynecologic history (Mezey et al 1980). Respect the patient's decision whether or not to answer questions. An overly enthusiastic, insensitive practitioner may create feelings of conflict and cause the patient embarrassment.

Subjective information

Table 12-1 shows subjective data for assessing urinary function.

Table 12-1. **Subjective information for assessing urinary function**

Question	Normal range	Symptom pursuit
1. About how often do you pass urine during the day? During the night?	q 3–4 hr 1–2 times	Diuretic use Urinalysis for bacteria Intake of caffeine or other irritants Intake before going to bed
2. Are you able to postpone voiding or is the sensation too urgent?	Can postpone 5 min	
3. Do you have trouble starting to void?	Some hesitancy may exist past age 60.	Check for prostatic hypertrophy
4. Have you noticed decreased force of the urine stream?		

continued

Table 12-1. (Continued)

Question	Normal range	Symptom pursuit
5. Has there been any change in urine		
Color?	Golden yellow	Urinalysis for bacteria, blood, pus
Odor?		Urinalysis for acetone
Amount?	500 ml minimum	Fluid intake and loss
		24-hr specimen
		Blood chemistry for clearance of urea, creatinine
		Electrolytes
		Urinalysis for casts
6. Do you have any trouble controlling your urine?		
When did it start?		Use bladder record (see Fig. 12-4) for a week
What do you think caused it?		Check for cystoceles
Describe what happens (time, frequency day and night, amount of urine, its relationship to coughing, sneezing, and laughing).		
Does this interfere in any way with your daily life?		
Home circumstances: difficult to get to toilet, help at home, support from relatives?		Home visit to assess adequacy
Disabling conditions:		
Vision?		Eye examination
Mobility?		Walking and toilet aids needed
Manual dexterity?		Assess clothing for adaptive needs
Episodes of constipation?		Check for impaction
Recent psychological trauma?		
Orientation?		Mental status exam
Use of sedation, tranquilizers?		
How have you tried to handle this problem (protective pads, fluid restriction, activity restriction)?		
7. (For women) Have you felt any soreness, itching, or burning in your genital area?		Assess mobility, and personal hygiene
		Assess adequacy of vaginal secretions.
(For men) Have you noticed any change in the size of your scrotum and penis?		Examine for hernias, hydrocele, tumors.
8. Do you have any sexual difficulties or concerns that you'd like to discuss?		Option to discuss topic is the patient's.
Are you presently sexually active?		
If particular problems (see box, page 298) exist, what do you think may be the cause?		
Do you have any problems with family members objecting to your sexuality, feelings, and friendships?		Assess coping patterns and interactions with significant others

Objective data

Examination of women

During a physical examination, or while giving nursing care, note abnormalities in the genital mucosa such as whitish plaques, lesions, lumps, and signs of irritations or infection. As a result of relaxed pelvic muscles, the urethral meatus may be very near or within the vaginal opening. Also note any vaginal inflammation or profuse vaginal discharge, which should be cultured. Vaginal secretions are normally decreased because of low estrogen levels. Ask the patient to bear down and observe for urine leakage or bulging of mucosa into the vagina. Check the strength of the pelvic muscles by asking the patient to tighten the perineal muscle on the examining finger in the vagina. Any amount of pressure felt suggests some muscle tone (Gioiella and Bevil 1985).

Examination of men

The prostate gland as palpated through the rectal wall is normally smooth, firm, and about 1.5 inches in diameter. Observe the urethral meatus for discharge, irritation, or lesions (Gioiella and Bevil 1985).

Other observations

As the bladder fills, it becomes pear-shaped and rises into the abdomen, where it can be palpated. The bladder must contain at least 150 ml of urine to be palpated about 1 inch to 2 inches above the symphysis pubis at the midline. When the bladder contains more than 500 ml of urine, it is visible as a tense, bulging mass in the lower abdomen (McConnell 1985).

The nurse should also note signs of overhydration or dehydration, vital signs, and the general state of the patient's personal hygiene.

Laboratory data for nursing assessment

Most of the normal values on the serum chemistry are unchanged in elderly persons, except for slight increases in uric acid, potassium, and creatinine, and an increase in blood urea nitrogen (BUN) to a normal of 10–38 mg/100 ml. The normal ratio of creatinine to BUN is 15:1. When both rise and maintain this ratio, an excess of nitrogenous compounds in the blood is indicated, the result of impaired renal clearance. When only the BUN is elevated, dehydration is often the cause (Gioiella and Bevil 1985).

Urinalysis data also have the same normal values in elderly persons as in younger adults. It is difficult, however, to obtain an uncontaminated specimen from elderly women. It is important to carefully instruct the patient about cleansing procedures, and how to catch a midstream specimen. If the patient is unable to do this, the nurse should carry out the procedure. Catheterization is the only practical method of obtaining an uncontaminated specimen from the incontinent patient, even though the procedure carries a risk of infecting the urinary tract (Gioiella and Bevil 1985).

The aging renal and genitourinary tract and drugs

Drugs used to treat renal and genitourinary problems are shown in Table 12-2. After a drug is administered and reaches the bloodstream, its passage through the body will depend upon what sort of drug it is. Some drugs are immediately metabolized in the liver; others are bound to protein or tissues, or deposited in fatty stores; and some proceed straight to the kidneys and are excreted in the urine. Because glomerular filtration is reduced by half in elderly persons, drugs that are eliminated mainly by the kidneys have a long half-life. Some examples of such drugs are digoxin, procainamide (Pronestyl), nadolol (Corgard), clonidine (Catapres), the thiazide diuretics, penicillins, aminoglycoside antibiotics, sulfamethizole, and methotrexate. Other common problems such as dehydration and urinary-tract infections further reduce the rate of drug elimination. Therefore, when treating elderly patients smaller doses of such drugs should be given less frequently.

Nomograms and dosage guidelines for a number of drugs have been developed, based on the patient's creatinine-clearance test results. If this test is unavailable, dosages for elderly patients should be one-third to one-half the usual amount, given at less-frequent intervals, and gradually titrated, depending on blood levels or clinical response. Toxic effects and unintended side-effects may be more frequent, requiring close observation by the nurse for a longer period, and knowledge of the route of elimination of the drugs (Cape 1978; Wiener and Pepper 1985).

Diuretics are administered to a large majority of elderly patients, usually to treat congestive heart failure. Once the episode of congestive heart failure has been cleared, the dosage of the diuretics should be reduced. Failure to do this causes some elderly patients to become dehydrated, confused, and hypotensive on standing. The elderly are also susceptible to incontinence. Furosemide (Lasix), a frequently prescribed diuretic, is quick-acting and causes the production of large quantities of urine. In the older patient who has reduced bladder capacity and precipitancy of voiding, incontinence may result. Therefore, slower-acting drugs may be better tolerated (Cape 1978).

Drug dosages in renal failure

Decreased drug elimination by the kidney is the most important alteration seen in renal failure; however, absorption of the drug from the GI tract, distribution, and metabolism by the liver are also adversely affected by azotemia.

The selection of dose and interval that will produce a desired clinical effect in a patient with renal failure requires knowledge of the patient's creatinine clear-

Table 12-2. **Drugs used in treating renal and genitourinary problems**

Drugs	Effect/response in elderly	Nursing implications
Renal failure*		
Diuretics Furosemide (Lasix) Ethacrynic acid (Edecrin)	Increases renal tubule output of fluid, alleviates edema. Adverse: ringing in ears, hearing loss, electrolyte imbalance, incontinence.	Check intake and output, weight, serum electrolytes, and BUN.
Antiemetics Prochlorperazine (Compazine)	Decreases nausea, prevents vomiting. Adverse: jaundice, skin reactions, motor symptoms—may aggravate restless limb syndrome of uremia.	Give rectally or intramuscularly at the first sign of nausea. Check blood pressure and watch for postural hypotension.
Antacids Aluminum hydroxide (Amphojel) Aluminum carbonate (Basaljel)	Binds phosphate in the GI tract for elimination, as renal excretion is impaired. Adverse: constipation	Teach patient not to substitute antacids containing magnesium. Give stool softeners.
Sodium Polystyrene sulfonate (Kayexalate)	Binds potassium in the lower GI tract for excretion.	May need cleansing enema before administration. Give in warm enema, mix at bedside, have patient retain 1 hr. Check serum potassium levels and number of stools.
Anabolic steroids Androlone phenpropionate (Durabolin)	Improves anemia by promoting erythropoiesis. Adverse: edema, bleeding if patient is on anticoagulants, or has blood dyscrasias.	Check edema, urine and stool for blood, hematocrit, hemoglobin. Explain androgen effects to female patients.
Vitamin D	Prevention of osteoporosis caused by renal failure.	Check serum calcium and BUN. If BUN increases, stop drug. Teach patient not to use over-the-counter preparations that contain vitamin D.
Miscellaneous supplements: iron, vitamins, folic acid	Provide essential elements poorly absorbed or not included in dietary allowances.	Check serum levels, patient understanding, and compliance.

continued

Table 12-2. (Continued)

Drugs	Effect/response in elderly	Nursing implications
Urinary tract infection*		
Sulfas or antibiotics according to culture and sensitivity Trimethoprim Sulfamethoxazole (Bactrim) Amoxicillin (Amoxcil)	Kill organisms causing infection. Adverse: nausea, vomiting, allergic reaction, blood dyscrasias, neurologic symptoms.	Monitor intake and output, increase fluids to 2000 ml, give cranberry juice to acidify urine, re-culture urine in 7–14 days.
Nalidixic acid (NegGram)	Contraindicated in renal failure.	
Methenamine mandelate (Mandelamine)	Contraindicated in renal failure.	
Nitrofurantoin macrocrystals (Macrodantin)	Contraindicated in renal failure.	
Anesthetics Phenazopyridine hydrochloride (Pyridium)	Local anesthetic effect on mucosa of urinary tract; has no bacteriocidal effect. Adverse: blood dyscrasias; contraindicated in renal failure.	Instruct patient that urine will be orange-colored.
Incontinence†		
Anti-cholinergics Propantheline bromide (Pro-banthine) Tridihexethyl chloride (Pathilon) Dicyclomine hydrochloride (Bentyl)	Abolishes uninhibited bladder contractions and increases bladder capacity in uninhibited neurogenic bladder. Adverse: urinary retention, constipation, symptoms similar to those with atropine.	Increase fluid intake to minimize constipation. Examine over-the-counter drugs taken for anticholinergic effect that would be additive. Check for urinary retention.
Urinary retention†		
Cholinergics Bethanechol (Urecholine)	Increases tone and contraction of detrusor muscle of bladder in atonic neurogenic bladder and postoperative retention. Contraindicated in urinary tract obstruction with retention. Adverse: flushing, nausea, vomiting, headache, diarrhea, hypotension, asthmatic attacks, tachycardia or bradycardia, discomfort in bladder area.	Administer on empty stomach to minimize nausea. Check intake and output, blood pressure, pulse. Administer subcutaneously, never give intravenously or intramuscularly. Antidote is atropine.

* (Data from Wiener MB, Pepper G: Clinical Pharmacology and Therapeutics in Nursing, pp 491, 563. New York, McGraw-Hill, 1985)

† (Data from Brocklehurst JC: The genitourinary system—the bladder. In Brocklehurst JC: Textbook of Geriatric Medicine and Gerontology, 3rd ed, p 641. New York, Churchill Livingstone, 1985)

ance and of data on the usual half-life of the drug at the patient's level of renal function. Correct dosage is achieved usually by decreasing the amount of drug and lengthening the interval between doses.

The following principles will greatly reduce the incidence of adverse drug reactions in patients with renal failure:

- Do not give any drug unless specifically indicated. Sleeping pills, laxatives, and antacids, when ordered routinely, can have adverse effects.
- Be fully aware of the route of excretion and potential adverse effects of any drug used.
- Drugs which do not have guidelines for use in renal failure should not be used. Check all drug doses against published guidelines.
- Monitor drug blood levels, especially those with a narrow therapeutic index such as digoxin, gentamycin, phenobarbital, and phenytoin. Clinical monitoring of therapeutic effects and toxicity are also important.
- Note the amount of electrolytes in the drug preparation, especially sodium, potassium, magnesium, and phosphate, and include in the calculation of intake.
- Drugs that are dialyzable will need to be readministered at the end of dialysis (Wiener and Pepper 1985).

Nursing care plans

Medical diagnosis: Renal insufficiency or failure

1. Clinical nursing problem: Alteration in acid-base balance: ineffective renal clearance

Goal	*Nursing interventions*
Patient will maintain optimum acid-base balance.	1. Monitor blood-chemistry readings. 2. Observe for increase in rate and depth of respirations. 3. Administer bicarbonate or its precursors as ordered.

2. Clinical nursing problem: Fluid volume excess or deficit: ineffective renal regulation

Goal

Patient will maintain optimum fluid balance in intracellular and extracellular fluid compartments; ingested fluid volume will be equal to the volume of urine output.

Nursing interventions

1. Monitor vital signs.
2. Observe for signs of edema or dehydration.
3. Monitor fluid intake, output, and daily weight (in acute care: central venous pressure, pulmonary wedge pressure).
4. Monitor heart and lung sounds.
5. Monitor serum electrolytes, BUN, urine osmolality.
6. Administer diuretics or fluid replacement.

3. Clinical nursing problem: Alteration in electrolyte balance: ineffective renal clearance

Goal

Patient will maintain optimum serum electrolyte levels, and will verbalize self-care actions to prevent electrolyte imbalances.

Nursing interventions

1. Monitor blood chemistry data.
2. Observe for signs of imbalance in levels of sodium, calcium, potassium, and phosphate.
3. Administer electrolytes or electrolyte binders.
4. Teach self-care actions to prevent imbalances: foods rich in sodium, potassium, dietary restrictions, signs of electrolyte imbalance, effects of medications on electrolyte balance.

4. Nursing diagnosis: Alteration in nutrition (less than requirement) related to dietary restrictions

Goal

Patient will have sufficient personal or community resources to meet basic nutritional needs. Patient will verbalize dietary restrictions necessary to maintain health; and will maintain serum albumin levels within normal range for age.

Nursing interventions

1. Assess patient's resources for meeting basic nutritional needs.
2. Assess condition of mouth and teeth, and fit of dentures.
3. Make appropriate referrals for meeting basic nutritional needs.
4. Identify current dietary patterns, likes and dislikes.

continued

Nursing interventions

5. Teach and reinforce diet modifications: low protein, high calorie, small feedings, electrolyte content of various foods.
6. Provide optimal mealtime environment.
7. Monitor results of laboratory studies: serum albumin, total protein.
8. Monitor food intake.

5. Nursing diagnosis: Potential for injury related to altered sensory perception, secondary to ineffective waste clearance

Goal

Patient will verbalize self-care actions to compensate for decreased sensory perception.

Nursing interventions

1. Assess environment for hazards.
2. Teach safe self-care actions for bathing, application of heat, and performing domestic tasks.
3. Make appropriate referrals for correction of hazards in the patient's environment.

6. Nursing diagnosis: Knowledge deficit of disease process and therapy related to lack of instruction or motivation

Goals

Patient will verbalize the kidney functions that are impaired and the resulting physical symptoms.
Patient will participate actively in the desired self-care behaviors: dietary modification, fluid restriction, safety, access care if on dialysis.
Patient will verbalize the purpose and schedule for self-administration of medications; and if on dialysis, verbalize purpose of treatment, and related self-care actions.

Nursing interventions

1. Assess physical factors that are affecting ability to learn: fluid and electrolyte balance, azotemia, neurologic deficits.
2. Assess personal factors: age, intelligence, stage of adaptation to illness, language and cultural background, socioeconomic status, past experience and health habits, and support systems.
3. Plan teaching to meet individual needs with regard to disease process and symptomatology, self-care actions, medications, safety.
4. Use visual aids with large print to aid learning.

7. Nursing diagnosis: Noncompliance with recommended therapy related to changes in lifestyle

Goals	Nursing interventions
Patient will identify the barriers to compliance with the recommended program.	1. Assess for barriers to learning. (See Nursing Diagnosis #6, items 1 and 2, above.)
Patient will verbalize the benefits of compliance on health status, and will make an effective compromise between recommended self-care and personal needs	2. Solicit patient's point of view about the situation and recommended treatment.
	3. Encourage active involvement in making decisions about care.
Patient will have sufficient resources to make changes; and be prepared to give informed consent for life-prolonging treatment.	4. Modify recommendations to meet individual needs, present alternatives for choice.
	5. Provide simple, specific, written instructions.
	6. Give positive support for any changes made.
	7. Teach patient to increase awareness of bodily feedback (e.g., daily weights).
	8. Assess caregiver's need for relief from role.

Medical diagnosis: *Urinary incontinence*

8. Nursing diagnosis: Alteration in patterns of urinary elimination related to dysfunctional voiding pattern

Goals	Nursing interventions
Patient will eliminate or reduce incontinent episodes.	1. Assess for precipitating and contributing factors.
Patient will verbalize the cause of incontinence and rationale for treatment.	2. Reduce or eliminate any of these factors.
	3. Initiate a bladder-training program.
Patient will demonstrate the bladder training regime and verbalize measures to prevent complications.	4. Manage a meticulous skin-care program.
	5. Select and teach appropriate sanitary and hygienic methods to patient and family members.
Patient will have a residual urine of 30–50 ml or 15% of total bladder capacity.	6. Monitor voiding pattern and skin integrity.

9. Nursing diagnosis: Alteration in self-concept related to loss of control

Goals

Patient will verbalize the personal meaning of the problem to him or her.

Patient will verbalize positive, realistic perception of self.

Patient will manage the problem of incontinence in a manner that minimizes social embarrassment, and will be able to participate actively in social situations.

Nursing interventions

1. Elicit patient's view of the problem, its meaning, and identify the feelings associated with it.
2. Provide teaching about the high incidence of the problem, and methods available for coping with it.
3. Assist patient to choose methods of self-care that are personally and socially acceptable.
4. Assist patient to maintain good grooming and appearance.
5. Provide opportunities for social interactions and participation.
6. Instruct staff and family on the importance of touch and frequent positive messages to maintain patient's self-esteem.

10. Nursing diagnosis: Potential for alteration in skin integrity related to prolonged contact with urine

Goal

Patient will have intact skin and, if capable, will carry out self-care actions to prevent skin breakdown.

Nursing interventions

1. Set up a bladder-training program if feasible.
2. Initiate a schedule for frequent changing of protective padding and inspection of skin.
3. Select a skin-cleansing method and teach its consistent use to patient or caregivers.
4. Select a skin-protective agent and instruct patient or caregivers on its consistent use.
5. Observe for signs of vaginitis resulting from urinary incontinence.
6. Plan for alleviation of pressure on bony prominences at least every 2 hr.

11. Nursing diagnosis: Potential for infection related to indwelling catheters

Goals

Patient will have urinary output that is normal in content and quantity, surveillance cultures that demonstrate no growth, and normal vital signs.
Patient will verbalize self-care actions necessary for catheter maintenance

Nursing interventions

1. Select equipment that provides sterility and a closed system with no back-flow.
2. Insert the catheter under sterile conditions.
3. Instruct the patient and caregivers with regard to perineal care; positioning the tubing; emptying and recording output; and assessment of amount, color, and consistency of urine.
4. Assess vital signs, and signs and symptoms of infection.
5. Establish a plan for increased fluid intake.
6. Set up schedule for catheter irrigation, catheter replacement, urinalysis, culture and sensitivity, according to nursing service standards.
7. Monitor urinalysis (U/A) and cultures.

Medical diagnosis: *Urinary infection*

12. Nursing diagnosis: Alteration in patterns of elimination related to dysuria

Goals

Patient will experience a decrease in pain and discomfort.
Patient will identify self-care practices to prevent recurrences.

Nursing interventions

1. Assess intake and output patterns.
2. Observe for urinary retention.
3. Increase the dilution and acidity of urine by increasing fluid intake to patient's cardiovascular capacity; give cranberry juice twice a day.
4. Provide warm tub baths to alleviate discomfort.
5. Teach self-care actions to prevent infections: personal hygiene, increased fluid intake.

Medical diagnosis: Prostate tumor or prostatectomy

13. Nursing diagnosis: Altered sexual patterns related to surgical procedure

Goal

Patient will verbalize feelings in relation to sexual inadequacy or impotence.

Nursing interventions

1. Be aware of feelings of diminished self-esteem and image.
2. Spend sufficient time, allowing patient to verbalize freely.
3. Discuss altered sexual patterns with patient and with significant others or family members.
4. Allow patient time to grieve, and to become aggressive and angry in his response to another loss.
5. Arrange for counselling if appropriate.
6. Arrange for diversional activity (occupational and recreational therapy), making referral to Senior Citizens, and so forth.
7. Discuss the needs for intimacy and closeness that can still be met.

14. Nursing diagnosis: Knowledge deficit of disease, risks outcomes related to lack of instruction

Goal

Patient will be able to discuss the nature of the tumor and the need for surgical intervention.

Nursing interventions

1. Teach patient about development of prostate cancer and the aging immune system (see Chapter 9).
2. Explain the need for life-saving surgery and the inevitable impotency that will develop.
3. If appropriate, have surgeon intervene to discuss future possibility of penile prosthesis.
4. Bring family and significant others into discussion.
5. Assess coping patterns with new knowledge, asking for feedback and comprehension.

References

Brocklehurst JC: The genitourinary system—the bladder. In Brocklehurst JC: Textbook of Geriatric Medicine and Gerontology, 3rd ed, p 626. New York, Churchill Livingstone, 1985

Cape R: Aging: Its Complex Management. New York, Harper & Row, 1978

Carnevali D, Patrick M (eds): Nursing Management for the Elderly. Philadelphia, JB Lippincott, 1986

Clay E: Urinary continence/incontinence. Habit retraining: A tested method to regain urinary control. Geriatr Nurs 1:252–254, 1980

Gioiella EC, Bevil CW: Nursing Care of the Aging Client. Norwalk, Connecticut, Appleton-Century-Crofts, 1985

Karr JP, Murphy GP: Carcinoma of the prostate and its management. In Brocklehurst JC (ed): Urology in the Elderly, p 203. New York, Churchill Livingstone, 1984

Kart CS, Metress ES, Metress JF: Aging and Health: Biologic and Social Perspectives. Menlo Park, California, Addison-Wesley Publishing Co, 1978

Lye MDW: The milieu interieur and aging. In Brocklehurst JC (ed): Textbook of Geriatric Medicine and Gerontology, 3rd ed, p 216. New York, Churchill Livingstone, 1985

Millard RJ, Oldenburg BF: The symptomatic, urodynamic, and psychodynamic results of bladder re-education programs. J Urol 130:715–719, 1983

McConnell EA: Assessing the bladder. Nursing 85, 15:44–46, 1985

McCormick K, Burgio K: Incontinence: An update on nursing care measures. J Gerontol Nurs 10:17–23, 1984

McNeal JE: Aging and the prostate. In Brocklehurst JC (ed): Urology and the Elderly, p 201. New York, Churchill Livingstone, 1984

Mezey MD, Raukhorst LH, Stokes SA: Health Assessment of the Older Individual. New York, Springer Publishing, 1980

Riehle RA, Vaughan ED: Disease of the bladder. In Brocklehurst JC (ed): Urology in the Elderly, p 144. New York, Churchill Livingstone, 1984

Sourander LB, Rowe JW: The genitourinary system—the aging kidney. In Brocklehurst JC (ed): Textbook of Geriatric Medicine and Gerontology, 3rd ed, p 608. New York, Churchill Livingstone, 1985

Stanton SL: Surgical management of female incontinence. In Brocklehurst JC (ed): Urology in the Elderly, p 93. New York, Churchill Livingstone, 1984

Wells TJ: Social and psychological implications of incontinence. In Brocklehurst JC (ed): Urology in the Elderly, p 113. New York, Churchill Livingstone, 1984

Whitehead WE, Burgio KL, Engel BT: Behavioral methods in the assessment and treatment of urinary incontinence. In Brocklehurst JC (ed): Urology in the Elderly, p 74. New York, Churchill Livingstone, 1984

Wiener MB, Pepper G: Clinical Pharmacology and Therapeutics in Nursing. New York, McGraw-Hill, 1985

Yarnell JWG, Volye GJ, Richards CJ, Stephenson TP: The prevalence and severity of urinary incontinence in women. J Epidemiol Community Health 35:71–74, 1981

Jéanne Bauvette-Risey

Nervous system 13

Is cognitive impairment an inevitable consequence of aging? The suggestion is refuted by the existence of the many world leaders over age 65 who effectively command several countries in the world. In fact, 80% to 90% of the elderly population display no cognitive deficits in learning, memory, or abstract thinking (Cohen and Eisdorfer 1986).

However, neurologic *disease* is the major cause of disability in old age, and can include neurologic trauma, infections, deficiency states, and neoplasms. This chapter focuses on the three most common syndromes that occur among the elderly: stroke, Parkinson's disease, and Alzheimer's disease.

Normal aging of the nervous system is defined as the changes that occur in persons who are free of overt disease of the nervous system. Nurses must develop the skills required to distinguish between normal and abnormal neurologic functions, commensurate with a patient's age.

Age-related changes

From birth, nerve cells do not regenerate; they are never replaced, no matter what the cause of loss. The process of aging is little understood, but in the nervous system it is characterized by a steady loss of neurons, which begins as early as age 25 (Carter 1986). Studies have shown a small but consistent reduction in neurons from a maximum at physical maturity, declining in number through advanced age (Coull 1984a). The loss rate of neurons is not uniform throughout the brain's structure, nor does the process of neuronal loss take place at a steady

This chapter is dedicated to the memory of Dr. Jeffrey P. Ellison. He was a brilliant neurologist, a caring physician, and an advocate for neuroscience nursing.

rate. The areas of cortex that show the greatest age-related loss of neurons are the frontal poles (main area for cognition), superior portion of the temporal lobes (main area for audition), occipital poles (visual center), and prefrontal gyrus (sensory motor area) (Coull 1984a). Other areas may show almost no tissue loss, but demonstrate significant compromises in function.

With advancing years, the central nervous system (CNS) undergoes changes anatomically, histologically, and physiologically, but no one has yet determined a formula that explains how these changes progress with increasing chronologic age.

Anatomically, the brain loses water and weight with age, thus developing a narrowing of the convolutions and widening of the sulci. Histologic examinations demonstrate cellular degeneration and the presence of senile plaques.

Physiological and biochemical researchers have documented that with age neurons exhibit a decrease in glucose and cerebral oxygen consumption, amino-acid uptake, and protein synthesis. This decrease in protein synthesis is related to a decrease of sulfur and nitrogen in nerve cells. An increase in sodium concentration within the neurons leads to a slight decrease in nerve conduction velocity. There is also a demonstrated decrease in catecholamine concentration (Goldman 1979).

Whether the decrease in cerebral blood flow can be attributed to a pathologic origin or to normal aging remains controversial. The development of research concerning the neurotransmitters (dopamine, noradrenaline, serotonin, GABA, acetylcholine, and so forth) will be of great importance to understanding aging of the brain. Although neurotransmitters are thought by many to be the key to aging, it is not known if changes in neurotransmitters are a normal process of aging or are responsible for the pathology in dementia and other neurologic dysfunctions among the elderly.

The complexity of function of the nervous system has made it, as yet, impossible to develop a comprehensive view of the CNS aging process. It is difficult to identify which changes associated with age are due to disease and which, if any, are due primarily to the aging process.

Forgetfulness is a frequently heard complaint of elderly persons. Although the problem is complex, it must be noted that several aspects of learning and memory remain unchanged during normal aging. Specifically, immediate memory recall is well preserved, as is the retrieval of information from longterm memory storage (Katzman and Terry 1984). Verbal skills, including vocabulary and comprehension, are preserved. However, acquisition and memory of new information are impaired in normal aging. Of significance to the nurse who teaches patients is that although an elderly person may take longer to learn something new, the use of verbal repetition, mnemonic cues, and visual clues will usually result in retention of new information (Albert 1984; Katzman and Terry 1984). A normal elderly person can also interpet written informational instructions as well as a younger person.

One of the most significant age-related changes in the function of the nervous system is a slowing of certain behaviors (Katzman and Terry 1984). This occurs in simple motor tasks, such as running or the rate of finger tapping, and there is a continuous loss in the speed of learning, processing new information, and reaction to simple and complex stimuli. The degree of loss is based on a comparison between the elderly individual and a sedentary younger competitor. It is important to note that practice of specific tasks can increase the speed of performance.

Ordinary actions that show a decline in ability of up to 40% between the ages of 25 and 75 years include rising from a chair without support, putting on a shirt, buttoning a button, zipping garments, cutting with a knife, writing quickly, and standing on one leg with the eyes closed (Katzman and Terry 1984). In 40% to 60% of persons aged 75 years, compared with those aged 25 years, both the vibratory sense of the upper extremities and ability to flex the legs decline (Katzman and Terry 1984). People over age 80 may be able to walk, jog, and even do calisthenics but cannot safely stand on one leg with their eyes closed. Nurses who are assisting elderly patients should remind them to keep their eyes open when walking or stepping into or out of a car or bathtub. An elderly patient who wears an eye patch or keeps the eyes closed for some other therapeutic reason should be monitored closely for difficulty in maintaining balance.

Other observations indicate that the elderly have diminished energy, tend to be cautious, and show decreased initiative (Albert 1984). Elderly persons frequently complain of insomnia or disrupted sleep, and often experience change in sleep patterns. Typically, the total sleep time per night does not change, but the elderly person awakens more frequently and spends more time awake in bed.

With age, impairment of visual accommodation for near objects is almost universal; by age 70 most people require corrective lenses for distant vision. Adaptation to the dark diminishes with age; therefore most elderly people require greater illumination for accurate vision. Pupil size decreases and pupillary responses are diminished or even absent. Ocular motility tends to be slowed, and upward gaze is often limited.

Hearing is similarly diminished, beginning at about age 50. High-frequency sounds are chiefly affected, perhaps as the result of the acoustic trauma that is suffered over a lifetime. Concomitant declines in the senses of taste and smell have also been noted, but the frequency of this phenomenon has not been under study.

As neuronal alterations occur, certain variations that would be considered abnormal in younger people are considered within normal limits for elderly persons. These variations include irregular pupil outline; loss of muscle tone in the face, neck, and spinal musculature; loss of ankle jerks; loss of appreciation of tuning-fork vibrations at the ankle; and some loss of position sense in the toes. There is a general decrease in muscle bulk, particularly in the small muscles of the hands (Albert 1984).

Many of the changes that usually accompany aging—changes in vascular and cardiac reflexes, galvanic skin response, potency, micturition, and pupillary response—may be due to alterations in autonomic nervous system activity (Katzman and Terry 1984). A body of evidence suggests that sympathetic hyperactivity is commonly present, and may underlie the mild increase in plasma glucose often seen in normal elderly people (Katzman and Terry 1984).

Since there are so many "normal" variations in the manifestations of aging in the nervous system, the clinical significance of neurologic symptoms and findings becomes more difficult to resolve.

Assessment variables

Aging cannot be measured by years alone, yet some yardstick is necessary; the presented neurologic assessment in the elderly is based on experience with patients over the age of 65 (Carter 1986). Nurses must remember that no specific chronologic age comparison can be made to aging of the brain. Often when a history is investigated, the person over 65 years will relate the onset of symptoms to have been as early as 40 to 45 years of age.

Adding to the complexity of assessing the "healthy" aged nervous system is the fact that 75% of persons over age 65 have at least one serious chronic illness (Albert 1984), making it impossible to equate normal (average) function in the elderly with a state of health or absence of disease.

Examination of the nervous system

Mental status
    State of consciousness
    Orientation
    Information
    Memory
    Calculation
    Language function
    Special testing for aphasia, apraxia, or agnosis

Cranial nerves
    Sense of smell
    Visual acuity, visual fields, optic fundi, ocular motility, pupillary response
    Facial sensation, corneal reflexes, jaw movement, jaw jerk
    Facial movement and symmetry, taste
    Hearing (air, bone conduction), gag reflex, swallowing, phonation
    Sternocleidomastoid and trapezius movement
    Tongue motion

Motor and coordination
    Gait, station, walking on heels and toes, tandem gait
    Direct testing of strength, tone, and coordination in extremities

Reflexes
    Deep tendon reflexes, plantar reflexes, abdominal reflexes

Sensation
    Primary (touch, pinprick, vibration, and position sense)
    Cortical (face–hand, double simultaneous stimulation, and so forth)

The nurse is responsible for assessing the integrity of the patient's nervous system, based on the patient's history and performance. Although the nurse is not usually responsible for doing a complete neurologic examination, it is imperative to identify the relevance of all information documented by other health professionals, including physicians, physical and occupational therapists, speech therapists, dieticians, and other consultants. The nurse must be able to identify acute changes that require immediate medical or nursing intervention. Furthermore, the nurse must attempt to identify those features of the patient's condition that contribute to any disability in an effort to modify as much as possible problems that limit independence and personal satisfaction.

The complete neurologic evaluation of any adult includes a history, neurologic examination, and laboratory tests. Because specific details of the neurologic evaluation are not unique to the elderly, they are presented in the box on page 316, and can be reviewed elsewhere (Albert 1984; Hickey 1986; Mitchell et al 1984).

In addition to recording each neurologic complaint and obtaining the standard history, the nurse must carefully document the rate of decline of function and any past history of neurologic injury such as head injury; stroke; neuroinfections; and cranial, spinal, or peripheral nerve surgeries. A review of the neurologic system must also include episodes of loss of consciousness, use of alcohol or other drugs, and a specific review of cranial nerve, motor, and sensory functions.

The nurse must be prepared to deal with a number of special problems in obtaining the neurologic history of an elderly person. These problems are fully explained by Albert (1984), and should be reviewed by any nurse who plans to assess the elderly (see boxed material, below).

During the neurologic examination of the elderly patient, the nurse should focus on certain areas of special interest that may limit the elderly person's ability to function. These include memory function, vision and hearing, and gait. In a familiar environment, that patient should be able to manage personal, family, and financial affairs, maintain knowledge of world events, and keep up appropriately in conversations, card games, and other activities with contemporaries. Strub and

---

Pitfalls in the neurologic history of the aged

Paucity of accurate history resulting from memory loss

Varying expectations for the aged

Sudden change versus revealing events

Denial; excessive somatic concern

Impact of environment changes

Activity decline versus depression

Sensory deprivation

Black (1985) used the results of specific psychometric tests to objectively document mental deterioration, cognitive capacity, and affective disorders. Many clinicians (Cohen and Eisdorfer 1986; Kelly 1984; Strub and Black 1985) have outlined brief mental examination questionnaires that the nurse may use to assess mental status. Because the pathologic origins of visual and auditory impairments are frequently neurologic, an assessment of these functions must be included in a complete neurologic examination. The evaluation of vision and hearing is outlined in detail in Chapter 5 of this text.

Secondary to mental deterioration, impaired gait and movement are the most frequently noted neurologic disabilities associated with aging (Albert 1984). The average elderly person develops a hesitant, broad-based, small-stepped gait with stooped posture, but does not lose the ability to walk safely and independently. Mechanical impairment resulting from joint degeneration may lead to significant gait impairment and thus must be covered in the review of the patient's symptoms and in the examination. Degenerative changes of the cervical spine occur in more than 80% of persons age 55 and are found almost universally in persons over age 75. Although only 50% of the elderly develop any symptoms

---

Significant neurologic symptoms in the elderly

New or "different" headache

"Blackout spells"—loss or alteration of consciousness

Transient neurological event
    Brief episodes of visual loss
    Difficulty finding words
    Weakness of an arm or a leg
    Any other event of transient nature

Uncorrectable visual impairment—loss of visual acuity not easily restored by glasses

Numb hand or weak hand

Lethargy
    Increasing drowsiness
    Falling asleep at inappropriate times

Acute mental change
    Sudden decline of intellectual function

Focal deficits
    Loss of motor function
    Loss of speech
    Onset of severe tremor
    Loss of limb sensation
    Any other local or lateralized deficit

with cervical spondylosis, there is the possibility of severe complications including stroke, quadriplegia, and various compressed-cord syndromes (Smith 1968).

In reviewing the patient's history and physical examination, certain complaints or symptoms should alert the nurse to the probability of significant neurologic disease, as outlined in the box on page 318.

Stroke

Stroke is recognized clinically as a sensory, perceptual, communicative, or motor dysfunction related to impaired blood flow within a region of the brain. Stroke, or symptoms of a stroke are medical emergencies that require hospitalization, because correct treatment depends on accurate diagnosis through technology that currently is available only in hospitals (Hachinski and Norris 1985).

Stroke is the most common serious neurologic problem in the world; it is the third most common cause of death and is a major cause of disability in North America and much of Europe (Kurtzke 1980). Although no age group is spared, stroke is primarily a problem in the elderly population. Compared with its incidence in persons 55 to 59 years of age, stroke occurs five times more often among persons 70 to 74 years of age and 10 times more often among persons over age 75 (Hardin 1983).

Categories of stroke

The major categories of stroke in the elderly include: cerebral infarction resulting from atherosclerotic cerebrovascular disease (thrombosis); cardioembolic cerebral infarction (embolism); and intracerebral hemorrhage.

Thrombosis

In the elderly, the vast majority of strokes are due to cerebral infarctions related to cerebrovascular atherosclerosis resulting in an acute occlusion of a cerebral artery or arteriole (Coull 1984a). In atheroembolic infarction, degenerative changes within the thrombus, typically at the carotid bifurcation or involving the vertebral or basilar arteries, can encourage the formation of a friable thrombus, which embolizes distally into the cerebral circulation, causing a cerebral infarction.

Embolism

Because of the coexistence of significant cardiovascular and cerebrovascular disease in the elderly, cerebral embolism of cardiac origin is increasingly identified as a cause of stroke. About 75% of stroke victims have one or more signs of cardiac failure, atrial fibrillation, or an enlarged heart, as demonstrated by x-ray examination or electrocardiogram (ECG). Elderly patients whose routine resting and exertional ECGs show normal sinus rhythm (NSR) may be discovered at the time of transient cerebral ischemic attacks to have unsuspected transient cardiac dys-rhythmias. In a recent study, 74% of the elderly patients with a history of NSR who were studied were found on 24-hour ECG to have dysrhythmias sufficient to cause their transient cerebral attack (Carter 1986). These dysrhythmias included primar-ily atrial fibrillation, as well as asystole, sinus bradycardia, sinoatrial block, runs of atrial and ventricular ectopies, ventricular tachycardia, and various degrees of heart block.

Hemorrhage

The third most frequent cause of stroke in the elderly is intracerebral hemorrhage. Cerebral arteries are thinner than other arteries of equivalent size. When not af-fected by atherosclerosis, cerebral arteries appear almost transparent, illustrating their thinness and susceptibility to rupture. A variety of conditions may predispose to intracerebral hemorrhage, including hypertension, blood dyscrasias, anticoagu-lants, collagen vascular disease, hemorrhage into primary and metastatic brain tumors, mycotic aneurysms, and vascular malformations. In the elderly, however, in hemorrhages classified as stroke, hypertension is by far the most frequent cause identified.

Hypertension contributes to stroke through many mechanisms (Wolf and Kannel 1982). It leads to structural changes in the cerebral arteries, eventually impairs the brain's capacity for autoregulation, and also leads to cardiac failure.

In addition to thrombus, embolus, and hemorrhage, other possible causes of diminished cerebral blood supply in the elderly must be identified. Drugs may be responsible, particularly thiazide diuretics, reserpine compounds, and proma-zine derivatives, because of their hypotensive effects (Carter 1986). Anemia is often overlooked in the elderly; physical exertion or even standing for any length of time can produce signs of cerebral ischemia, particularly if the hemoglobin level is below normal. In addition, extension or full rotation of the head (for ex-ample, during a salon shampoo, when reaching for a high-shelved item, or be-cause of a quick head turn) interferes with vertebral artery flow if, as is common, cervical spondylosis is combined with degenerative arterial disease (Smith 1968).

Clinical presentation of stroke syndromes

In discussing the clinical presentations of stroke syndromes, three terms are gen-erally used: transient ischemic attack (TIA), reversible ischemic neurological defi-cit (RIND), and stroke.

Transient ischemic attack (TIA)

A TIA is an episode of temporary neurologic dysfunction of vascular origin with rapid onset and a duration of no more than 24 hours. The usual duration is 5 to 7 minutes (Jankovic 1982). The importance of a TIA is that it signals the possibility of an impending stroke and requires prompt, detailed investigation and treatment, preferably in a hospital setting. In any health-care setting the nurse may be the first to suspect that a patient is having a TIA, so nurses should be aware that a completed stroke usually occurs within the first to sixth month after the first TIA (Jankovic 1982). Because it cannot yet be predicted which TIAs will result in stroke, each TIA must be treated as a medical priority for preventing major stroke.

Reversible ischemic neurologic deficit (RIND)

The term RIND describes an episode of temporary neurologic dysfunction of vascular origin with a rapid onset, in which deficits persist for more than 24 hours but resolve completely within several days or weeks. Although the use of the term RIND is not without controversy, it has significance to medicine and nursing. In the past 10 to 15 years, many patients who were considered previously as having had strokes recovered total function over a period of weeks. Therefore, in clinical management, the potential for reversible neurological deficits requires physicians and nurses to initiate and extend the acute phase of stroke therapy. No longer can clinicians manage stroke as a process of aging that requires no acute intervention. No longer should a patient who is experiencing symptoms of stroke be managed at home or in an extended-care facility unless he or she is moribund as the result of other medical conditions. Recognition of RIND mandates that neuroscience gerontologic nurses assume an aggressive attitude in the management of elderly stroke patients.

Stroke

A completed stroke is the result of a thrombotic, embolic, or hemorrhagic event in which maximum neurologic dysfunction is acquired at the onset. The deficits stabilize and may show improvement over days, weeks, or months, but a plateau is reached with permanent residual deficit. Even in the presence of a medical diagnosis of completed stroke, the nurse must be alert to the need for a complete diagnostic workup and ongoing accurate nursing assessment. This procedure will maximize patient recovery and identify those patients who may regain function. In addition, as the president of the local American Heart Association Stroker's Club stated, ". . . just because I've had one stroke and survived doesn't give me any immunization from having another stroke." Therefore, the cause and possible correction of every cerebrovascular episode must be pursued until all possibilities are exhausted. This quote also reminds nurses of their responsibility to educate all patients, with and without a history of stroke, on the risk factors related to stroke prevention. These factors are covered in the assessment section below.

An in-depth discussion of the ways in which stroke symptoms are based on their anatomic presentation is beyond the scope of this text. However, a brief overview of the typical presentations of strokes involving the anterior and posterior circulations, as well as strokes in general, is presented in Table 13-1.

Table 13-1. **Stroke syndrome presentations**

Stroke in general	Anterior circulation, carotid distribution		Posterior circulation, vertebrobasilar distribution
	Right hemisphere	Left hemisphere	
Paralysis (?)	Paralyzed (L) side	Paralyzed (R) side	Bilateral alternating or "crossed" motor and sensory symptoms
Quality control deficits	Memory deficits (performance)	Memory deficits (language)	
Memory deficits (general)	Spatial–perceptual (deficits)	Speech language (deficits)	Ataxia
Decreased retention	Behavior style: quick, impulsive	Behavior style: slow, cautious	Vertigo
Old versus new learning (deficits)	Hemianopia		Dysarthria
Generalization deficits	Impaired judgment	Hemianopia	Dysphagia
Emotional lability	Lack of insight	Extreme awareness of deficits	Diplopia
Sensory deprivation effects	Neglect of involved extremities		Bilateral visual blurring
	Easy distractability		
	Short attention span		

Assessment variables

Stroke implies a sudden and potentially devastating vascular syndrome. This diagnosis requires a complete history, physical examination, and diagnostic tests to determine cause and potential treatments.

Transient ischemic attacks are underestimated by patients and health-care professionals because they are brief and rarely disabling. They, too, should be investigated scrupulously because they often signal impending, but avoidable, disaster.

Although several diagnostic procedures are necessary for definite pathologic diagnosis, a precise and complete interview discussing symptoms, contributing risk factors, and past health history gives the clinician the most significant information. A patient who is experiencing a stroke or symptoms of a stroke may not be able to talk, and therefore family members or other caregivers become paramount in providing vital information regarding presenting symptoms. In the initial interview, the nurse should include questions relating to weakness or sensory disturbance involving any part of the patient's body; difficulties with speech, reading, writing, or comprehension; seizures; loss of consciousness; disturbance of memory; visual symptoms such as diplopia or loss of vision in one or both eyes; vertigo; and impairment of hearing or balance.

To investigate possible causes of stroke symptoms, the nurse should note what the patient was doing when symptoms occurred, and detail the onset, as

Table 13-2. **Clinical manifestations found in the early stages of stroke**

Clinical manifestations	Thrombosis	Embolism	Hypertensive hemorrhage
Prior warning	Yes (Transient Ischemic Attacks [TIA] in 50% of patients)	No	No
Activity at onset	Anytime; more often during rest or sleep, or shortly after awakening	Often during physical exertion	Anytime
Initial loss of consciousness	Uncommon with carotid infarct Sometimes with vertebrobasilar infarct	Uncommon	Common
Headache	Sometimes	Sometimes	Very common
Nucchal rigidity	No	No	Yes
Signs of increased intracranial pressure	Rare	Rare	May be present

well as the duration and progression of symptoms. It is important to detail specifically the very first symptom (which is not necessarily the most dramatic one) because this clue may identify the cause as infarction (thrombosis, embolism) or hemorrhage (Table 13-2). If several attacks have occurred, each episode should be reviewed to determine patterns indicative of carotid, vertebral, or cardiac origin.

Risk factors

Of paramount importance is a review of the risk factors of stroke specific to the individual patient. Atherosclerosis, hypertension, and heart disease are the most important risk factors related to stroke syndromes (Hachinski and Norris 1985). In addition, diabetes mellitus, cardiac arrhythmias, coagulopathy, anemia, cancer, and migraine headaches are systemic diseases related to increased stroke risk.

Mounting evidence implicates lifestyle as a strong determinant in the development of circulatory disorders. This finding suggests that the nurse is increasingly responsible for teaching patients behavior-modification techniques in stroke prevention. A decreasing level of physical activity, increasing experience of stress, and high-calorie, high-lipid diets result in obesity and hypertension, thus raising the risk of stroke. Smoking, a strong contributor to ischemic heart disease, is currently identified as only a weak risk factor for stroke. (However, this should not deter the nursing profession from fulfilling its responsibility to campaign against smoking as a major contributor to other systemic illnesses.)

Additional predisposing historical factors to be reviewed include any history of head trauma, family history of strokes or hematologic disorders, or use of anti-coagulants, sedatives, or diuretics, which may induce postural hypotension.

In conjunction with the history, a complete neurologic examination is imperative in patients suspected of stroke symptoms. Details of a complete neurologic examination are outlined in the box on page 316.

It is important to identify the following key points during the evaluation of the stroke patient. The nurse must accurately assess and record the patient's blood pressure in both arms. A difference of 20 mmHg in systolic pressure between the two arms is important because it may indicate subclavian steal syndrome (Hickey 1986). Hypertension, whether systolic or diastolic, has already been identified as the greatest but most treatable factor for all types of stroke syndromes. Hypotension is also an important cause of brain ischemia; however, in cases of an acute stroke event the patient should not be made to stand as a way to facilitate blood pressure evaluation lying and standing, which could demonstrate orthostatic drop. A consequence of infarction or hemorrhage is that the normal autoregulation of cerebral blood flow is impaired, and even a moderate decrease in blood pressure may result in reduction of cerebral perfusion and extension of the stroke. Therefore, after an acute stroke or suspected stroke symptoms, the patient should remain supine for several days until cerebrovascular stability improves and cardiovascular integrity is determined (Hachinski and Norris 1985).

Palpation of the carotid arteries is an unreliable measure of their patency and risks bradycardia or dislodgement of atheroma or thrombus. Auscultation of the carotid arteries may yield some useful information, although its clinical significance is not well understood. The presence of carotid bruits suggests a turbulent flow, usually resulting from irregularities in the lumen of the artery. Bruits may be audible in asymptomatic persons or may be absent in severely diseased blood vessels. Noninvasive diagnostic tests (Yatzu 1984) such as oculoplethysmography, ophthalmodynamometry, cerebral blood flow measurements, ultrasound imaging, and digital vascular imaging prove most helpful in accurately determining vessel patency and potential need for more invasive testing, such as angiography. Because palpation and auscultation of cerebral vessels can lead to serious complications (Jankovic 1982), and because other reliable tests are available, I do not recommend palpation and auscultation as routine nursing assessment procedures.

As the patient is examined, a pattern of symptoms related to anatomic involvement should develop if a true cerebrovascular event has occurred (Albert 1984; Fowler and Fordyce 1974; Linde 1986) (see Table 13-1). Nurses who assess the condition of stroke patients should remember that only seven of ten stroke patients manifest paralysis (Hachinski and Norris 1985). Therefore, a careful complete neurologic assessment must be carried out in the presence of any neurologic dysfunction, so that a stroke diagnosis is not missed.

Experts and technology

The rationale for mandatory hospitalization of all patients with stroke symptoms is that the expertise and technology for accurate diagnosis and treatment are currently available only in the hospital setting (Hachinski and Norris 1985). Certainly, a CAT scan can rule out hemorrhage, and laboratories are available for rapid and frequent monitoring of hemoglobin, hematocrit, electrolytes, clotting factors, and so forth. If the stroke patient develops secondary pulmonary, cardiac, or neurologic complications, the availability of critical-care specialists is crucial. But— who are the "experts" in the clinical management of stroke? Obviously the neurologist, cardiologist, and radiologist who work in close relation to one another and the patient are able to maximize collaboration and quickly initiate therapies to optimize patient recovery. However, an expert who is cited with greater frequency in medical literature is the acute-care nurse. In identifying "experts," Hachinski and Norris (1985) state, "Potentially reversible deterioriation in the acute stroke patient is detected earlier by attentive nurses than by any cardiac or cerebral monitoring systems yet devised." They add, "Continuous observation and standardized neurologic assessment by skilled personnel show more sensitivity in detection of early clinical deterioration than does any laboratory test yet devised." Clearly, both statements set the tone for nurses to be knowledgeable in stroke pathophysiology and to be able specifically to accurately assess and document the findings.

How does the nurse continue to evaluate and record findings in the patient with stroke symptoms? Although nothing can entirely take the place of narrative nursing documentation, neurologic assessment flowcharts such as the Canadian Neurological Scale (Cote et al 1986) allow the nurse to follow up a stroke patient's symptoms and previous assessment findings in a comprehensive format. The Glasgow Coma Scale, which was never intended for all neurologic assessment documentation, is inadequate in stroke documentation because it omits critical variables such as vision, language and speech deficits, sensory impairments, and memory deficits.

Information concerning the pharmacologic treatment of stroke is presented in Table 13-3.

Parkinson's disease

Parkinson's disease (PD) is the second most common neurologic disorder in the elderly. It is a movement disorder resulting from abnormalities in the extrapyramidal motor system, basal ganglia, and associated pathways. The disease is predominantly associated with the substantia nigra (SN), and the caudate, putamen, globus pallidus, and claustrum of the striatum (Figure 13-1). Deficiencies in the SN are believed to be responsible for the primary symptoms of PD, which include tremors, muscle rigidity, slowness, poverty of movement, and difficulty balancing and walking.

Table 13-3. **Pharmacologic treatment of stroke**

Drug	Effect/response in the elderly	Nursing implications
Warfarin (Coumadin)	Coumadin produces anticoagulant effect by interfering with the action of vitamin K necessary for the production of blood clotting factors. Onset of action 1–3 days *after* initial dose. Takes about 5 days of drug therapy to reach steady state. Side-effects include hematuria, bruising, minor or major hemorrhage from any tissue or organ.	Monitor prothrombin time (PT) daily during initial therapy. Give dose at same time daily (5 pm at our institution—to accommodate lab results). Observe for side-effects. Educate patient and family in drug precautions, including diet, concomitant medications, dental services, observation for bleeding.
Aspirin	Antiplatelet agent; inhibits platelet adhesion and aggregation. Determined most effective in men presenting with TIAs.	Observe for signs of gastric side-effects. Educate patient and family in drug and its precautions.
Dipyridamole (Persantine)	Antiplatelet agent; inhibits platelet adhesion. Side-effects include headache, dizziness, nausea, flushing, weakness, syncope, mild gastrointestinal discomfort, skin rash.	Observe for side-effects. Educate patient and family in drug and its precautions.

(Data from Brocklehurst JC: Geriatric Pharmacology and Therapeutics. Boston, Blackwell Scientific, 1984)

Messages pass between the SN and the striatum through the aid of dopamine (DA), a neurotransmitter. Dopamine has an inhibitory effect on the extrapyramidal system, thus refining the control of voluntary movement. This discovery has led to the use of Levodopa, the primary drug therapy for PD.

In addition to DA deficiencies in the striatum, PD may result from a DA deficiency in other parts of the brain. Dopamine deficiencies in the neocortex and in the hippocampus may cause the secondary symptoms of PD, which include depression, senility, postural deformity, and difficulty speaking (Lannon et al 1986). Parkinson's disease can also impair the autonomic nervous system, resulting in forced eyelid closure, difficulty swallowing, dizziness on standing, oily skin, impotence, constipation, drooling, and difficulty breathing (Lieberman et al 1985).

A second neurotransmitter, acetylcholine (Ach), which has an excitatory effect on neurons, appears to contribute to the symptomatology of PD. The level of Ach is normal in patients with PD. For the striatum to function, however, a balance between DA and Ach is necessary. As a result of dopamine deficiency in PD, the DA–Ach balance is disturbed. This disturbance further aggravates the disease symptoms.

The use of drugs that increase dopamine (Levodopa), and drugs that block the action of acetylcholine (anticholinergics) partially restores the balance. With the advent of antiparkinsonian drug therapies in the 1970s, more patients with PD

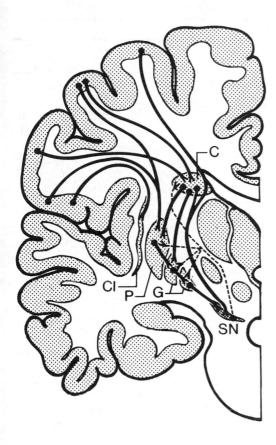

Figure 13-1. *The symptoms of Parkinson's disease result from the loss of dopaminergic neurotransmitters in the substantia nigra* (SN), *the striatum* (C, *caudate;* P, *putamen;* G, *globus pallidus;* Cl, *claustrum*), *and the cortex.*

are able to avoid invalidism and institutional care. The nurse's goal is to maximize the PD patient's independence for as long as possible and to educate patient and family in the disease process and drug therapies as prescribed (Table 13-4).

In the elderly patient population, the second most common cause of parkinsonian features is drugs given for sedation, particularly haloperidol (Haldol) and the phenothiazines (such as Thorazine) (Jancovic 1984). Since Haldol and Thorazine are used in treating the elderly, nurses must be alert to assess and report symptoms of PD if they occur as side-effects of medications.

Assessment variables

Parkinson's disease is a slow, progressive, degenerative illness. No specific biochemical or other diagnostic test pinpoints the disease process. Therefore, a diagnosis is based on the history and neurologic examination, including evaluation of symptoms and their severity. The patient's earliest observations may be nonspecific and include weakness, tiredness, and fatigue. More specific complaints may include tremor of the hands at rest, a change in speech, difficulty turning while in bed or walking, and decreased arm swing while walking (Lieberman et al 1985).

Table 13-4. *Pharmacologic treatment of Parkinson's disease*

Drug	Effect/response in the elderly	Nursing implications
Combination of levodopa and carbidopa (Sinemet)	Most frequently used form of Levodopa. Given to replace decreased or absent dopamine while preventing or diminishing side-effects of levodopa. It is usually given with carbidopa. Dosage variable: increasing until symptoms are relieved or side-effects appear. Same serious side-effects, decreased benefit as L-dopa, decreased benefits on longterm use. Serious side-effects: nausea, vomiting, hypotension, dizziness, confusion, dry mouth, cardiac dysrhythmias, constipation, abnormal involuntary movements (dyskinesias), decreased appetite, hallucinations, delusions, end-of-dose deterioration, and clinical fluctuations. Benefits are decreased with longterm therapy (3–5 yr), requiring drug holiday (Lannon et al 1986). Levodopa does not slow down underlying neuronal degeneration. Phenothiazines, phenytoin, and papaverine may reduce or reverse effects of Sinemet. Pyridoxine (vitamin B_6) should definitely be avoided, and should not be given with carbidopa. Observe patient if concomitant administration necessary.	Maintain accurate record of administered doses and adjustments. Monitor blood pressure and heart rhythm frequently during initial therapy and during dosage alterations. Assess and record patient symptoms for reversal with medication dosage. Avoid multivitamins that contain pyridoxine.
Levodopa (Levodopa)	Levodopa is given to replace decreased or absent dopamine in the central nervous system. Dosage variable: based on increasing dose until symptoms are relieved or side-effects appear. Serious side-effects: nausea, vomiting, hypotension, dizziness, confusion, dry mouth, cardiac dysrhythmias, constipation, abnormal involuntary movements (dyskinesias), decreased appetite, hallucinations, delusions, end-of-dose deterioration, and clinical fluctuations. There are decreased benefits with longterm therapy (3–5 yr), requiring a drug holiday (Lannon et al 1986). Levodopa does not slow down underlying neuronal degeneration. Phenothiazines, phenytoin, and papaverine may reduce/reverse effects of levodopa. Observe patient if concomitant administration necessary.	Monitor blood pressure and heart rhythm frequently during initial therapy and during dosage alterations. Assess and record patient symptoms for reversal with medication dosage.
Benztropine (Congentin) Trihexyphenidyl (Artane) Biperiden (Akineton)	Anticholinergics—used to block the action of the neurotransmitter acetylcholine, thus enhancing balance between dopamine and acetylcholine. Each agent used independently; one agent's effectiveness does not negate trying another. Effective against rigidity and tremor; not effective against bradykinesia or difficulty in balancing or walking. Side-effects include dryness of the mouth, blurred vision, mental changes, difficulty voiding, or constipation.	Monitor urinary output. Monitor bowel habits; encourage exercise, fluids, and roughage to prevent constipation.

continued

Table 13-4. (Continued)

Drug	Effect/response in the elderly	Nursing implications
Bromocriptine (Parlodel)	Dopamine agonist—mimics the effects of dopamine. Useful in treating all of the primary symptoms of Parkinson's disease. Can be used in conjunction with any of the other antiparkinsonian agents. Side-effects include orthostatic hypotension, psychiatric problems, digital and coronary vasospasm, erythromelalgia, and nausea and vomiting.	Monitor blood pressure with patient lying, sitting, standing. Expensive.

(Data from Brocklehurst JC: Geriatric Pharmacology and Therapeutics. Boston, Blackwell Scientific, 1984; Lannon MC et al: Comprehensive care of the patient with Parkinson's disease. J Neurosci Nurs 18:121–123, 1986)

Other early symptoms may include difficulty in starting to walk; difficulty in getting into and out of a car or chair; a change in handwriting; depression; or drooling, especially at night (Lieberman et al 1985). The cardinal symptoms are bradykinesia, rigidity, tremor at rest, and postural instability.

Bradykinesia (disturbance in movement) is the most disabling of the major symptoms. Deliberate, slow movement can progress to episodes when no movement is possible. The person has difficulty varying the velocity of movement, particularly when trying to increase speed. Reaction time is slower; delayed reactions during conversation may give the impression that the patient does not hear well or does not understand what is being said (Lannon et al 1986). The nurse must allow the patient time to complete a task or respond to a question. Added stress and increased effort result in even slower movement. Visual, auditory, and proprioceptive cues may be useful in facilitating movement and response (Lannon et al 1986). Tasks that require repeated movements, such as writing, result in decreased amplitude with each successive trial. Lack of automatic movements makes certain functional skills (such as rising from a chair) difficult. *"Freezing"* (akinesia) is the term that describes the difficulty a patient with PD may have in performing two movements simultaneously. The nurse may observe this phenomenon as the patient attempts walking through a doorway, in narrow passages, on inclines, or when the floor changes color or texture.

Rigidity (often referred to as "lead pipe" muscle rigidity) is the most common symptom of PD. The "cog-wheel" component of rigidity that the nurse feels when putting a limb through passive range of motion is actually the contraction of the antagonist muscles coupled with increased tone (Lewis 1985). The rigidity is present when the limbs are still and increases with movement.

Rigidity by itself is not disabling. The muscles that are most affected by rigidity are the two-joint flexor muscles. Rigidity of trunk muscles results in decreased trunk rotation and extension, and leads to difficulty in rolling over, coming to a sitting position, and standing up. Rigidity of the facial muscles results in "masked facies," the staring appearance of persons with Parkinson's disease.

Intercostal muscle rigidity can lead to restricted chest wall expansion and altered respiratory function. Difficulty with chewing and swallowing results from facial and pharyngeal muscle rigidity. Hypophonia and difficult articulation may be due to rigidity of vocal cords and associated structures. Truncal rigidity causes problems with balance and posture (Lewis 1985). While maximizing the patient's mobility and independence, the nurse must also be astutely aware of the need for safety precautions through routine skin inspections, pulmonary and nutritional assessments, and an evaluation of the patient's limitations in ambulation related to rigidity.

Tremor is rarely a disabling symptom, and is present in about 75% of PD patients. Tremor appears in the hands and sometimes the feet of limbs at rest. In the hands, the term "pill-rolling" is used to describe the observed tremor. Usually this tremor decreases when the hands are stretched out in front of the patient, when the hands are moving, and while the patient sleeps. It is aggravated when the patient feels nervous, frightened, angry, or otherwise stressed and lessens in intensity in a calm and relaxed situation. Although the presence of tremor can be very disconcerting to the patient and caregivers, current clinical studies indicate that patients with marked tremor have a better prognosis than patients with marked bradykinesia or rigidity (Jancovic 1984).

Postural instability results from loss of postural and balance reactions. These decreased responses to movement can produce an increased fear of falling and apprehension about walking outside or in crowded areas (Lannon et al 1986).

Mental status changes were originally said to be absent in PD, but now many authors think that dementia is a frequent feature (30–50%) of the disease (Boller 1983; Jancovic 1984). Furthermore, the dementia found in PD patients is similar in its qualitative aspects, as well as in its course and progression, to the dementia of Alzheimer's disease (Lieberman et al 1985). Many studies suggest that Alzheimer's disease and PD are indeed associated by a common pathogenetic mechanism—alteration in neurotransmitter activity.

There is no specific therapy for the dementia associated with PD, but PD patients with dementia tolerate all antiparkinsonian drugs poorly. In addition to their dementia, they frequently develop the side-effect of a toxic confusional syndrome consisting of delusions, hallucinations, and aggressive behavior. The toxic confusional syndrome, but not the dementia, is reversible when the drug is discontinued. Any antiparkinsonian drug should be used cautiously and at a lower dose in the demented PD patient (Lieberman et al 1985).

Most of the symptoms of PD can be significantly reduced when the patient responds to current medical therapies. Because of the possibility of associated dementia, speech therapy, physical therapy, and occupational therapy should be used to educate the PD patient about the disease early in the disease process, even before the patient actually experiences functional limitations. Thus, in the presence of subsequent dementia, the patient will be able to use already learned adaptive behavior and will not be impeded by the eventual inability to learn new information.

Alzheimer's disease

An estimated 19% to 20% of the population over age 65 have significant cognitive dysfunction of dementia (Cohen and Eisdorfer 1986). These dementing illnesses are categorized as two types: reversible dementias, and nonreversible dementias. Causes of reversible dementia include depression, metabolic toxic reactions, medication-induced toxicity, and vitamin deficiency. An estimated 30% to 40% of persons referred with memory disturbances have a treatable dementia. The restoration of full cognitive function in this population of reversible dementias, however, appears to be contingent on prompt diagnosis and treatment. Delayed treatment increases the probability that some of the lost functions will not be recovered (Cohen and Eisdorfer 1986).

Depression is the most frequently occurring reversible cause of dementia in the elderly and the most common psychiatric disturbance. It has been documented in more than 44% of the elderly (Carter 1986). The elderly depressed person can demonstrate behavioral changes, easy fatigability, apathy, social withdrawal, self-care neglect, and decreased appetite. Depression can also be manifested as disturbances of memory, inattention, or disorientation, which further complicates the diagnosis of dementia. Although depression is covered elsewhere in this text (Chapter 15), it should be noted here that the increased frequency for another primary illness (such as stroke [Hatcher et al 1985], Parkinson's disease [Lieberman 1983], or Alzheimer's disease [Lieberman 1983]) limits the recovery of the patient. Therefore, the patient's entire recovery may be enhanced by rapid identification of the depressive components of all diseases, followed by appropriate therapy.

The most common form of nonreversible dementing illness in the elderly population is primary neuronal degeneration of the Alzheimer's type (50–70%) (U.S. Department of Health and Human Services 1984). Other frequent causes of irreversible dementia include multi-infarct dementia, mixed dementia, and other dementias associated with Parkinson's disease, multiple sclerosis, Huntington's disease, Crutzfeld-Jacob disease, Pick's disease, syphilis, and alcohol abuse.

The cause(s) of Alzheimer's disease (AD) still eludes researchers, although several causative theories are being actively investigated (Kelly 1984; U.S. Department of Health and Human Services 1984). These theories include accumulation of aluminum deposits in neuronal nuclei, immunologic changes, active and latent viruses, and alterations in the cholinergic neurotransmitter system. This last theory is receiving the most attention. The brains of AD patients have been confirmed to have a profound decrease in activity of the enzyme choline acetyltransferase (CAT). This is a key ingredient in the chemical process that produces acetylcholine, a neurotransmitter involved in both learning and memory. Acetylcholine is not the only neurotransmitter system affected in AD, but it does appear to be the one most consistently and severely damaged.

Early and accurate diagnosis is difficult. Because relatively little information is available on the natural history of the disease in its early phases, nurses must make diagnoses based on clinical deficits as they appear. Initially, patients complain of forgetting where they have placed familiar objects and forgetting names they formerly knew well. After this problem, they may demonstrate decreased facility in remembering names of people who have just been introduced or may retain very little information after reading a passage in a newspaper. A patient may have no recall of some events and yet recall others well. These difficulties become evident to intimates. Decreased performance may be manifested during demanding situations at the workplace, or the person may become seriously lost when traveling to an unfamiliar location. This confusion is accompanied by mild to moderate anxiety.

The duration of each phase of illness is not specific. When a more serious decline is evident, the patient has significant concentration deficits and decreased knowledge of recent events. The ability to travel alone to new places is notably curtailed, although traveling to familiar locations may pose no problem. The person may have difficulty managing personal finances and performing complex tasks accurately and efficiently. Denial is often the dominant defense. The person withdraws from social activity, develops a flattened affect, and loses initiative, tact, and judgment, yet still may be able to function safely in a limited, familiar environment with familiar routines.

As the disease progresses to the next phase, the AD patient can no longer survive without some assistance. He or she will forget his or her address, telephone number, or names of close family members; but will retain his or her own name and those of spouse and children. Ability to tend to personal care remains intact, although difficulty in selecting the proper clothes to wear is a common problem. Even in this phase, there may be episodes of lucidity.

As decline continues, the patient may occasionally forget the name of his or her spouse and becomes largely unaware of all recent events and experiences. Typically, these persons are unaware of their surroundings, the year, and the season. Nocturnal sleep is severely disturbed in AD; the periods of sleep that are most refreshing almost completely disappear in the severe stages of the disease. This diurnal rhythm disturbance and a decreased stress threshold are thought to be primarily responsible for the nocturnal wandering of some patients. Episodes of incontinence may occur. Personality and emotional changes may include delusional and paranoid behavior, such as accusing a spouse of being an imposter or talking to imaginary figures. Obsessive symptoms such as repetitive washing of dishes may appear. The AD patient may also exhibit anxiety, agitation, newly manifested violent and abusive behavior, or the inability to retain a thought long enough to pursue a purposeful course of action.

Ultimately, all verbal abilities are lost. The patient is incontinent of urine, requires assistance with all aspects of personal care, and may lose the ability to walk (Dodson 1984).

Alzheimer's disease is a progressive disorder with a downward course requiring different services at different stages. It is estimated that more than one million people with AD are maintained at home, with the burden of caretaking resting on women—daughters, daughters-in-law—and wives who are themselves aging. Because the person with AD functions better and longer in familiar surroundings, it is important to promote care at home. But as is frequently observed by health-care professionals, "Alzheimer's causes more damage to the family than any other disease." Most stressful to the caretaker are the patient's catastrophic reactions, overt sexual behavior, incontinence, combativeness, violence, and abrupt mood swings.

The importance of care of the caregiver cannot be overemphasized (Mace and Rabins 1981; Williams 1986). Caregivers need factual information about the degenerative clinical presentations of AD. They need creative ideas and support to minimize, when possible, the impact of the disabilities of the AD patient. Members of community-sponsored AD support groups are often effective in working together to develop innovative approaches to care problems. It is the nurse's responsibility to be insightful and nonjudgmental in approach, to be an effective listener, and to support the patient and caregivers with accurate information and counsel. When the caregivers determine that institutional care is the only alternative for their family member, assistance, referral, and emotional support are appropriate nursing interventions.

Assessment variables

AD is a progressive, at present incurable, degeneration of the brain, causing marked changes in mental capability and personality.

It is unusual for patients with AD to exhibit focal neurologic abnormalities. Most patients have generalized and progressive dementia without signs of systemic disease. Perhaps the most characteristic feature is the absence of significant medical or focal neurologic abnormalities in the presence of severe dementia.

At present, AD is conclusively diagnosed only on autopsy or biopsy where anatomic changes specific to AD are observed in clinically demented patients. In the future, however, studies of cerebrospinal fluid and blood may be used to evaluate the levels of neurotransmitters. For example, it is already possible to examine cerebrospinal fluid levels of choline and acetylcholine and the hormone cortisol and growth hormone, which are thought to be at least partly under cholinergic neurotransmitter control.

The diagnosis of AD is made in progressively dementing persons in whom other known causes for cognitive and memory impairment have been excluded (Coull 1984b). Tools for the diagnosis include the history, with specific review of activities of daily living (ADL); physical examination; neurologic and psychiatric evaluations; mental status examinations and psychometric tests; laboratory studies of blood and urine; and a CT scan. Even with all these studies, it is still difficult to differentiate AD from multi-infarct dementia, depression, or other functional disorders.

One of the first goals in the nursing assessment of patients suspected of having AD is to measure the decline in intellectual function that occurs as the patient becomes ill (Palmateer and McCartney 1985). Apparently, little, if any, loss occurs in the normal elderly person when intelligence is measured in terms of stored information. In normal elderly persons, most verbal abilities are maintained and may even increase in the later years of life. This is especially true for persons of intellectually high or average ability (Botwinick 1985).

The most prominent features in AD are the cognitive dysfunctions including deficits in attention, learning, memory, and expressive and receptive language (Coull 1984b). Frequently, impairments in focal skills such as calculation, judgment, abstraction, and orientation are reported. Early in the disease course, only one or two cognitive functions may fail.

Intellectual losses

The intellectual process requires the constant use of memory. Memory is the recollection of words, concepts, faces, names, and objects—all the elements of life's experiences. Decline in memory function is readily detected early in the course of dementia and therefore tests of verbal learning and memory at the initial stage are very useful. To live without memory is to live always in the immediate present.

Affective losses

Affective losses are a second major category of symptoms to be explored with patient and family. The patient with AD loses his or her learned social skills, including the ability to communicate effectively. Relationships with family and friends become impaired. Inept social behavior and personality change occur, including paranoid ideation, aggression, and alterations in sexual behavior.

Conative losses

A third category of symptoms to be observed and discussed are conative losses. Conative implies the ability to plan, initiate, and carry through to a goal anything that is voluntary. Thus, the AD patient loses the ability to program his or her brain and body actions to do anything voluntarily. The patient knows what he or she wants to do, knows that he or she should be able to do it—indeed, knows that it was once a common action—but now cannot perform simple tasks such as tying shoes or making coffee. The history may reveal that after distraction the patient is later able to complete the initial task.

Lowered stress threshold

The presenting symptom in AD patients that is probably most difficult to define, yet that causes greatest problems for caregivers, is a progressively lowered stress threshold, which results in dysfunctional behavior, catastrophic reactions, and nocturnal wandering (Hall 1986). The causative factor is thought to be inability on the part of the AD patient to express himself or herself and adequately cope with the environment because of a decline in functioning neurons. Thus, the patient who is cognitively and socially inaccessible responds to overstimulation, fatigue, or change in environment with a sudden behavioral change that can occur at any time, depending on existing stressors. These dysfunctional behaviors can present threats to patient or caregiver safety, disrupt planned group activities, or be exhausting to family and caregivers, especially if the patient wanders at night.

Pharmacologic treatment of Alzheimer's disease

The effectiveness of drug therapy for AD has been disappointing. No drug has been developed that consistently retards or reverses disease progression, enhances intellectual function, or improves clinical condition.

Cerebral vasodilators such as papaverine hydrochloride (Pavabid), niacin, isoxsuprine hydrochloride (Vasodilan), cyclandelate (Cyclospasmol), nylidrin (Arlidin), and ethaverine (such as Ethatab) have been used based on a formerly held, now disproven, theory that dementia was secondary to cerebral arteriosclerosis or cerebral ischemia.

Ergoloid mesylates (such as Hydergine) are the only drugs in the United States currently approved by the Federal Drug Administration for use in "individuals over sixty who manifest signs and symptoms of an idiopathic decline in mental capacity," certainly a euphemism for AD. The drug improves functional status test scores but this is not often clinically discernible. This drug does not effectively improve daily living skills, intelligence or psychological test scores, nor does it delay disease progression.

Other drugs currently in use to control behavioral complications such as verbal outbursts, wandering, and physical attacks include thiothixene (Navane), loxapine (Loxitane), and thioridazine (Mellaril).

No drug has been confirmed to reverse or retard the disease process (Brocklehurst 1984, Kelly 1984).

Nursing care plans

Medical diagnosis: Stroke, TIA

1. Clinical nursing problem: Alteration in cerebral tissue perfusion: stroke, TIA

Goal

Patient will maintain or regain neurologic function.

Nursing interventions

1. Assess and record signs of decreased cerebral tissue perfusion
  • Consciousness (response to voice, noise, pain; orientation)

continued

Nursing interventions

- Mentation (attention; affect; language—spontaneous speech, naming, comprehension, reading, writing, spelling; spatial perception; memory—recent and remote; intellect—fund of knowledge; social awareness and judgment; abstract thinking).
- Movement: Head (extraocular movement; eating—chewing and swallowing; facial expression and symmetry; articulation, phonation).
- Movement: Body (muscle strength; symmetry; involuntary movements; coordination; abilities in ADL).
- Sensation (visual acuity; hearing; pain and temperature; touch; position sense).
- Integrated regulation (breathing, circulation; temperature control; ingestion and digestion; elimination; sexual response).
- Coping with disability.

2. Identify and control factors that contribute to decreased cerebral tissue perfusion
   - Body positions
   - Medications
   - Dehydration
   - Hypertension or hypotension
   - Hypoxia or hypercapnea
   - Deep hip flexion
   - Valsalvar maneuvers
   - Negative tone of voice
   - Negative conversation

3. Institute measures to promote cerebral tissue perfusion
   - Maintain adequate respiratory status
     a. Mouth care
     b. Suction machine at bedside (if decreased level of awareness, depressed gag reflex)
     c. Suction PRN (*only* as needed)
     d. Monitor arterial blood gases
   - Monitor, record, effect needed hydration

continued

Nursing interventions

- Monitor effective heparin therapy (when ordered)
    a. Infusion starts and restarts should be done within 30 min.
    b. IV-push orders should be handled STAT.
    c. Notify physician of any interruption in infusion >30 min
    d. Monitor PTT at least daily (no heparin should be initiated until after cerebral hemorrhage is ruled out)
- Monitor effective oral anticoagulant or antiplatelet therapy when ordered.
- Monitor lab values (PTT, PT, electrolytes, glucose, hemoglobin, hematocrit, etc.).
- Until vasomotor stability confirmed, maintain head of bed flat (may turn side to side).

2. Nursing diagnosis: High risk of respiratory impairment related to ineffective airway clearance, impaired gas exchange, dysphagia, paresis, plegia

Goals

Patient will maintain maximum pulmonary function.
Patient will have a decreased risk of aspiration.

Nursing interventions

1. Monitor respiratory rate, pattern, quality, airway patency, arterial blood gases, chest x-ray, breath sounds.
2. Encourage deep breathing, position change; discourage coughing.
3. Monitor for restlessness.
4. Test for gag and swallow reflex.
5. Observe for nausea and vomiting and keep NPO if nausea and vomiting occur.
6. Suction PRN.
7. Monitor for calf tenderness, redness, high pCO_2, low pO_2, chest pain.
8. Maintain oxygen flow rate as ordered.
9. Avoid administration of tranquilizers, sedatives, narcotics, which may depress respiration and mentation.

3. Nursing diagnosis: Alterations in nutrition (less than body requirements) related to facial paresis, plegia, dysphagia, altered awareness

Goals	Nursing interventions

Goals

Patient will maintain adequate nutrition.
Patient will have decreased risk of aspiration.

Nursing interventions

1. Assess ability to swallow, cough and gag reflex, level of alertness, extent of facial and extremity weakness.
2. Weigh patient at least weekly.
3. Provide adequate assistance in feeding.
4. Evaluate and document patient's ability to eat ordered diet.
5. Collaborate with speech and language pathologist and occupational therapist for patient with swallowing difficulties.
6. Observe for nausea and vomiting and keep NPO if it occurs.
7. Monitor solid and liquid food intake.
8. Collaborate with physician and dietician as indicated.
9. If facial paresis present, place food on back of tongue and on the side of face that patient is still able to control.
10. Inspect affected facial paretic orifice for food particles.
11. Assure good oral hygiene before and after each meal.

4. Nursing diagnosis: Uncompensated cognitive deficits related to inattention to stimuli on affected side; lack of awareness of impairment or physical limitations; inability to follow left-right commands; inability to recognize body parts, objects, and persons; memory deficit; impaired judgment; lack of insight.

Goals

The patient will not sustain injury caused by cognitive deficits.
Patient and family will use compensation techniques to facilitate patient function.

Nursing interventions

1. Structure environment to ensure safety, consistency, and minimal distractions.
2. Use repetition, verbal cues, and memory aids.
3. Avoid left–right directions.
4. Encourage the patient to look at the affected body parts.
5. Keep affected body parts on the midline and within the patient's sight.
6. Teach safety awareness and compensation techniques to patient and family.

5. Nursing diagnosis: Alterations in sensory perceptions related to impaired vision, impaired proprioception, altered touch, impaired hearing, altered pain perception, altered temperature.

Goals	Nursing interventions
Patient will not sustain injuries related to sensory deficits.	1. Assess and document sensory awareness (vision; awareness of the location of body and body parts; hot and cold; sharp and dull; response to pain, response to sound and speech).
Patient will maintain and optimize unaffected sensory functions.	2. Institute proper safety precautions.
Patient will adapt skills to compensate for sensory deficits.	3. Provide sensory stimulation (familiar smells, music, voices, photographs, touch, changes in light, and so forth)
	4. Encourage family to participate in sensory stimulation program.
	5. Arrange bed with personal-care articles, food tray, window view on unaffected visual field side (acute phase).
	6. Approach patient on unaffected visual field side for assessment and conversation (acute phase).
	7. Carry out interventions listed above (5 and 6) on affected visual field side; encourage "scanning" (post-acute phase).
	8. Describe where body parts are when moving patient.
	9. Have patient wear prescribed eyeglasses and hearing aid as per routine and during therapies.
	10. Avoid use of extremes of hot and cold in foods, bath water.

6. Nursing diagnosis: Impaired communication related to impaired verbal language, written language, speech and writing programming, altered articulation, inability to write and make gestures.

Goals	Nursing interventions
Patient will communicate that needs are being met.	1. Assess ability to comprehend, speak, read, and write.
Patient will demonstrate an increased ability to understand.	2. Provide an alternate method of communication appropriate to specific needs and

continued

Goals

Patient will demonstrate improved ability to express himself or herself.
Patient will express decreased frustration with communication.
Patient will demonstrate ways to maximize ability to communicate.

Nursing interventions

abilities (writing pad and pencil; word board; flip chart; word computer; sign language [*i.e.,* eye blinks, head nods, gestures, pantomime]).
3. Assess ability to hear and see.
4. Encourage patient to wear prescribed eyeglasses and hearing aid.
5. Speak slowly, distinctly, and calmly.
6. Have only one person speak at a time.
7. Listen attentively.
8. Use simple, single words.
9. Give only one direction at a time.
10. Provide sufficient light and remove distractions.
11. Allow time for thought comprehension.
12. Acknowledge patient's frustration.
13. Include family in communication re-training.
14. Consult speech and language pathologist.
15. Teach and follow through with techniques to improve speech.

7. Nursing diagnosis: Impaired physical mobility related to altered awareness, paresis, plegia, bedrest, lack of awareness of body parts.

Goals

Patient will maintain full range of motion in all extremities.
Patient will maintain required bedrest without developing problems of immobility.
Patient will maintain proper body alignment.
Patient will progress in mobilization when neurologically stable.
Patient and family will understand the rationale for interventions and restrictions in activity.

Nursing interventions

1. Assess and document motor function of face and each extremity on admit and at least every 4 hr.
2. Position and support head and extremities in normal body alignment.
3. Support affected arm with hand and arm raised slightly higher than heart level.
4. Range of motion to paretic extremities and feed every 4 hr.
5. Range of motion to all extremities at least every shift.
6. Coordinate range of motion and exercise plan with physical therapist and occupational therapist.

continued

Nursing interventions

7. Use trochanter roll along the outer aspect of the paretic thigh when patient is lying on back.
8. Keep patient flat or *only* slightly elevate head of bed when patient is on back (to decrease hip flexion contractures).
9. Use footboard.
10. Involve family and patient in exercise program.
11. Begin range of motion on admission (no deep hip flexion exercises).

8. Nursing diagnosis: Ineffective individual coping related to altered body image; loss of independence; economic stressors; loss, grieving, or alteration in family role

Goals

Patient will verbalize feelings related to his or her emotional state.
Patient will recognize and maximize personal strengths.
Patient will develop coping skills in light of disabilities.

Nursing interventions

1. Assess ability to understand.
2. Identify previous activities.
3. Have continuity of care and caregivers.
4. Answer questions honestly and offer information.
5. Involve patient and significant others in care, daily planning, and decision making as much as possible.
6. Encourage independence, diversional activities.
7. Support planning for a realistic lifestyle that is within limitations but fully using capabilities.
8. Explore sources of support—significant others, family, clergy, professional counseling.
9. Refer to community support groups.

9. Nursing diagnosis: Knowledge deficit of risk factors, disease process, medications, altered techniques of ADL, longterm care, and economics related to lack of instruction.

Goals	*Nursing interventions*
Patient will actively participate in prescribed health behavior.	1. Identify causative and contributing factors for patient's and family's lack of knowledge.
Patient will experience less anxiety related to the fear of the unknown.	2. Reduce or eliminate barriers to learning.
	3. Establish a teaching plan.
Patient will describe the disease process, signs, symptoms, risk factors, and prescribed medical therapy for stroke or TIA.	4. Individualize the teaching program based on patient's intellectual or physical impairments.
	5. Repeat teaching program several times with patient and family to maximize learning.
	6. Give patient written, easy-to-read information for future reference.
	7. Establish a routine of medication administration, using aids based on patient's needs (*e.g.*, Coumadin calendar, pill organizers, large-type labelling, buddy system).
	8. Refer patient and family to American Heart Association, National Stroke Association, or local support groups.
	9. Refer to Chapter 3 for further suggestions.

(Data from Carpenito LJ: Nursing Diagnosis: Application to Clinical Practice. Philadelphia, JB Lippincott, 1983; Doenges ME, Jeffries MF, Moorhouse MF: Nursing Care Plans: Nursing Diagnoses in Planning Patient Care. Philadelphia, FA Davis, 1984; Gee ZL, Passarella PM: Nursing Care of the Stroke Patient—A Therapeutic Approach. Philadelphia, AREN-Publications, 1985; Hickey JV: The Clinical Practice of Neurological and Neurosurgical Nursing. Philadelphia, JB Lippincott, 1986; Joint Committee to Revise STANDARDS of Neuroscience Nursing Practice: Process and Outcome Criteria for Selected Diagnoses. Kansas City, American Nurses' Association, 1985; Linde M: Cerebrovascular Accidents. In Carnevali DZ, Patrick M (eds): Nursing Management for the Elderly. Philadelphia, JB Lippincott, 1986)

Medical diagnosis: Parkinson's disease

10. Nursing diagnosis: Impaired physical mobility related to disturbance in free-flowing movement, muscular rigidity, tremors, muscular weakness and fatigue, loss of postural reflexes

Goals	*Nursing interventions*
Patient will maintain maximum independent function.	1. Ambulate with patient.
	2. Encourage patient to lift feet and take large steps when walking.
Patient will not develop complications of immobility.	3. Range of motion to all joints.

continued

Nursing interventions

4. Consult with a physical therapist or occupational therapist.
5. Establish activity baseline.
6. Allow sufficient time for daily-care activities (do not rush).
7. Simplify environment: reduce stress, encourage use of hands unless tremor is extreme, avoid situations that create frustration and failure.
8. Involve patient and family in individualized activity program and identification of short-term and long-range goals.
9. Assist with fine and gross motor activities as needed.

11. Nursing diagnosis: Impaired communication (written or spoken) related to decreased volume, slowness of speech, inability to move facial muscles, decreased tongue mobility, micrographia, inability to write

Goal

Patient will be able to communicate needs effectively

Nursing interventions

1. Assess level of difficulty.
2. Encourage verbalization, recognize patient frustration.
3. Allow patient time to express himself or herself.
4. Encourage performance of face and tongue exercises.
5. Massage facial and neck muscles.
6. Consult speech pathologist early in course of disease.
7. Encourage patient to take deep breaths when speaking.
8. Suggest use of gestures if patient is unable to speak.
9. Provide electric typewriter if patient is unable to write.
10. Anticipate needs and help when needed.

12. Nursing diagnosis: Potential for injury related to rigidity, loss of postural reflexes, bradykinesia, uncontrolled forced eyelid closure, orthostatic hypotension

Goals	*Nursing interventions*
Patient will not sustain injury.	*1.* Assess safety risk.
Patient will be given a safe environment.	*2.* Supervise ambulation.
Patient and caregiver will identify and correct safety hazards in environment.	*3.* Monitor blood pressure with patient lying and standing.
Patient will accept needed assistance to maintain safety.	*4.* Encourage patient to sit or stand slowly.

13. Nursing diagnosis: Self-care deficit related to carrying out ADL.

Goal	*Nursing interventions*
Patient will maintain maximum independent function.	*1.* Arrange patient's room for optimal self-care.
	2. Provide assistance as needed to maintain hygiene.
	3. Consult with an occupational therapist.
	4. Allow sufficient time for patient to complete own care.

14. Nursing diagnosis: Potential for respiratory impairment related to decreased secretions, restricted chest wall expansion, dysphagia, or inactivity

Goals	*Nursing interventions*
Patient will breathe without difficulty.	*1.* Assess respiratory function.
Patient will not develop aspiration pneumonia.	*2.* Encourage deep breathing, coughing.
	3. Provide humidity if needed.
	4. Encourage turning; turn every 2 hr if patient unable to do so unassisted.
	5. Administer chest physiotherapy as needed.
	6. Assess swallowing: hold foods and fluids if aspiration suspected.

15. Nursing diagnosis: Alteration in nutrition (less than body requirements) related to dysphagia, drooling, difficulty chewing, medication side-effects of nausea or vomiting, or decreased appetite

Goals

Patient will maintain an adequate caloric and fluid intake.
Patient will have decreased risk of aspiration.

Nursing interventions

1. Monitor swallowing ability.
2. Provide soft–solid and thick liquid diet.
3. Avoid thin liquids.
4. Provide small frequent feedings.
5. Massage facial and neck muscles before meals.
6. Place patient in upright position for meals.
7. Provide suction for increased secretions.
8. Maintain calorie counts.
9. Weigh every Monday.
10. Consult occupational therapist, speech therapist, and dietician.

16. Nursing diagnosis: Depression related to disease process, loss of self-image, loss of independence, chronicity of illness, medication, side-effects

Goals

Patient will express feelings to significant others.
Patient will participate in care planning.
Patient will cope and adjust to physical limitation.

Nursing interventions

1. Encourage independence and self-care.
2. Avoid unattainable goals.
3. Emphasize capabilities rather than limitations; avoid overprotection.
4. Minimize emotional stressors.
5. Plan rest periods to increase effectiveness of planned activities.
6. Allow verbalization about fears and concerns, loss of function, self-esteem, and sexuality.
7. Discuss symptoms and methods to effectively compensate.

17. Nursing diagnosis: Alteration in urinary elimination related to disease process, side-effect of medication, or immobility resulting in incontinence

Goals	*Nursing interventions*
Patient will achieve normal urinary elimination. Patient will not develop complications of altered urinary function.	1. Maintain fluid intake of 3000 cc/day unless contraindicated. 2. Assess color, clarity, and quantity of urinary output. 3. If night incontinence occurs, restrict fluids after supper until morning. 4. Refer to Chapter 12, Nursing Care Plans, #8.

18. Nursing diagnosis: Alterations in bowel elimination (constipation) related to decreased bowel sounds, gastrointestinal discomfort, nausea and vomiting, decreased appetite

Goal	*Nursing interventions*
Patient will achieve or maintain normal bowel habits.	1. Increase fluid intake. 2. Increase fiber in diet. 3. Increase mobility. 4. Add bulk to diet: prune juice, fruit, leafy vegetables, bran, methylcellulose. 5. Give stool softeners, laxatives, suppositories as needed. 6. Establish a bowel routine. 7. Refer to Chapter 10, Nursing Care Plans, #1.

19. Nursing diagnosis: Potential for impaired skin integrity: drooling, incontinence, immobility, diaphoresis, and seborrhea

Goals	*Nursing interventions*
Patient will be free of skin lesions. Patient will participate in a treatment plan to prevent skin breakdown.	1. Inspect skin daily: identify problems. 2. Have patient shower or bathe as needed. 3. Apply lotion or prescribed medication to areas of dermatitis. 4. Encourage use of lightweight clothes. 5. Avoid prolonged periods of activity because of heat intolerance. 6. Refer to Chapter 4, Nursing Care Plans, #3.

20. Nursing diagnosis: Impaired home maintenance related to inability to be independent in self-care activities

Goals	Nursing interventions
Patient or caregiver will identify factors that restrict self-care and home management. Patient or caregiver will demonstrate the ability to perform skills necessary for the care of the patient at home. Patient or caregiver will express satisfaction with home situation.	1. Use pressure-relief devices in bed and chair as needed. 2. Turn and position patient every 2 hr. 3. Massage bony prominences every 2 hr and as needed. 4. Begin discharge planning at hospital admission. 5. Involve patient, family, and all team members in discharge planning. 6. Consult social service worker. 7. Consult home health agency. 8. Refer care-giver to a Parkinson's support group.

21. Nursing diagnosis: Knowledge deficit of disease process and medications related to lack of instruction.

Goal	Nursing interventions
Patient and caregiver will verbalize understanding of the disease process and medications.	1. Obtain database, record teaching plan. 2. Provide written and verbal information regarding the disease process and current treatment. 3. Provide information on local support groups and national organizations. 4. Provide information on medication, diet, home exercise, speech therapy, and assistive devices for discharge planning.

(Data from Carpenito LJ: Nursing Diagnosis: Application to Clinical Practice. Philadelphia, JB Lippincott, 1983; Doenges ME, Jeffries MF, Moorhouse MF: Nursing Care Plans: Nursing Diagnoses in Planning Patient Care. Philadelphia, FA Davis, 1984; Gioiclla EC, Bevil CW: Nursing Care of the Aging Client: Promoting Health Adaptation. Norwalk, Connecticut, Appleton-Century-Crofts, 1985; Joint Committee to Revise STANDARDS of Neuroscience Nursing Practice: Process and Outcome Criteria for Selected Diagnoses. Kansas City, American Nurses' Association, 1985; Lannon MC, Thomas C, Bratton M et al: Comprehensive care of the patient with Parkinson's disease. J Neurosci Nurs 18:121–131, 1986)

Medical diagnosis: *Alzheimer's disease*

22. Nursing diagnosis: Ineffective rest and activity pattern related to decreased stress threshold, sensory overload, neuronal degeneration, wandering behavior, loss of therapeutic sleep pattern

Goals

Patient will demonstrate an optimal balance of rest and activity.

Patient will demonstrate decreased symptoms of sensory overload.

Patient will demonstrate a decrease in wandering behavior.

Nursing interventions

1. Provide "time-outs" during daily schedule to avoid and control stress-related behavior.
2. Reduce or eliminate environmental distraction and sleep interruptions.
3. Identify factors that prevent or inhibit sleep.
4. Identify techniques to induce sleep.
5. Provide comfort measures to induce sleep.
6. Allow patient to wear clothes and shoes during rest periods if it will decrease anxiety.
7. Minimize potential hazards in the environment.
8. Provide safe environment in which patient may wander.
9. Provide patient with proper identification on his or her person.
10. Avoid use of restraints.

23. Nursing diagnosis: Deficit in diversional activity related to decreased attention span, cognitive losses

Goal

Patient will participate in activities coinciding with abilities.

Nursing interventions

1. Plan appropriate brief activities based on cognitive abilities.
2. Provide simple, brief instructions, one step at a time.
3. Provide distraction techniques to allow patient to refocus on task.
4. Recognize the patient's inability to participate in a diversional activity.

24. Nursing diagnosis: *Alteration in self-care capacity related to impaired judgment, impaired cognition, conative losses.*

Goals

Patient will maintain independence as much as possible.

Patient will receive needed assistance in self-care activities.

Nursing interventions

1. Keep instructions simple; repeat them frequently.
2. Avoid distractions in all activities.
3. Encourage attention to the task.
4. Be alert for fatigue (increases confusion).
5. Allow sufficient time for care activities.
6. Provide privacy during care activities.
7. Give the patient verbal cues as to what is expected of him or her.
8. Give positive reinforcement for successes.
9. Make a structured, consistent program for care activities (decrease confusion).
10. Encourage patient to wear prescribed adaptive devices, (*e.g.,* eyeglasses, dentures, hearing aid).
11. Provide all care that patient is unable to do or complete.

25. Nursing diagnosis: *Alteration in thought processes (catastrophic reactions, dysfunctional behavior, paranoia, and delusions) related to neuronal degeneration, inability to evaluate reality, decreased stress threshold*

Goals

As much as possible, patient will be aware of reality, based on the stage of disease presentation.

Patient will demonstrate fewer episodes of stress-related behavior.

Patient will experience positive feedback in response to positive behaviors.

Nursing interventions

1. Approach patient in a slow, calm manner.
2. Delete caffeine from food and beverages
3. Eliminate noise, extra people, clutter from living environment.
4. Eliminate misleading stimuli (*e.g.,* television, pictures that provoke negative behavior).
5. Maintain consistency and continuity in daily schedule and living space.
6. Address patient by surname preceded by "Mr.," "Mrs.," "Miss," or "Ms."
7. Give simple, short directions, step by step.
8. Use positive feedback (*e.g.,* hug, smile, words) to reinforce positive behavior.

continued

Nursing interventions

9. Provide "time-outs" during daily schedule to avoid and control stress-related behavior.
10. Recognize patient's inability to participate in an activity.
11. Label room, drawers, belongings with patient's name to decrease confusion of ownership.
12. Allow idiosyncratic behavioral actions (*e.g.,* hoarding objects that do not pose safety hazard or inconvenience to others).
13. Use validation and reminiscence therapies to encourage positive participation and reality awareness.
14. Do not challenge patient's response errors unless patient expresses awareness of errors or if a safety hazard exists.
15. Protect patient, self, and others if patient displays violent behavior.

26. Nursing diagnosis: Uncompensated cognitive deficit related to neuronal degeneration, memory deficit, impaired judgment, impaired problem solving, lack of insight

Goals

Patient will sustain no injury caused by cognitive deficit.
As much as possible, patient will maintain optimal contact with reality, based on the stage of disease presentation.
Patient will enjoy preserved remembrances.
Patient's needs will be met.

Nursing interventions

1. Structure the environment to ensure safety, consistency, privacy, minimal distractions.
2. Provide clues to orientation using repetition, verbal clues, memory aids, clocks, calendars, note cards.
3. Give positive reinforcements for successes.
4. Indulge in reminiscence; supply with mementos.
5. Evaluate continually the appropriateness of reality therapy, based on disease presentation.

27. Nursing diagnosis: Potential for injury related to memory deficits, conative losses, impaired problem solving, lack of insight, wandering behavior, catastrophic reactions, dysfunctional behaviors

Goals

Patient will not sustain injury (item 1).
Caregiver will be aware of and correct environmental hazards.

Nursing interventions

1. Patient-oriented interventions as follows
   • Be attentive to nonverbal physiologic symptoms related to unrecognized physical needs
   • Establish a routine schedule for baseline health assessments.
   • Have patient dress according to physical environment
   • Encourage patient to use prescribed adaptive devices (*e.g.*, eyeglasses, hearing aid, walking devices)
   • Assure adequate nutritional intake and proper medication administration
   • Provide a safe environment
2. Environment-oriented interventions as follows
   • Teach caregivers to be alert for and correct hazardous environmental factors
   • Initiate health and safety teaching for caregivers
      a. Install socket covers to prevent accidental electric shocks
      b. Install specially designed locks ("child-proof") to prevent patient from opening closets where corrosive liquids, medications, sharp items, and so forth, are stored
      c. Place on home exterior "Fire Rescue" stickers identifying that special evacuation will be needed
      d. Recognize patient's inability to act appropriately in emergency situations.
      e. Review with caregiver how to administer antidotes for poison ingestion.
      f. Identify poison control and other emergency phone numbers for the caregiver's quick reference.

28. Nursing diagnosis: Social isolation related to degenerative illness, dysfunctional behaviors, change in habitat

Goals

Patient's needs for affection, love, and acceptance will be met (item 1).
Patient's own sexual needs will be met in an acceptable manner (item 2).

Nursing interventions

1. Patient-oriented interventions as follows
   • Assist patient with physical appearance
   • Assure modesty in public
   • Demonstrate affection, caring, through your actions
   • Use touch therapeutically
   • Allow patient to use preserved social skills
2. Spouse-oriented interventions as follows
   • Teach partner the need for hygiene before intercourse if patient is incontinent and sexually involved with mate.
   • Teach spouse and caregivers to avoid and protect themselves from unacceptable sexual advances through distraction and removal of self from environment.
   • Provide privacy during self-expression for sexual release (*e.g.*, masturbation, disrobing).

29. Nursing diagnosis: Alterations in family processes related to family member with chronic degenerative disease process

Goals

Caregivers will verbalize feelings to nurse and to each other.
Caregiver(s) will participate in the care of the ill family member.
Caregiver(s) will seek appropriate external resources when needed.
Caregiver(s) will maintain a system of mutual support for each member.

Nursing interventions

1. Identify stressors in the family unit.
2. Create a private and supportive environment for family and caregivers.
3. Promote family and caregiver strengths.
4. Intervene when family weaknesses dominate.
5. Assist family with an appraisal of the situation.
6. Provide family with anticipatory guidance as illness continues.

7. Refer family to community and national support groups.

(Carpenito LJ: Nursing Diagnosis: Application to Clinical Practice. Philadelphia, JB Lippincott, 1983; Doenges ME, Jeffries MF, Moorhouse MF: Nursing Care Plans: Nursing Diagnoses in Planning Patient Care. Philadelphia, FA Davis, 1984; Hall GR: A conceptual model for planning and evaluating nursing care of the client with Alzheimer's or a related disorder. Lecture before the American Association of Neuroscience Nurses. Denver, Colorado, April 15, 1986; Joint Committee to Revise STANDARDS of Neuroscience Nursing Practice: Process and Outcome Criteria for Selected Diagnoses. Kansas City, American Nurses' Association, 1985; Mace N, Rabins P: The 36-Hour Day. Baltimore, Johns Hopkins University, 1981; Palmer MH: Alzheimer's disease and critical care. J Gerontol Nurs 9:86–90, 1983; Yurick AG, Robb SS, Spier BE: The Aged Person and the Nursing Process, 2nd ed. Norwalk, Connecticut, Appleton-Century-Crofts, 1984)

References

Albert ML: Clinical Neurology of Aging. New York, Oxford University Press, 1984

Boller F: Alzheimer's disease and Parkinson's disease: Clinical and pathological associations. In Reisberg B (ed): Alzheimer's Disease: The Standard Reference. New York, Free Press, 1983

Botwinick J: Intellectual abilities. In Birren JE, Schaie KW (eds): Handbook of the Psychology of Aging. New York, Van Nostrand Reinhold, 1985

Brocklehurst JC: Geriatric Pharmacology and Therapeutics. Boston, Blackwell Scientific, 1984

Carpenito LJ: Nursing Diagnosis: Application to Clinical Practice. Philadelphia, JB Lippincott, 1983

Carter AB: The neurologic aspects of aging. In Rossman I (ed): Clinical Geriatrics. Philadelphia, JB Lippincott, 1986

Cohen D, Eisdorfer C: Dementing disorders. In Calkins E, Davis PJ, Ford AB (eds): The Practice of Geriatrics. Philadelphia, WB Saunders, 1986

Cote R, Hachinski VC, Shurvell BL et al: The Canadian Neurological Scale: A preliminary study in acute stroke. Stroke 17:731–737, 1986

Coull BM: Cerebrovascular disease. In Cassell CK, Walsh JR (eds): Geriatric Medicine, vol 1. New York, Springer-Verlag, 1984a.

Coull BM: Neurologic aspects of dementia. In Cassell CK, Walsh JR (eds): Geriatric Medicine, vol 1. New York, Springer-Verlag, 1984b

Dodson J: The slow death: Alzheimer's disease. J Neurosci Nurs 16:270–274, 1984

Doenges ME, Jeffries MF, Moorhouse MF: Nursing Care Plans: Nursing Diagnoses in Planning Patient Care. Philadelphia, FA Davis, 1984

Fowler RS, Fordyce WE: Stroke: Why Do They Behave That Way? Dallas, American Heart Association, 1974

Gee ZL, Passarella PM: Nursing Care of the Stroke Patient—A Therapeutic Approach. Philadelphia, AREN-Publications, 1985

Gioiella EC, Bevil CW: Nursing Care of the Aging Client: Promoting Health Adaptation. Norwalk, Connecticut, Appleton-Century-Crofts, 1985

Goldman R: Decline in organ function with aging. In Rossman I (ed): Clinical Geriatrics, 2nd ed. Philadelphia, JB Lippincott, 1979

Hachinski VC, Norris JW: The Acute Stroke. Philadelphia, FA Davis, 1985

Hall GR: A conceptual model for planning and evaluating nursing care of the client with Alzheimer's or a related disorder. Lecture before the American Association of Neuroscience Nurses. Denver, Colorado, April 15, 1986

Hardin WM: Neurological aspects. In Steinberg FU (ed): Care of the Geriatric Patient in the Tradition of EV Cowdry. St Louis, CV Mosby, 1983

Hickey JV: The Clinical Practice of Neurological and Neurosurgical Nursing. Philadelphia, JB Lippincott, 1986

Jancovic J: Parkinsonian disorders. In Appel SH (ed): Current Neurology, vol 5. New York, John Wiley & Sons, 1984

Jankovic J: Differential diagnosis of stroke. In Meyer JS, Shaw T (eds): Diagnosis and Management of Stroke and TIAs. Menlo Park, California, Addison-Wesley, 1982

Joint Committee to Revise STANDARDS of Neuroscience Nursing Practice: Process and Outcome Criteria for Selected Diagnoses. Kansas City, American Nurses Association, 1985

Katzman R, Terry R: The Neurology of Aging. Philadelphia, FA Davis, 1984

Kelly WE (ed): Alzheimer's Disease and Related Disorders: Research and Management. Springfield, Illinois, Charles C Thomas, 1984

Kurtzke JF: Epidemiology of cerebrovascular disease. In Seikert RG (ed): Cerebrovascular Survey Report. Bethesda, Maryland, National Institute of Neurology and Communicative Disorders and Stroke, 1980

Lannon MC, Thomas C, Bratton M et al: Comprehensive care of the patient with Parkinson's disease. J Neurosci Nurs 18:121–131, 1986

Lewis CB: Aging: The Health Care Challenge. Philadelphia, FA Davis, 1985

Lieberman AN, Gopinathan G, Neophytides A, Goldstein M: Parkinson's Disease Handbook: A Guide for Patients and Their Families. New York, American Parkinson Disease Association (PAR-446), 1985

Linde M: Cerebrovascular accidents. In Carnevali DZ, Patrick M (eds): Nursing Management for the Elderly. Philadelphia, JB Lippincott, 1986

Lucas MJ, Steele C, Bognanni A: Recognition of psychiatric symptoms in dementia. J Gerontol Nurs 12:11–15, 1986

Mace N, Rabins P: The 36-Hour Day. Baltimore, Johns Hopkins University Press, 1981

Mitchell P, Ozura J, Cammermeyer M, Woods NF: Neurological Assessment for Nursing Practice. Reston, Virginia, Reston Publishing, 1984

Palmateer LM, McCartney JR: Do nurses know when patients have cognitive deficits? J Gerontol Nurs 11:6–16, 1985

Palmer MH: Alzheimer's disease and critical care. J Gerontol Nurs 9:86–90, 1983

Smith BH: Cervical Spondylosis and Its Neurological Complications. Springfield, Illinois, Charles C Thomas, 1968

Strub RL, Black FW: The Mental Status Examination in Neurology. Philadelphia, FA Davis, 1985

U.S. Department of Health and Human Services: Task Force on Alzheimer's Disease. Washington DC, U.S. Department of Health and Human Services, September 1984

Williams L: Alzheimer's: The need for caring. J Gerontol Nurs 12:21–28, 1986

Wolf PA, Kannel WA: Controllable risk factors for stroke: Preventive implications in trends of stroke mortality. In Meyer JS, Shaw T (eds): Diagnosis and Management of Stroke and TIAs. Menlo Park, California, Addison-Wesley, 1982

Yatzu FM: Cerebrovascular disease. In Appel SH (ed): Current Neurology, vol 5. New York, John Wiley & Sons, 1984

Pain in elderly patients   *14*

The pain experience

Pain comprises sensation and reaction. It threatens well-being. It holds unique connotations for each person, based on previous experiences with pain, its significance, and the resulting outcome (surgery, continued suffering, or relief). Other factors influencing response include the person's general state of health and restedness, available resources, response from others, and the presence of other stressors.

Pain itself is a stressor that provokes physiological and psychological changes designed to help the person prepare to meet or avoid a crisis. Some of these changes, caused by the sudden release of epinephrine, norepinephrine, and cortisol into the bloodstream, include increased pulse rate, respiration, and blood pressure, accompanied by anxiety and increased vigilance. Blood flow is directed away from the periphery of the body and toward the internal organs. In the elderly, physical, sensory, and cognitive impairment makes coping with stress less effective (Hussian 1981).

Research and observations have shown that pain in general is a phenomenon that is not well understood nor well responded to by many people, including professional health-care providers. Assessments of pain are omitted commonly and patients are undertreated for acute pain. Chronic pain sufferers fare worse.

Pain in the elderly

Pain is a difficult experience for almost all people, but it is especially hard for the elderly. Their memories of their previous painful experiences that have been suffered over the years shape current pain experiences. They have proportionately more chronic illnesses, which may be painful in themselves and which may be treated by a number of drugs given concurrently. They may have suffered a number of losses (well-being, resources, support persons) and pain represents another loss that is akin to grief. Anger is experienced early in grief work. Depression is a consequence of suppressed anger. The elderly are subject to the stereotypic views of others who may see them as different, difficult, or childish. They, like children, suffer from the misconception of health-care providers that pain is not keenly perceived in the very young and old, and so pain may go untreated or undertreated.

Age-related changes

Age-related anatomic and physiological changes have particular relevance to the management of pain by the administration of drugs. Although age-related changes are highly individual, affecting some people more than others and acting at varying rates, the nurse needs to be aware of what some of the changes may be (Kenny 1985; Oles 1983; Pagliaro and Pagliaro 1983; Reidenberg 1982; Simonson 1985).

First, body mass and circulating blood volume are reduced in the elderly. Blood becomes more concentrated, which can result in an enhanced drug effect or even toxicity. Proportionately more fat is deposited. Fat-soluble drugs (*e.g.,* barbiturates) are released slowly, prolonging the action of the drug. A reduction in albumen allows some drugs (*e.g.,* meperidine) that bind to protein to remain unbound in the plasma, causing increased sensitivity, greater respiratory depression, and even the idiosyncratic reactions of confusion and central nervous system (CNS) stimulation. Not only are there changes that affect the distribution of drugs within the body and interfere with their pharmacologic action or cause adverse responses, metabolism and elimination may also be affected. Most analgesics are metabolized in the liver and excreted by the kidney. Both function more slowly and less efficiently, prolonging the action of analgesics and other drugs, increasing the risk of reactions.

Simonson (1985) identified five factors that signal a patient at high risk for drug reactions:

1. Being over 75 years of age
2. Being small in stature
3. Receiving an excessive number of drugs, with a change noted with introduction of the new drug
4. Having renal dysfunction
5. Taking high-risk drugs (sedatives, narcotics)

The number of nerve receptors in the aged body is decreased; and many elderly patients are reluctant to complain of pain. In addition, research has demonstrated a greater duration of narcotic analgesia in the elderly (Bellville et al

1971: Kaiko 1980; McCaffery 1985). These observations have led to the theory that the pain threshold (level of noxious stimulation needed to be identified as painful) rises with age. However, careful assessment in which specific questions are asked is necessary to determine the patient's true state of comfort (Malseed 1985) and need for analgesia. The dosage must be determined with care to ensure that the dose and frequency of administration are adequate for pain relief without risking overdosage. Equally important, because of skin and receptor changes, the application of heat must be made with caution.

In spite of reduced gastrointestinal motility and regional blood flow, and gastric acidity, oral analgesics seem to be effectively absorbed (Reidenberg 1982). Giving analgesics with food reduces gastric irritation. Because of reduced tissue mass, injected medications may be poorly absorbed or cause irritation. Be sure the tissue is adequate to accept the fluid or use another route.

Because the elderly have a greater number of drug reactions and interactions and are more sensitive to their effects, the nurse must monitor their progress with analgesics (especially narcotics) very carefully. It helps to keep a record of blood pressure, pulse, respiration, estimate of pain intensity, and state of alertness in relation to the drug given. Adverse effects must be documented. Such a record in collaboration with the physician is useful in making necessary changes in the regimen. It may be necessary to change a drug, or reduce the dosage and/ or extend the intervals between administrations to promote effective relief while minimizing the risk of adverse reactions. Table 14-1 presents information on major drugs used in pain management and nursing implications associated with their use in elderly patients.

Assessment parameters

Elderly patients may complain bitterly about pain, or they may suffer in silence, especially if they feel resigned to receiving inadequate treatment or lack of supportive response when they do report pain.

In assessing the elderly who may have sensory or cognitive impairment, it is important first to gain their attention, to be sure they understand what is being asked. The assessment should be thorough and not rushed, to allow the patient time to answer accurately. A complete assessment is necessary whenever pain is first detected or is reported as changed. It is important to realize that acute and chronic pain may coexist. Both need to be assessed.

To detect complications or worsening of the painful condition, the nurse needs to note if the pain is new or a change in one previously reported.

In all interactions with the patient, the nurse must respect the reports of pain, and work with the person to achieve relief. To doubt a report only creates an adversary relationship, which is nonproductive and adds to the person's suffering. On admission, a pain history that identifies the patient's coping strategies and their effectiveness is helpful in maximizing the patient's input in the care plan.

Text continues on p 362

Table 14-1 **Major drugs used in pain management**

Nonnarcotics

Drug	Effect/response in the elderly	Nursing implications
Acetaminophen (Tylenol)	Acetaminophen is used for the relief of mild to moderate pain. Absorbed by the GI tract, metabolized by the liver, and excreted by the kidney—all influenced by the aging process. Hypersensitivity reactions may occur. Other adverse effects include CNS stimulation, liver toxicity, renal damage, blood dyscrasias. Because of ready drug availability and presence of chronic pain, acetaminophen is frequently taken in excessive dosages.	Anticholinergics, antacids, and narcotics may reduce absorption. Teach to avoid indiscriminate use.
Aspirin	Aspirin is used for mild–moderate pain and inflammatory conditions. Absorbed from the GI tract, metabolized by the liver, and excreted by the kidney. Like acetaminophen, aspirin is readily available and frequently is over-used by those with chronic pain. Toxic effects of aspirin include angioedema, rhinitis, nasal polyposis, bronchial asthma, and gastrointestinal ulceration and hemorrhage. Other possible reactions include abdominal pain, nausea, tinnitus, deafness, shock, and coma. Reduces platelet aggregation.	Do not use if acid odor is present. Use with caution, especially in diabetics because glucose metabolism may be affected. Give with food; keep hydrated. Monitor response. Watch for fluid-base imbalance. Use with caution in patients who are bleeding or are taking anticoagulants. Avoid aspirin in patients receiving methotrexate to prevent over-suppression of bone marrow.
Choline magnesium trisalicylate (Trilisate)	This nonsteroidal, anti-inflammatory combination of choline and magnesium salicylates is used to treat the mild to moderate pain of patients with osteo- and rheumatoid arthritis. Absorbed from the stomach and excreted by the kidneys. Hypersensitivity may occur. Does not cause platelet aggregation.	Reduce dosage if tinnitus occurs. Use with caution with renal impairment, gastric distress, anticoagulants, steroids, butazones, or alcohol.
Methyl salicylate (Oil of wintergreen)	Methyl salicylate is applied locally in liniments and ointments to relieve pain by counter-irritation. Absorbed in significant amounts by the skin.	Teach to avoid application to irritated skin.

continued

Table 14-1 (Continued)

Nonnarcotics

Drug	Effect/response in the elderly	Nursing implications
Phenylbutazone (Butazolidin)	Phenylbutazone is a nonsteroidal anti-inflammatory drug useful in arthritis. Absorbed from the GI tract, metabolized slowly by the liver, and excreted by the kidney. A potent drug that can cause the following side-effects: GI distress, rash, vertigo, blurred vision, insomnia, nervousness, and water and electrolyte retention. Adverse effects are ulceration and hemorrhage of the GI tract, blood dyscrasias, bone marrow depression, hypersensitivity reactions, renal damage, metabolic acidosis, thyroid hyperplasia, liver toxicity, hypertension, pericarditis, cardia decompensation, optic neuritis, retinal hemorrhage, deafness, CNS agitation, and psychotic depression.	Give with food or antacids. Restrict salt intake. Monitor closely. Examine stools for blood. Observe for interactions with warfarin, oral hypoglycemics, and sulfonamides. Do not give to non-alert patients. Teach patient to take drug as ordered and to stay under medical supervision. If no favorable response is obtained after 1 wk, use of drug should be discontinued.
Ibuprofen (Motrin)	A nonsteroidal, anti-inflammatory drug used for those with arthritis to reduce pain and stiffness. Relieves mild to moderate pain. May be used with gold salts and/or corticosteroids. Absorbed in the stomach and eliminated by the kidney. Ibuprofen inhibits platelet aggregation. Ready availability may result in excessive use in chronic pain.	Watch for gastric distress and hemorrhage and blurred vision. Monitor fluid intake–output. Do not give to those who are aspirin-sensitive or who react to other nonsteroidal anti-inflammatory agents. Use with caution in patients with cardiac decompensation or hypertension. Do not use with anticoagulants.
Indomethacin (Indocin)	Indomethacin, a nonsteroidal anti-inflammatory drug, is absorbed from the GI tract, metabolized in the liver, and excreted in urine and bile. This potent drug can cause GI ulceration and hemorrhage, hepatitis, pancreatitis, blood dyscrasias, bone marrow depression, renal impairment, CNS stimulation with headache, drowsiness, vertigo, confusion, psychic disturbances and convulsions, and corneal deposits.	Do not give if allergic to aspirin. Use with caution in patient with psychosis, Parkinsonism, coagulation defects, and epilepsy. Give with food. Restrict salt intake. Monitor closely. Do not give with oral anticoagulants. Watch for interactions with probenecid. Be aware that indomethacin may mask symptoms of infection. Teach patient to take medication as ordered and to stay under medical supervision, and to avoid hazardous activities because of drowsiness or dizziness.

continued

Table 14-1 (Continued)

Nonnarcotics

Drug	Effect/response in the elderly	Nursing implications
Morphine	Morphine is used to relieve moderate to severe pain. Absorbed from the GI tract at a variable rate, metabolized in the liver, and excreted in bile and urine. Like all opiates (narcotics), morphine causes tolerance and dependence, and in certain persons, addiction. Elevates mood and causes respiratory depression, constipation, increased intrabiliary pressure, hypotension, bronchoconstriction, and in some persons, hypersensitivity reactions. Brompton's mixture includes oral morphine. It is used with progressive cancer pain.	Have the patient lying or sitting to receive the first dose. Monitor blood pressure, pulse, respiration, and state of alertness. Counteract constipation. Patient may respond to smaller doses at longer intervals; monitor response to enable pain relief with minimal risk of reaction.
Codeine	Codeine is a narcotic used to treat moderate pain.	Less likely to cause nausea, vomiting, and dependence. Counteract constipation. Monitor respirations; watch for atelectasis. Teach patient to avoid hazardous activities (driving).
Hydromorphone (Dilaudid)	Hydromorphone is about 6 times more potent than morphine, but has decreased sedative, hypnotic, and gastric distress effects.	Keep patient sitting or lying down. Monitor closely for respiratory depression. Counteract constipation.
Levorphanol (Levo-Dromoran)	This drug is about 5 times more potent than morphine on an mg : mg basis and has a strong sedative effect.	Keep patient sitting or lying. Monitor closely, especially respirations.
Meperidine (Demerol)	Meperidine is used for moderate to severe pain and it counteracts anxiety. Toxic to the CNS, this drug may cause dizziness, tremors, and uncoordinated muscle movements.	Keep patient sitting or lying. Do not give with barbiturates. Use with caution in presence of renal impairment. If parenteral, give deep intramuscularly to avoid tissue damage, rotate sites. Monitor blood pressure, pulse, respiration, and state of alertness.
Oxycodone (Percocet, Percodan)	Percocet contains acetaminophen. Percodan contains aspirin. Oxycodone is more potent than codeine.	

continued

Table 14-1   (Continued)

Narcotic agonists–antagonists

Drug	Effect/response in the elderly	Nursing implications
Butorphanol (Stadol)	Butorphanol has an analgesic (agonist) action and is a weak narcotic antagonist. Causes less respiratory depression.	Keep patient sitting or lying. May precipitate a withdrawal reaction if given to patients on longterm narcotic therapy. May increase blood pressure in hypertensives. Use with caution in those with liver impairment.
Pentazocine (Talwin)	This narcotic agonist–antagonist may cause hypersensitivity reactions. Limited use for cancer pain, psychotomimetic effects with higher dose. Available only in combination with naloxane, aspirin or acetaminophen. May cause physical dependence.	Give deep intramuscularly and rotate sites to decrease tissue damage with injection. Monitor respirations.

(Data From Goldstein FJ: Narcotic analgesics and age-associated changes of non-narcotic analgesics. In Goldberg PB, Roberts J (eds): Handbook on Pharmacology of Aging. Boca Raton, Florida, CRC Press, 1983; Malseed RT: Pharmacology: Drug Therapy and Nursing Considerations. Philadelphia, JB Lippincott, 1985)

It is essential that the nurse take time to assess the pain accurately so that pain management can be effective. Assessment of pain should include the categories presented below.

Type of pain

It is acute? progressive? chronic? These types of pain are dissimilar, with each requiring a different plan for care. One or more type of pain may coexist in the same person. *Acute pain* is usually caused by obvious pathology or trauma and steadily decreases after treatment. Because it is short-lived, there is less hesitancy to order adequate doses of analgesics. Health-care workers and relatives are usually supportive and empathetic. Acute pain has some value as an indicator of tissue injury. *Progressive pain* is that which steadily worsens, as in some patients with terminal carcinoma. It serves no useful purpose and causes much suffering. Progressive pain usually requires the use of increasingly more potent analgesics. Because it may last for months, health-care providers hesitate to use adequate doses of analgesics. Dosage must be carefully titrated to achieve pain relief in a patient still alert enough to function. *Chronic pain* lasts longer than two months, often resisting relief in spite of treatment. Often no obvious pathology is found. Physicians are reluctant to order potent analgesics lest the patient become dependent. The patient is often depressed and pain-centered, which drives social support away. These patients especially need nurses who understand and can be helpful.

Location and movement of pain

Where is the pain? Does it move? Some pain can be localized; in other cases it may be diffuse. A painful muscle can be identified easily; an inflamed viscus may cause diffuse abdominal pain. Some pain radiates outward from the source; some projects along a nerve; some is felt in a distant place and is termed "referred" pain. Description of location and movement is necessary in identifying the source of the problem. Elderly patients may have some difficulty in localizing pain. They should be encouraged to point to the painful part.

Characteristics of pain

Is the pain sharp and shooting? Is it dull and aching? Cramping? Burning? Note and record the words used by the patient to describe pain. Such observations are helpful in clarifying the diagnosis.

Intensity of pain

On a scale of 0–10 (with 0 indicating no pain and 10 the worst possible) how severe is the pain? The use of an intensity scale helps to establish a common baseline for comparison of reports. To say a person's pain is "bad" is to provide useless data. To say, "It is 8 on a 10-point scale" gives a basis for accurate comparisons and enables the effectiveness of the pain treatment to be evaluated. It is essential that all personnel use the same scale of the many that are available. Patients seem to like the concept of a scale and are reliable in its use.

Accompanying symptoms with pain

Is there nausea? Syncope? Sweating? Confusion? Restlessness? In elderly patients, confusion or restlessness may be the only evidence of pain. In patients who have cognitive impairment, nurses' observations of symptoms and behavior are essential.

Mood associated with pain

Is the patient anxious? Depressed? Anxiety is more typical with acute pain and is evidence of activation of the sympathetic nervous system. Relaxation strategies are appropriate means of anxiety reduction. Reduction of anxiety usually results in pain reduction. While the fight-or-flight syndrome resulting from stimulation of the sympathetic nervous system may be less intense in the elderly, anxiety does occur and compounds the distress caused by pain. Depression often accompanies progressive and chronic pain, induced, no doubt, by the many severe losses these patients report. Divorce is not uncommon when one spouse has suffered pain that is steady and prolonged. The price taken over the years in financial resources, friends, comfort, productivity, activity, and self-esteem takes its toll. The mood changes and personality characteristics typical of some patients with chronic pain usually revert to normal when pain is relieved.

Nursing management

The nurse is in a pivotal position for influencing the pain experiences of elderly patients. Of prime importance is the establishment of a climate in which the patient feels secure and respected. Such a climate enables the person to retain self-control, to avoid increasing anxiety or deepening depression. The patient with pain needs to talk about the experience and the feelings it engenders—the anger, the frustration, the fear.

The nurse also needs to teach what sensations to expect with potentially painful procedures and how to stay in control of the pain. Most elderly patients continue to learn and gain insight. Teaching should be geared to the individual's level of interest and ability, with allowances made for any problems with vision or hearing. Teaching must be specific, with examples and demonstrations, be presented at a slow pace to give time to learn, and be repeated for reinforcement (Pierce 1980).

Making the patient physically comfortable, changing the patient's position, or initiating activity, and ensuring hydration and nutrition are prerequisites for achieving pain relief. Another prerequisite is the suggestion of relief. The patient needs to know what to expect of medications and other pain relief measures so that the belief system can be used to enhance the relief.

Many patients are helped to reduce their pain by using guided imagery and progressive muscle relaxation exercises. These provide more than distraction; they are, in fact, self-hypnotic technics that produce a light trance and counteract the stress response. Patients who have cardiac arrhythmias, severe asthma, extreme mood alterations, or cognitive dysfunction are not candidates for these strategies.

Both strategies encourage mental and physical relaxation by (1) placing the person in a quiet environment in a comfortable, supported position, (2) coaching the patient to close his or her eyes and take two to three deep cleansing breaths, letting go of tension. In guided imagery the person is assisted to imagine a favorite place and "walk" into it, observing in detail whatever is there, using all the senses. In a beach scene, the call of the gulls and the crashing waves can be heard; salt tang can be smelled; sand and water can be felt and seen. A script designed for the patient can be read or reproduced on a tape. It should take approximately 20 minutes and can be used two to three times a day.

Progressive muscle relaxation assists the patient to relax groups of muscles in sequence, starting from the head and moving to the toes or vice versa. Telling the patient the part is limp, heavy, and warm encourages relaxation as vasodilation occurs. Each part of the body is scanned and deliberately relaxed. It is not necessary for the patient to contract the muscles first because most patients in pain already have tensed muscles. At the end of these strategies, patients must be assisted to return to an alert state. Usually counting back from five to one will be effective; if the trance was deep, counting backward from ten will be necessary.

Elderly patients who are not candidates for these strategies can be helped with distraction. Often they have already learned to distract themselves by reading, watching television, and doing puzzles or crafts. They need to be helped to find interesting activities they can do to help distract attention from the pain.

Nursing care plans

Medical diagnosis: *Cholecystitis, cholelithiasis, cholecystectomy*

1. Clinical nursing problem: *Alteration in comfort: acute pain*

Goals

Preoperatively: Patient will know what to expect regarding surgery, pain, and the postoperative course.

Postoperatively: Patient's pain will be controlled (items 3 and 4).

Nursing interventions

1. Teach patient what procedures will be performed and when, the sensations that may be experienced, and how to cooperate in postoperative care. Instruct him or her about turning, deep breathing, coughing, and ambulating. Invite input into a plan for pain management. Let patient know pain reports will be heeded.
2. Help reduce anxiety by interaction and giving support.
3. Give adequate amounts of analgesics at regular intervals to stay on top of the pain for the first few days as ordered; when change to oral analgesics, use equi-analgesic chart to be sure dosage is adequate and safe.
4. Encourage use of relaxation strategies and other coping techniques.

Medical diagnosis: *Osteoarthritis of vertebral column*

2. Nursing diagnosis: *Alteration in comfort related to chronic pain*

Goal

Pain will be reduced enough to allow patient to assume usual activity and roles and to prevent as much disability as possible.

Nursing interventions

1. Encourage rest periods alternated with activity.
2. Teach the proper use of body mechanics, the avoidance of stooping and lifting, support while at rest.
3. Teach the proper use of supports and walking devices.
4. Teach to use medications only as ordered at regular intervals. Be sure medications are clearly identified and easily opened. Teach what signs indicate the need to report to the physician.
5. Teach how to use treatments ordered, such as stimulation of pain inhibitory fibers by transcutaneous nerve stimulator and/or the careful application of heat.
6. Teach patient to relax using progressive muscle relaxation or guided imagery.
7. Encourage distraction through meaningful activities.
8. Reinforce other effective coping strategies used by the patient.
9. Help patient to see meaning in the prolonged suffering as related to spiritual or philosophical views. Finding some positive meaning improves coping.
10. Encourage social interactions.

Medical diagnosis: *Adenocarcinoma of the rectum with metastasis to the liver*

3. Clinical nursing problem: *Alteration in comfort: progressive pain*

Goal

Patient will have minimal or no pain while remaining alert enough to interact with others and function in care—as evidenced by verbal report and observed activity.

Nursing interventions

1. Maintain comfort through bathing, massaging back, turning—all of which stimulate large pain inhibitory nerve fibers.
2. Encourage activity as tolerated.
3. Identify coping strategies that patient uses effectively and facilitate usage.

continued

Nursing interventions

4. Teach how to relax using progressive muscle relaxation or guided imagery.
5. Accept pain reports and assess for changes in characteristics or location.
6. Medicate *before* pain peaks, preferably at fixed intervals rather than as needed. Do not be overly concerned with dependence.
7. Keep a record of vital signs, state of alertness, and pain as a basis for changes in drug order and collaboration with the physician.
8. Help patient with grief work; reinforce faith.

References

Bellville JW, Forrest WH, Miller E, Brown BW: Influence of age on pain relief from analgesics. JAMA 217:1835–1841, 1971

Goldstein FJ: Narcotic analgesics and age-associated changes of non-narcotic analgesics. In Goldberg PB, Robert J (eds): Handbook on Pharmacology of Aging. Boca Raton, Florida, CRC Press, 1983

Hussian RA: Geriatric Psychology. New York, Van Nostrand Rheinhold, 1981

Kaiko RF: Age and morphine analgesia in cancer patients with postoperative pain. Clin Pharmacol Ther 28:823–826, 1980

Kenny RA: Physiology of aging. Clin Geriatr Med 1:37–59, 1985

Lewis CB: Aging, the Health Care Challenge. Philadelphia, FA Davis, 1985

Malseed RT: Pharmacology: Drug Therapy and Nursing Considerations. Philadelphia, JB Lippincott, 1985

McCaffery M: Narcotic analgesia for the elderly patient. Pain Research News 4:2, 1985

Oles KS: Pharmacokinetics of commonly used drugs in the elderly. In McCue JD (ed): Medical Care of the Elderly. Lexington, Mass, Collamore Press, 1983

Pagliaro LA, Pagliaro AM (eds): Pharmacologic Aspects of Aging. St. Louis, CV Mosby, 1983

Pierce PM: Intelligence and learning in the aged. J Gerontol Nurs 6:268–270, 1980

Reidenberg MM: Drugs in the elderly. Med Clin N Amer 66:1073–1089, 1982

Simonson W: Medications and the Elderly. Rockville, Maryland, Aspen Publishers, 1985

Suggested readings

Boss GR, Seegmiller JE: Age-related physiological changes and their clinical significance. Geriatr Med 135:434–440, 1981

Hayflick L: The cell biology of aging. In Geokas MC (ed): Clin Geriatr Med 1:15–27, 1985

Faherty BS, Grier MR: Analgesic medication for elderly people postsurgery. Nurs Res 33:369–372, 1984

Ingham R, Fielding P: A review of the nursing literature on attitudes toward old people. Int J Nurs Stud 22:171–180, 1985

NIH: Pain in the elderly. JAMA 241:2491–2492, 1979

O'Malley K, Kelly JG: Pharmacological consequences of aging. In Bergener M, Ermini M. Stahelin HB (eds): Thresholds in Aging. New York, Academic Press, 1985

Wachter-Shikora NL: The elderly patient in pain and the acute care setting. Nurs Clin N Am 18:395–401, 1983

Weiner MB, Brok AJ, Snadowsky AM: Working with the Aged. Englewood Cliffs, New Jersey, Prentice-Hall, 1978

Psychosocial Care　　　　　　*15*

The older adult has a long history that spans many years. Their lives have been marked by time and shaped by coping patterns developed in reaction to historic events and situations: two world wars, a severely depressed economy, the ravages of disease, and the presence of epidemics without cure. *Survivors* is an appropriate term for the current population of elders.

Now, in the midst of coping with chronic disease and the inherent losses associated with old age, the elderly are still in the role of survivors, and look to health-care professionals for assistance. The elderly, more than persons in other age groups, have a long, emotionally charged history that must be considered in their nursing care.

Age-related changes

Development stages

During the latter stages of development, the elderly person faces a variety of stressors that require adaptive responses. Erikson (1980) described eight stages of ego development from infancy to old age. Each of his stages represents a developmental task reflective of a choice of crises in the expanding ego. The tasks in adult life begin with *intimacy versus isolation.* Failure to develop intimacy may result in isolation. A person who is stuck at this stage of development may not be able to develop close relations with others and may be at risk for dysfunctional social relations or abusive "love" relations, or may enter adult life without intimacy or attachments. This type of person may live with, but never love, another.

The next adult life task is *generativity versus stagnation.* The adult seeks to find a vocation or avocation as a means to help others and to contribute to society. Through helping and giving of self, the person learns and experiences caring.

The final stage of adulthood described by Erikson is ego-*integrity versus despair*. The elderly adult reviews his or her life to create a sense of uniqueness, accomplishment, and life integration. Often, the elderly adult finds himself or herself to have grown old with unresolved goals, and then will become frustrated over the future. If the person is unable to satisfactorily resolve this conflict, despair may develop. He or she will feel unhappy and bitter about life; many life experiences will be regretted and the approach of death dreaded.

Havighurst (1973) views old age as a period in which the person is confronted with a series of adjustments—adjusting to decreasing strength and health; adjusting to retirement and reduced income; and adjusting to the death of a spouse or significant other. The elderly person is also expected to establish an explicit affiliation with members or his or her age group, meet social and civic obligations, and maintain satisfactory physical living arrangements. According to Havighurst (1973), achieving these tasks constitutes a major step toward attaining and maintaining psychological health and well-being.

Maintenance of psychosocial well-being for the elderly requires continued education, learning, and adaptation. These processes require effort and energy. Often the elderly patient will respond to illness with a diminished interest in life; however, this generalization does not apply universally. The elderly are a heterogeneous group. Adaptive responses may range from diminution, depression, denial, and withdrawal to enhanced life satisfaction, high morale, high self-esteem, and continued physical functioning. It is the latter attitudes that the nurse can work to promote.

Health-care workers will not only encounter elderly patients at various stages of adult development, but will work with them in a variety of clinical settings. These may include the patient's home, physician's office, extended-care facility, or general hospital. Of all possible sites for clinical interaction, the general hospital probably evokes the greatest stress.

In the past, the typical health-care regimen was directed primarily to the physical needs of patients. More recently, attention has been focused on the patient's psychosocial, and mental and emotional needs. Each patient admitted to an acute care facility brings with him or her not only a physical or mental illness, but also a long history of coping strategies that will influence the entire course of hospitalization, or longterm care adjustment. It is paramount that the nurse recognize the importance of assessing previous coping strategies and reinforcing those strategies that produce positive outcomes.

Physiologic changes

The presentations of problems for which an elderly person might be hospitalized are often quite different from those in younger patients. The new problem is usually superimposed on existing signs, symptoms, and disease. The occurrence of mental confusion represents a prime example of how a new health problem can be superimposed upon an existing problem. The nurse faces multiple difficulties in trying to determine which adaptations resulted from illness or aging, which are normal or abnormal, and which are resolving or evolving (South Texas Geriatric Education Center 1986). The correlations between physical dysfunction and mental dysfunction in the elderly are further examined by reviewing specific body systems and associated mental–emotional alterations. The alterations include changes in mentation, nutrition, sleep, mood tone, and functional ability.

Research studies have found that cerebral blood flow and metabolism are significantly reduced with aging. As a result of these changes, varying degrees of confusion and memory loss may be seen in elderly persons. The confusional state may lead to shunning and stigmatizing by peers and other persons, resulting in additional social isolation, feelings of loneliness, and aloneness (Goldman 1979). Nurses play a key role as advocates to protect the elderly from mental and physical harm. Through accurate assessment, supervision of aides, and care planning, the nurse can develop a comprehensive reality-orientation program aimed at reducing confusion and increasing socialization.

Changes in appetite and nutrition have been correlated with problems of loss, grief, isolation, alcoholism, and depression in the elderly. Changes in gastrointestinal metabolism, however, may account for many elderly persons' lack of interest in food and subsequent problems with malnutrition. Lowered basal metabolism, delayed emptying of the stomach, limited activity, and lack of a companion with whom to enjoy a meal may have considerable effect on appetite.

Psychosocial care requires careful planning. When a nurse is already feeling the pressure of too much to do in too little time, the added burden of planning for nutritional and psychological support may seem unrealistic. Yet, there are occasions when the impact of psychosocial factors on the clinical course of physical health problems consumes more time, energy, and resources than either problem alone. Time spent in psychological support at the outset of an elderly person's nursing care can produce important effects that will benefit the entire health-care process.

With aging, the deeper sleep levels become less prominent and brief arousals are more frequent. A common misconception is that the elderly stay awake all night; this is untrue. Despite frequent periods of wakefulness, actual reduction of sleep time is minimal (Goldman 1979). The elderly and care-givers of the elderly need to know that the frequent periods of wakefulness are typical and usually do not impair the total period of sleep. Many elderly persons nap or dose during the day and thus have difficulty sleeping at night.

Expressions of dissatisfaction with sleep may really reflect that the elderly patient is bored. Much of responsive boredom is the result of a feeling of predictability about one's life, and simple changes such as a change of scenery may be all that is needed to relieve boredom. Changing the pictures on the patient's walls may help. Novelty may be added to the environment by giving access to entertainment devices such as handheld video games. Keeping a game at the patient's bedside will give him or her the opportunity to allay boredom during the frequent periods of wakefulness. Studies have shown that daytime exercise increases tolerance for environmental monotony and enhances sleep and feelings of self-esteem (Weinstein 1985). If it is known that a patient has frequent periods of wakefulness, the care plan should reflect this and include nursing interventions for both night and day.

If insomnia is a primary complaint, it should be investigated as a symptom of depression. Determine if early morning wakefulness occurs and if it is accompanied by anxiety or diaphoresis. Nursing measures to deal with frequent wakefulness include instructions to avoid caffeinated beverages after 6 pm, provision of adequate stimulation during the daytime hours, and performance of a thorough assessment for the presence of depression (see Figure 15-1).

The brain neurotransmitters include acetylcholine, epinephrine and their precursors, and metabolites (for more detailed information refer to Chapter 13, *Nervous System*). Investigations have shown that, with age, monoamine oxidase (MAO) and serotonin increase and norepinephrine decreases (Goldman 1979). Depression in the elderly has been linked with decreased stores of catechols in the brain. The increase of MAO and decrease of norepinephrine with aging are offered as one explanation for the depression and apathy frequently associated with elderly patients.

It is generally thought that 15% to 20% of the elderly suffer from depression severe enough to require psychiatric intervention (Shamoian 1985). From 75% to 80% of depressed patients, however, can be helped. Emphasis should be placed on early and accurate assessment. Nurses might respond to the need for intervention with various adjunctive therapies. Music has been used as therapy historically, and has long been valued as a physical, mental, and emotional stimulus (Glynn 1986). Reminiscence therapy may facilitate the life-review process while giving the elderly patient the pleasure of recounting happy past events. This therapy may also enhance self-esteem, and lead to a more comprehensive data collection.

Changes in vision and hearing may cause problems with self-concept, independent living, and continued employment. By age 40 or 50, the ability to shift vision from far to near objects is often sufficiently impaired to make corrective lenses a necessity. After age 50, the loss of visual acuity tends to accelerate and problems tend to be compounded (South Texas Geriatric Education Center 1986).

Additionally, the need for increased intensity of light doubles with each 13-year age increase after age 50. The elderly person's life is further complicated by decreases in depth perception and the ability to distinguish colors, especially blues and greens. Dark adaptation will take 1 minute for a 30-year-old, but for a 75-year-old it may take 10 minutes (Goldman 1979). Altered dark adaptation can cause problems with maneuvering in dimly lit spaces and this difficulty may lead to falls, severe bruising, and, often, broken bones.

Inappropriate use of colors in the elderly person's environment can place him or her at greater risk. For example, the standard admission kit for a hospital or nursing home contains a blue or green plastic water pitcher. The male patient is also provided with a plastic disposable urinal of the same color, making a matching set. It should come as no surprise that an 80-year-old man whose vision is dimmed by cataracts will mistake the water pitcher for the urinal (Henthorn 1980). Such a person is then wrongly labeled as "confused."

Psychosocial Assessment

1. Demographic/Social

   Name _____

   Date _____

   Occupation _____

   Address _____

   How long at present address _____

   Living with whom _____

   Marital status   S   M   D   W

   Children

       (How often do you see them?) _____

   Friends

       (How many do you see in a week?) _____

   Activities engaged in daily _____

   Next of kin _____

   Education _____

   Sources of income _____

       (Are they satisfactory for your needs?) _____

2. Medical History

   Physical problems

   a. Visual deficit   Yes   No   Type

   b. Hearing deficit   Yes   No   Type

   c. Acute or chronic medical problems

       Diabetes   Yes   No

       Heart disease   Yes   No

       Cancer   Yes   No

       COPD   Yes   No

       Stroke   Yes   No

       Other

   d. Hospitalization for physical problems _____

   _____

   e. Medicines currently taking, including over-the-counter drugs_____

   _____

Figure 15-1. Psychosocial assessment form.

continued

f. Are these being taken as prescribed? _____

_____

g.｜Allergies _____

_____

h. Sleep pattern _____

_____

i. Appetite and eating habits _____

_____

3. Psychiatric History

　　Previous psychiatric treatment　　Yes　　No

　　Reason for treatment _____

_____

　　Type of treatment _____

　　Date of hospitalization for psychiatric problems _____

　　Last seen for treatment _____ Where? _____

　　Alcohol _____ Type _____ Daily consumption _____

　　Last use _____

　　Illicit drug use _____ Type _____ Daily consumption _____

　　Last use _____

Figure 15-1. (*Continued*)

4. Mental status

Behavior		Appearance		Communication	
Cooperative	____	Unkempt	____	Normal conversation	____
Hostile	____	Appropriatcly dressed	____	Logical	____
Agitated	____	Personal care & hygiene	____	Confused	____
Anxious	____	Adequate	____	Mute	____
Restless	____	Inadequate	____	Aphasic	____
Fearful	____			Rapid speech	____
Suspicious	____			Perseverative speech	____
Suicidal ideation	____			Slurred speech	____
Homicidal ideation	____			Other	____
Combative	____				
Delusional	____	Memory		Mood	
Hallucinating	____	Impaired	____	Euphoric	____
Oriented	____	Appears intact	____	Depressed	____
Disoriented	____			Satisfied	____
Alert	____			Happy	____
Drowsy	____			Crying	____

Insight ____ Good ____ Fair ____ Poor

Judgment ____ Good ____ Fair ____ Poor

Affect

Appropriate ____

Inappropriate ____

Acute psychological distress   Yes ____ No ____   Other ____

5. Additional comments: _____

_____

_____

6. Nursing diagnosis: _____

_____

_____

_____

_____

(Developed by Jeanne A. Thomaston (RNC, MA),

Coordinator, Mental Health Evaluation Clinic

VA Medical Center, New Orleans, 1987)

Figure 15-1. (Continued)

The elderly patient experiencing varying degrees of hearing loss is often angered, frustrated, fearful, embarrassed, suspicious, withdrawn, and mislabeled (Maguire 1985). Many people do not know they have a hearing problem, because the loss occurs gradually over a long period of time. The ability to hear and understand speech may be significantly impaired by age 70, and background noises reduce the ability to hear a conversation. The elderly person may stop trying to hear what is being said by others and withdraw. Threats to personal independence because of hearing loss may greatly distress the patient and his or her family (Williams 1986).

Age-related psychosocial changes may result from internal or external stressors. Several internal stressors have been presented. Retirement is an external stressor with tremendous psychosocial impact on the elderly. The change of status from worker to retiree is often viewed negatively by the patient. The person's self-view might become one of "liability" instead of "asset." The patient's self-perception and preparation for retirement can have a significant impact on future adaptation.

LeBray (1984) identified eight potential problem areas for the retiree: the retirement event, social relations, disability, forgetfulness, death of a spouse, loneliness, diminished resources, and adaptation. Some of these factors are unique to growing older; all may pose problems for the person contemplating retirement.

Two major public health problems affecting elderly persons are the effects of mental health status and the psychosocial influence of retirement on the course of physical health (Cohen 1986).

For many elderly persons, retirement signifies the cessation of full-time, meaningful employment. Psychosocial research shows retirement to be a complex process for which many persons are unprepared. For some, the cessation of full-time employment may leave more time for socializing with friends outside the work environment. Usually, retirement marks the end of many meaningful social relationships. The ability to maintain social interests and to establish new relationships is significant in positive aging and mental health.

Loneliness (the subjective sense of being alone) in combination with the death of a spouse and retirement can be the straw that breaks a person's capacity to maintain an independent level of functioning. Suicide may become the solution; it is an especially common action for white men who are widowers. The events surrounding the suicide or attempted suicide may also be the events that first bring the patient and family to the attention of health-care professionals. A relationship with a suicidal patient can be extremely fatiguing to the nurse and other health-care team members. Nurses must be responsive to the patient's needs, as well as their own; however, the therapeutic plan must be patient-based and not nurse-dominated. At this point, nursing interventions are usually supportive, providing assistance in problem-solving and decision-making, or when distress is increasing. Structuring activities clearly is an important supportive strategy. The patient needs to know that the nurse will do whatever is possible to help, and that the patient is expected to be an active participant.

Assessment variables

The evaluation and care of elderly patients with psychosocial, behavioral, and medical problems requires good nursing care skills. Emphasis should be placed on a systematic nursing-care-plan approach with a sustained effort being made to develop health assessment and management skills for nurses who provide care for elderly patients.

Comprehensive psychosocial assessment of the elderly patient requires a critical and accurate evaluation. Valid and reliable assessment tools can be used to determine the course of treatment and outcomes. Five fairly sophisticated and refined assessment tools, which provide data relative to mental health and illness, are briefly reviewed in Table 15-1. These are the Geriatric Depression Scale (Yesavage and Brink 1983), Mini-Mental State (Folstein et al 1975), Self-Esteem Scale (Rosenberg 1965), Life Satisfaction Indices (Neugarten et al 1961), and the Revised Philadelphia Geriatric Center Morale Scale (Lawton 1975). Each assessment tool is brief, appropriate for use with elderly patients, and usually can be completed within 10 minutes to 15 minutes. Use of standardized assessment tools may

- Identify information relevant to the development of an initial plan of care
- Detect, by means of screening, the presence of psychological alterations
- Aid in evaluating the risk for later adjustment difficulties
- Aid in monitoring and documenting progress
- Provide quantifiable data supporting the effect of psychological alterations on physical status (Dush 1986)

The ability to accurately assess psychosocial functioning of patients is essential to both the prescription of appropriate psychosocial interventions and the evaluation of the effectiveness of those interventions (Dush 1986).

The psychiatric history and behavioral assessment provide the nurse with the beginning information to develop a psychosocial nursing care plan and to prevent further morbidity. This history should be incorporated into the health history if additional psychosocial information is needed and the patient has noticeable psychological deficits.

Depression

True depression in the elderly is the great imitator, and can itself be mistaken for other diseases. The interplay of coexisting physical and mental disorders complicates the appropriate assessment and diagnosis of depression. For example, depression may produce lethargy and sluggishness, and thus masquerade as hypothyroidism. Conversely, occult carcinoma may make its presence known by

Table 15-1. *Geriatric psychosocial assessment tools*

Geriatric Depression Scale (GDS)	15 questions Measures depression in the well, ill, or the cognitively impaired (Yesavage and Brink 1982)
Mini-Mental Status (MMS)	11 questions A quantitative assessment of cognitive performance. Identifies patients with cognitive disturbances (Folstein et al 1975)
Self-Esteem Scale (SES)	10 items A self-reporting test that reveals the extent of a person's self-acceptance. (Rosenberg 1965; Coopersmith 1967; Goldberg and Fitzpatrick 1980)
Life Satisfaction Index A (LSIA) Life Satisfaction Index B (LSIB)	A 20-item attitudinal scale 12 open-ended questions These tools can be used together; those scoring above 12 have greater life satisfaction. (Neugarten et al 1961)
Philadelphia Geriatric Center Morale Scale (PGCMS)	17 close-ended questions Measures morale under personality factors: agitation, attitude toward one's own aging, and loneliness. High morale responses are indicated by asterisks on the scoring key. (Lawton 1975)

inactivity, loss of appetite, and a vague loss of "get up and go," thus appearing to be depression (Coni et al 1977). The only presenting symptoms of depression may be a self-described feeling by the patient of being "low," or "just bad," although symptoms can include anorexia, insomnia, self-neglect, a state of withdrawal, and possibly mimicking of dementia.

The intense discomfort and demoralization of the depressed patient are most distressing to care-takers. But not only does depression cause morbidity, it may also increase mortality (Avery and Winokur 1976), and because it can be treated, it is imperative that it be recognized and documented. Only through careful, detailed assessment can the nurse bring maximum benefit to patients and make optimum use of available resources.

Self-esteem

Self-esteem is a person's self-evaluation, expressing an attitude of approval or disapproval, and indicating the extent to which the person believes himself or herself to be capable, significant, successful, and worthy (Coppersmith 1967). For the elderly patient, multiple role losses and feelings of uselessness can have a significant impact on how he or she now sees himself or herself in society. The Self-Esteem Scale (SES) can be helpful to the nurse's assessment (see Table 15-1). This tool may have some correlation with the Neugarten's Life Satisfaction Indices. Although the test is over 25 years old, it is still highly rated.

Morale

The morale level of elderly persons is one indicator of their qualify of life. Social gerontologists usually describe morale as outlook on life, or a person's assessment of quality of life. Psychiatric symptoms such as depression, fear, and paranoia are considered symptomatic of low morale (Goldberg and Fitzpatrick 1980). Low morale, lower expressed satisfaction with life, and lowered sense of contentment are also related to decreased social interaction, power, and health, and an increase in the number of hospitalizations.

People who are sick or physically disabled are less likely to express satisfaction with life or be motivated toward a positive outlook. Some studies suggest that less life satisfaction and lowered morale result from the pain, confinement, and uncertainty that accompany ill health.

Life satisfaction, as defined by Neugarten and coworkers (1961), has five component parts. The components are zest versus apathy, resolution and fortitude, congruence between desired and achieved goals, self-concept, and mood tone. *Zest versus apathy* refers to enthusiasm of response and degree of ego-involvement. *Resolution and fortitude* involves the extent to which persons accept responsibility for their lives. For example, a person may feel that life has dealt him or her a hard blow, but he or she is able to recover and continue life. *Congruence between desired and achieved goals* refers to the accomplishment of those things regarded as important. The *self-concept* component rates a person's physical, as well as psychological and social qualities. *Mood tone* assesses the person's attitudes and others' reactions to him or her.

Physical assessment

The medical section of the assessment provides an overview of physical problems, hospitalizations, as well as medications, allergies, and chronic diseases. The medication section may take up a major portion of the assessment because many elderly persons routinely take multiple, diverse medications. While listing these, the nurse should be alert to the interacting side-effects that can mimic psychiatric disturbances (*e.g.,* digitalis toxicity, antihypertensive depression). If the medications are not immediately available for recording, have one of the patient's significant others bring them to the hospital.

Use and abuse of psychotropic drugs and alcohol

The over-age-65 population is the largest user of prescription medications in the United States today. From 20% to 25% of all prescription drugs are given to the elderly, who make up roughly 11% of the total population (Ebersole and Hess 1981). Psychotropic (psychoactive) drugs constitute the major portion of prescription drugs used by the elderly, and sedatives and hypnotics constitute the third most common class (Salzman 1985). The incidence of psychotropic drug prescription ranges from 30% of elderly patients who are hospitalized for medical–surgical care, to as many as 92% of institutionalized elderly patients (Salzman 1984). The institutionalized elderly receive psychoactive drugs 17 times more frequently than other persons of their age. There are several reasons postulated for this situation: institutionalization may create great mental distress; the aged with mental or emotional problems may be more likely to be institutionalized; and drugs may be used for purposes of control (Zawadski et al 1978).

Surveys suggest that clinical depression may affect nearly one million elderly Americans and is the most common psychological disorder of advanced age (Salzman 1985). Depression is often a predictable part of physical disease, such as pancreatic cancer, hypoendocrine and hyperendocrine function, nutritional depletion, Parkinson's disease, and other neurologic disorders. Medications that are commonly prescribed for the elderly for treatment of physical disease may also aggravate depression. Drugs that are typically implicated are antihypertensives, sedatives, narcotics, antihistamines, and psychotropic drugs such as sedatives, antianxiety agents, and antidepressants (Salzman 1985).

Anxiety often accompanies depression in elderly adults because often they have much to worry about. Illness, financial insecurity, social isolation, aloneness, criminal attacks, physical abuse, accidents, and the approach of death may each serve as a stressor around which anxiety can develop. When anxiety interferes with the elderly person's ability to cope or obtain pleasure, then treatment with antianxiety drugs may be indicated. It should be kept in mind that some elderly patients are more sensitive to both the clinical and toxic effects of the antianxiety agents, benzodiazepines. Behavioral changes such as agitation and wandering can become prominent, and decline in memory function and symptoms resembling mild dementia may occur. These effects tend to intensify in the evening (Salzman 1985).

Researchers have noted that the elderly brain appears to be more responsive to psychotropic agents because of progressive loss of cortical neurons, accumulation of lipofuscin, and changes in number of receptors, neuronal metabolism, and blood flow. Because elderly people tend to tolerate psychotropic drugs less well than younger adults, doses of psychotropic medications should be started low and increased slowly.

Three major categories of psychoactive drugs are used to treat psychological problems in the elderly: antipsychotic agents, antidepressant agents, and antianxiety agents (see Table 15-2). The nurse must always remember that alcohol may interact with, and enhance the toxicity of these agents, and result in death (Brocklehurst 1984).

According to Guttman and colleagues (1977), many psychotropic drug users express a low level of life satisfaction. Their major concerns center around getting chores done, obtaining appropriate benefits, and establishing human contact.

Text continues on p 383

Table 15-2. *Selected psychotropic drugs*

Antipsychotic agents

Major classes and chemical types	Effect/response in the elderly	Nursing implications
Phenothiazines Thioridazine (Mellaril) (Other trade brands: Thorazine, Prolixin, Stelazine, Trilafon)	A 100-mg oral dose produces peak plasma concentration within 1–4 hr. Enhances motor coordination. Reduces anxiety and agitation. Improves logical thinking. Increases the incidence of orthostatic hypotension. Increases the incidence of Parkinson-like symptoms and effects.	Monitor for therapeutic effect. Monitor for potential drug interactions. Assess for adverse effects (*e.g.,* tardive dyskinesia). Urinary retention and constipation are frequent complaint; appropriate teaching is indicated. Monitor levels of sedation and hypotension. Observe patients for signs and symptoms of urinary retention and aggravation of glaucoma. Monitor patients for: • Decubitus ulcer formation, resulting from akinetic effects and reduced body motility • Drowsiness and hypotension • Accidental hypothermia resulting from drug influence on thermal regulation (Shields 1972)
Butyrophenones Haloperidol (Haldol)	See above	Tends to cause marked extrapyramidal symptoms. Other side-effects tend to be mild.

continued

Table 15-2. (Continued)

Antidepressant agents

Major classes and chemical types	Effect/response in the elderly	Nursing implications
Tricyclics Imipramine (Tofranil) (Other trade brands: Elavil, Sinequan)	May take up to 3 wk to reach therapeutic levels. Alters mood and may cause increased confusion and sedation. Improves psychomotor alterations (*e.g.,* slow speech, wringing hands, pacing). Adverse responses include anticholinergic psychosis, tachycardia, blurred vision, urinary retention, orthostatic hypotension.	Initial dose should be ½ to ⅓ of the usual adult dose. Therapy with an agent should be carried out for at least 4 wk before changes are made. Orthostatic hypotension is one of the more common and serious side-effects. Increased compliance noted with h.s. administration. Monitor for drug side-effects: constipation, dry mouth, urinary retention, blurred vision, congestive heart failure, dizziness from hypotension, mood swings, headache.
MAO Inhibitors Isocarboxazid (Marplan) (Other trade brands: Nardil, Parnate)	May cause bile stasis within the liver, resulting in an inflammatory reaction. Excessive central nervous system (CNS) stimulation produces tremors, insomnia, hyperreflexia, hyperpyrexia, agitation, convulsions.	Teach patient to avoid foods with significant amounts of tyramine: cheese, processed meats with tenderizers, beer, soy sauce, raisins, red wine.

Antianxiety agents

Major classes and chemical types	Effect/response in the elderly	Nursing implications
Benzodiazepine Chlordiazepoxide (Librium) (Other trade brands: Valium, Dalmane, Tranxene, Serax)	Reduces anxiety and promotes sleep. Promotes muscle relaxation. Variable half-life ranges from 23–99 hr, depending on the specific metabolite. May cause excessive sedation, ataxia, and confusion. Patients are at risk for toxicity resulting from altered distribution and elimination of the drug.	Use with great caution. Evaluate patient for desired effects. Evaluate for drug intoxication: excessive sedation (hangover effect), ataxia, confusion, aggressiveness, depression. Evaluate effectiveness of patient teaching. Monitor for drug interactions: increased effects with alcohol and Tagamet; initial daily dose: 10 mg or less.

continued

Table 15-2. (Continued)

Antianxiety agents

Major classes and chemical types	Effect/response in the elderly	Nursing implications
Propanediols		
Meprobamate (Miltown) (Other trade brand: Equina)	Causes sedation. Relieves anxiety and tension.	Monitor for drug side-effects: anxiety, agitation, jaundice, edema, nausea, vomiting, confusion, hyperthermia. Teach patient not to use with alcohol or to drive when taking the medication.
Barbiturates		
Secobarbital (Seconal) (Other trade brands: Nembutal, Luminal)	Produces rapid relaxation and sleep, used to treat insomnia.	Assess patient for paradoxical excitement or confusion. Monitor for overdosage: respiratory depression.
Antihistamines		
Hydroxyzine HCl (Atarax) (Other trade brands: Benadryl, Vistaril)	Also used as an antispasmodic and antiemetic. Drowsiness is common early in treatment.	Evaluate therapeutic drug effect. Monitor for drug side-effects: sedation, ataxia, dry mouth, blurred vision, hypotension, bradycardia, diarrhea (Perry et al 1981). Instruct patient not to use alcohol or drive.

They are inclined toward alcohol consumption and take more drugs than other elderly people.

Alcoholic beverages may be taken alone, or in combination with other drugs, to ease psychological pain or chronic physical pain. They may also be used to obliterate feelings of loneliness and to decrease anxiety (Ebersole and Hess 1981). Alcohol in combination with psychotropic drugs increases the risk of drug overdose, abuse, trauma, and death. The elderly alcoholic who presents in an emergency room may be improperly assessed, with alcoholic symptoms being attributed to "old age," chronic illness, social isolation, senility, malnutrition, or physical deterioration (Ebersole and Hess 1981).

Precautions must be taken to avoid this error.

Nursing care plans

Medical diagnosis: Reactive depression

1. Nursing diagnosis: Dysfunctional grieving related to retirement

Goal

Patient will be able to cope with feelings of loss.

Nursing interventions

1. Focus on patient's feelings.
2. Allow patient to ventilate feelings of loss by focusing on a period of life that was happy.
3. Use reminiscence therapy to explore post-retirement experiences, using open-ended questions (*e.g.,* Tell me about your work. . . . What did you like most?)
4. Allow for grief reactions of crying and anger.
5. Explore alternatives to work: gradual retirement, or leisure activities (*e.g.,* racketball, volunteer work, walking, tennis, woodcarving, needlepoint).
6. Involve patient in a group when able to discuss feelings on one-to-one basis.

2. Nursing diagnosis: Self-care deficit related to poor self image and inability to value self

Goal

Patient will assume responsibility for self care and activities of daily living (ADL)

Nursing interventions

1. Establish routines for the day, keeping to the schedule, (*e.g.,* bathing, eating, dressing, walking).
2. Observe sleeping habits, allowing only for one short nap each day.
3. Maintain balanced diet and encourage choices in food.
4. Explain the importance of exercise in well-being, encourage daily walking.
5. Encourage and praise independent behavior.

3. Nursing diagnosis: Fluid volume depletion related to malnutrition or loneliness

Goal	Nursing interventions

Goal

Patient will maintain fluid volume balance, as well as emotional balance.

Nursing interventions

1. Monitor intake and output every 3 hr.
2. Maintain infusion lines as appropriate.
3. Develop a list of patient's favorite foods.
4. Consult with dietician regarding frequent, small feedings.
5. Offer fluids by mouth every 2 hr; even between 6 am and 8 pm. Vary flavors and temperatures.
6. Afternoon snack should be mainly protein content, this enhances sleep.
7. After 6 pm, avoid caffeine drinks in effort to prevent incontinence.
8. Assist with toileting every 2 hr as needed.
9. Assist with grooming as needed.
10. Arrange opportunities for dialogue, twice a day. Plan should include formal and informally scheduled periods.
11. Use the Morale Scale, MMS, GDS, SES, or LSI (see Table 15-1) to assess patient's condition and progress throughout course of the hospitalization. Suggested intervals are on admission, after 3 days, and before discharge.
12. If a hypnotic is needed, suggest the use of L-tryptophan. This amino acid promotes sleep with few or no side-effects.
13. Before discharge, patient should consult with medical social worker.
14. If patient is interested, contact a community support group or self-help group for hospital visitation and follow-up (Carpenito 1983).
15. Reminiscence should be encouraged, about 60–90 min, twice weekly. Informal sessions may be arranged as indicated by the interviewer or patient.

Medical diagnosis: *Alcohol abuse or cirrhosis*

4. Nursing diagnosis: Severe anxiety related to nonspecific life dissatisfaction

Goal

Patient will reduce level of severe anxiety.

Nursing interventions

1. Use a calm, deliberate approach.
2. Ensure a safe environment—remove obvious physical threats.
3. Remain with patient or have a family member (chosen by the patient) stay with him or her.
4. Allow for uninhibited self-expression by the patient. Avoid making judgmental statements.
5. Use basic comfort measures:
   • Reposition every 1–2 hr if not self-initiated
   • Oral hydration if allowed
   • Assist with toileting as needed—patient may be unable to communicate the need.
6. Monitor and reduce environmental stimuli—lower lights and noise.
7. Approaches to patient need to be relatively consistent—short, directed commands.
8. Monitor vital signs every two hours during severe crisis, advance vital signs as level of anxiety decreases.
9. As anxiety level approaches moderate-mild state, arrange for psychiatric nursing follow-up (Carpenito 1983).
10. Allow patient to ventilate feelings, cry, talk.
11. Encourage ambulation, take walks with patient.
12. When anxiety level is diminished enough for learning to take place, direct interventions toward the subjects of the dysfunctional coping and abuse of alcohol.

Medical diagnosis: *Fractured humerus*

5. Nursing diagnosis: Fear related to physical abuse by a family member

Goal

Patient will experience an increase in psychological and physiological comfort.

Nursing interventions

1. Perform accurate assessment, both physical and emotional, and document.
2. Using data as a guide, contact police and protective services, informing them of the findings.
3. Do not leave patient unattended in presence of potential abuser.
4. Use facilitative communication techniques; do not probe.
5. Monitor visitors closely.
6. Use group psychotherapy to rebuild self-esteem and morale (use inpatient or community group.)
7. Assist patient to identify allies within the family constellation.
8. Allow time to discuss fears.

Medical diagnosis: *Acquired immune deficiency syndrome*

6. Nursing diagnosis: Social isolation related to ageism and homosexuality

Goal

Patient will cope with feelings of isolation and prognosis.

Nursing interventions

1. Use unbiased, nonjudgmental approach in caring.
2. Structure nurse–patient visits every 2–3 hr for at least 10 min.
3. Engage patient in dialogue on topics of interest.
4. Teach the patient progressive muscle relaxation techniques.
5. Listen attentively when patient describes past abuses.
6. Assist patient in contacting community agencies that provide social services.
7. Allow time for discussion of fears and anxieties.
8. See Chapter 16, *Caring for the dying elderly and their families.*

Medical diagnosis: Metastatic cancer

7. Nursing diagnosis: Powerlessness related to debilitating disease and rigid medical regimen

Goal

Patient will be able to make decisions about health care without fear of reprisal.

Nursing interventions

1. Keep interactions patient-focused (not family-focused or physician-focused).
2. Validate with patient inferences made about patient's verbal and nonverbal behaviors.
3. Accurately document subjective concerns, fears.
4. Provide timely and accurate information. Document all teaching.
5. Assure patient, through action, that nursing care and services will not be terminated.
   - Answer call light as quickly as possible
   - Visit patient at least 4 times per shift
   - Teach patient about other care options
6. Act as patient advocate:
   - State patient position accurately
   - Do not impose own values
   - Do not coerce the patient, intentionally or unintentionally.
7. Maintain an informed, yet unbiased, view throughout interactions.
8. Patient may experience ambivalence. Nursing approach must be consistent. Do not be manipulated.
9. Allow patient to participate in decision-making process (*i.e.,* expressing times for treatment and possible rejection of future treatment).
10. See Chapter 16, *Caring for the dying elderly and their families.*

8. Nursing diagnosis: Spiritual distress related to ridicule over religious rites and rituals

Goal

Patient will continue throughout the hospitalization those religious practices not detrimental to personal health (Carpenito 1983).

Nursing interventions

1. Assess nature of religious practices.
2. Identify and document in the patient's record any use of "by mouth" and "topical" ceremonial substances; these may adversely interact with other treatments.
3. Schedule time, as needed, for practice of religion.
4. Allow patient to share relationship between rites/rituals and health promotion.
5. If appropriate, use religious belief to facilitate discharge planning.
6. Document response to religious rites and rituals.

Medical diagnosis: Gun shot wound/attempted suicide

9. Nursing diagnosis: Dysfunctional grieving related to death of spouse

Goal

Patient will be able to resolve grief.

Nursing interventions

1. Physiological variables must be stabilized. Monitor vital signs (VS) wound, laboratory values, infection.
2. Designate a staff member to work with patient throughout hospitalization (example: a primary nurse).
3. The nurse will provide the initiative that the patient may lack. Use simple, precise directions.
4. Use actions instead of words to express concern:
   • Do not overwhelm patient with conversation
   • Visit patient every hour for 5 min (purpose: Just sit with the patient).
   • Meet with family or significant others to identify present and future strategies

continued

Nursing interventions

5. Enhance the therapeutic environment:
   • Room with sunshine
   • Use various colors; avoid drab blues (example: bright magazine pictures posted on a wall, change scenes every other day.
   • Soft, lively music; avoid television (may be too depressing).
   • Allow for open expression of grief.
6. Provide family, significant others with a list of community agencies providing counseling services free of charge, or on a sliding scale.
7. Assist with grooming and toileting as needed.
8. Arrange opportunities for dialogue, twice a day. Plan should include formal and informal periods each shift.
9. Use the Morale Scale, MMS, GDS, SES, or LSI (see Table 15-1) to assess current condition and progress throughout the course of the illness. Suggested intervals are on admission, after 3 days, and before discharge.
10. Contact psychiatric nurse therapist on hospital day 2 for appropriate plan development and follow-up.

Medical diagnosis: *Breast cancer/mastectomy*

10. Nursing diagnosis: Disturbance in self-concept related to breast amputation

Goal

Patient will be able to accept altered body image.

Nursing interventions

1. Allow patient to cry.
2. Sit with patient and facilitate expression of concerns.
   • Metastatic disease process
   • Age changes
   • Mutilation of body
   • Altered self-concept
   • Altered sexuality

continued

Nursing interventions

3. Contact American Cancer Society.
   • Arrange for a visit by a Reach for Recovery volunteer

4. Provide literature and information on programs for survival.

5. Instead of usual exercise, have patient exercise by putting on and taking off favorite articles of clothing. May assist the patient as needed.

6. Urge the patient to dress in street clothes instead of hospital pajamas.

7. Act as patient advocate:
   • Before operation, discuss with physician possibility of banking patient's nipple.
   • Discuss benefits of breast implants.

8. Provide patient with a list of community self-help groups, (*e.g.,* American Cancer Society "I Can Cope," and Reach for Recovery).

9. Encourage participation in self care/ADL activities.

10. Discuss breast prosthesis or breast implantation.

References

Avery D, Winokur G: Mortality in depressed patients treated with electroconvulsive therapy and antidepressants. Arch Gen Psych 33:1029–1037, 1976

Brocklehurst JC: Geriatric Pharmacology and Therapeutics. Oxford, Blackwell Scientific Publications, 1984

Carpenito L: Nursing Diagnosis: Application to Clinical Practice. St. Louis, JB Lippincott, 1983

Cohen G: The interface of mental and physical health phenomena in the elderly. In Geriatric Education—New Knowledge, New Settings, New Curricula: Conference Report. Bethesda, Maryland, U.S. Department of Health and Human Services, 1986

Coni N, Davison W, Webster S: Lecture Notes on Geriatrics. Oxford, London, Blackwell Scientific Publications, 1977

Coopersmith S: The Antecedents of Self Esteem. San Francisco, WH Freeman, 1967

Dush M: The health adjustment scale: Preliminary analyses. The Hospice Journal 14:33–54, 1986

Ebersole P, Hess P: Toward Health Aging. St. Louis, CV Mosby, 1981

Erikson E: Identity and Life Cycle. New York, Norton, 1980

Folstein M, Folstein S, McHugh P: "Mini-mental state." A practical method for grading the cognitive state of patients for clinician. Psychiatr Res 12:189–198, 1975

Glynn N: The therapy of music. J Gerontol Nurs 12:6–10, 1986

Goldberg W, Fitzpatrick JJ: Movement therapy with the aged. Nurs Res 29:339–346, 1980

Goldman R: Aging changed in structure and function. In Carneval DL, Patrick M (eds): Nursing Management for the Elderly, pp 53–79. Philadelphia, JB Lippincott, 1979

Granick S: Psychologic assessment technology for geriatric practice. J Am Geriatr Soc 31:728, 1983

Guttman D, Sirratt J, Carrigan Z: A study of legal drug use by older Americans. In Smith DE, Anderson S, Brexton M et al (eds): A Multicultural View of Drug Abuse. Cambridge, Massachusetts, Schenkman Publishing, 1977

Havighurst RJ: History of developmental psychology: Socialization and personality development through the lifespan. In Baltes PB, Schaire KW (eds): Life Span Developmental Psychology. New York, Academic Press, 1973

Henthorn BS: An ecological view of gerontological mental health. In Lancaster J (ed): Community Mental Health Nursing. St. Louis, CV Mosby, 1980

Lawton MP: The Philadelphia Geriatric Center Morale Scale: A revision. J Gerontol 30:85–89, 1975

LeBray PR: Psychological aspects of patient evaluation. In Cassel CK, Walsh JR (eds): Geriatric Medicine, Vol II: Fundamentals of Geriatric Care. New York, Springer-Verlag, 1984

Maguire G: Care of the Elderly: A Health Team Approach. Boston, Little, Brown and Co, 1985

Mitchell P, Loustau A: Concepts Basic to Nursing. New York, McGraw-Hill Book, 1981

Neugarten BL, Havighurst RJ, Tobin SS: The measurement of life satisfaction. J Gerontol 16:134–143, 1961

Rosenberg M: Society and the Adolescent Self Image. Princeton, New Jersey, Princeton University Press, 1965

Salzman C: Clinical Geriatric Psychopharmacology, p 241. New York, McGraw-Hill, 1984

Salzman C: Geriatric Psychopharmacology. Annual Reviews, 36217–36228, 1985

Shamoian CA: Assessing depression in elderly patients. Hosp Community Psychiatry 36(4):338–339, 1985

Shields E: Therapy and the Aging Individual (unpublished). Community Health Service, Health Services and the Mental Health Administration, USDDHEW, Washington, D.C., 1972

South Texas Geriatric Education Center: Psychological aspects of aging. GEC Scholars Program. San Antonio, Texas, University of Texas Health Science Center, 1986

Weinstein K: The restless mind. Feeling Great Feb:64–67, 1985

Williams TF: The impact of scientific advances on educational programs. In Geriatric Education—New Knowledge, New Settings, New Curricula: Conference Report. Bethesda, Maryland, U.S. Department of Health and Human Services, 1986

Yesavage J, Brink T: Development and validation of a geriatric depression screening scale: A preliminary report. J Psychiatr Res 17:37–49, 1983

Zawadski R, Glazer G, Lurie E: Psychotropic drug use among institutionalized and non-institutionalized Medicaid aged in California. J Gerontol 33:825–834, 1978

Betty Miller

Caring for the dying elderly and their families

Overview

All humans have two common experiences: birth and death. Historically, birth has been viewed as a positive happening, and death has been shrouded in mystery and sadness. Death reinforces the knowledge that each person is part of a whole and, as an individual, is mortal. Death should be viewed as the last life experience. As such, it offers an opportunity of continued growth for the dying person, as well as for care-takers. In death, as in birth, we share a common humanity.

Many studies have been done on the attitudes of Americans toward their own deaths. The following are some quoted observations:

> *My death is probable but only in a dim, distant fashion . . . I reason that my death is not only probable, but certain, but my imagination fails to picture such an event except in a crude fashion which is forced and artificial (Bomberg and Schilder 1933).*
>
> *The inevitable consequence of this apparently perennial contradiction between the individual's rational recognition of the inevitability of death and his concomitant inability to feel death's reality seems indeed to be the simultaneous maintenance of attitudes of acceptance and denial (Dumont and Foss 1972).*

The views and practices of society concerning death have changed dramatically in the course of the twentieth century. During the early 1900s birth and death were accepted as a natural part of life. People who became ill were treated at home. When their condition became terminal, they died at home, usually in the bed in which they were born, surrounded, in a familiar environment, by their family, loved ones, and friends. Practices that evolved over the decades that followed changed this situation. Technological advances demanded more centralized services, with a concomitant decrease in home visits by physicians. Hospitals, and extended-care facilities evolved (and the subsystems within these systems), much assisted by federal funding sources. Two-income households began to appear, and there was a decreased presence of extended families and in the number of children couples chose to have. The economy moved from an agricultural to an industrial one, then became service and information-oriented. Complex urban areas developed and attracted large numbers of people, which increased the demand for support systems outside the home.

Elderly and aging persons were removed from the environment of younger family members, and death became feared because people were rarely exposed to it. Societal attitudes toward the elderly have become negative as well. The elderly are seen as having no value, as no longer productive, and face forced retirement at age 65. Laws do exist to help safeguard the health of persons incapable of caring for themselves, but there is no way to enforce them. The elderly comprise 25% of all suicides (National Center for Health Statistics 1978). These statements may be startling—but they are no more than accurate reflections of the changes taking place in American society.

Hospitals and nursing homes have emerged as the places in which people are now admitted for acute, chronic, and long-term illness care. They are also the places in which elderly persons now die. Alternatives for these arrangements are limited, and are dictated by the social and economic factors already cited.

Until recently, access to services and duration that the services could be used were limited. Admissions to and care of dying persons in acute-care hospitals are governed by Medicare/Medicaid and private insurers' definitions of *acute care*. Unless their criteria are met, agencies or providers of care are not reimbursed. Third-party reimbursement has literally dictated the settings in which the care is to be given. As a result, instead of people dying at home, as was true in the 19th and early 20th centuries, 70% to 80% of all deaths occur in hospitals or institutions (Newsweek 1978; Ogg 1980). Almost 75% of these deaths each year are those of people who are over 65 years of age (Ogg 1980). Consider also that medical and nursing education has avoided teaching how to care for dying persons in general, much less for elderly dying patients (Dumont and Foss 1972). The achievement of a cure has been the emphasis in education of health professionals, with the effect that if cure is not possible, a feeling of failure results, with the pervading idea that "there is nothing more that can be done." At this point, the dying person has been placed "out of sight and out of mind." Uncertainty, avoidance, and isolation become their constant companions.

Unique needs of the dying

Until a few years ago, no one dared ask dying patients what they wanted or were feeling. Kubler-Ross began interviewing terminally ill patients in 1965, and as a result of her studies and those of the work of other researchers who were concerned for the welfare of dying patients, more information exists on the needs of this population. Kubler-Ross identified stages that the dying share: denial, anger, bargaining, depression, and acceptance (Kubler-Ross 1969).

The unique needs of the dying patient may be summarized:

Freedom from the noxious symptoms of the illness

The need to be with family and friends in familiar surroundings

Involvement in decision-making

Honest and frequent communication

A need to maintain his or her own identity and role

Freedom from heroic measures that become more of an obstacle to the quality of life than the disease

Need for a staff that understands and helps the patient work through anger and depression in coming to terms with dying

Avoidance of unattended bereavement that results in physical or psychological impairment to the survivors. These address the more basic issues of quality of life of the dying (Pegels 1980).

Usually, the nurse assists the patient and caregiver as they pass through the various stages, and sometimes as they repeat stages. The principles that should guide the nurse through this very difficult time are the following: allow them to proceed at their own pace; provide a supportive environment; and use appropriate counseling techniques of listening, being nonjudgmental, accepting their feelings and thoughts as their own, and never trying to superimpose upon them a more "acceptable" expression. *Never, never force patients through the emotional stages of death and grief as written in textbooks.* These stages provide only a framework within which guidance can be sought to assist nurses to assist patients and caregivers and to anticipate their needs. *Each patient's death is uniquely his or her own, as was his or her life.*

Factors that affect the dying elderly

It is important to understand the unique needs of the elderly patient who is dying. The following observations, offered by several authors, help clarify these unique needs (Clayton 1974; Earl et al 1976; Garfield 1978; Helsing et al 1981; Kneed et al 1981; Pegels 1980):

The chance is greater that important support groups will not be present, or if present, will be unable to physically care for the needs of the elderly patient who is dying.

The elderly live on fixed incomes and this population has fewer two-income families. Not all elderly persons can be categorized in this way, but the chance is greater for this to be the case.

The chance is greater for complicating chronic conditions to be present and to cause multiple problems to deal with besides the task of facing death.

The bereaved elderly have an increased chance of illness and death occurring within two years of the death of their spouses.

Self-concept

A dying person's view of self changes radically. No longer can he or she participate in previous activities, because of physical limitations and because people do not "expect" him or her to continue to do so. Others begin to relieve the dying person of "unneeded, burdensome" responsibilities. These efforts are well-meaning, but may create distress because the dying person is already facing many changes in the content of his or her life. This is doubly burdensome for the elderly dying patient because there may already have been adjustment to the limitations of chronic illnesses, as well as those of normal aging. This elimination of responsibility can be devastating, especially to those who have been decision-makers. They are left with only their dying as a focus for their attention. The nurse should think of it this way: the *who* we are is very much related to the *what* we do each day. If a person has nothing to do, then who is he or she? This outlook can lead a patient to despair and hopelessness, two emotions that nurses must assist dying patients to avoid. There are two types of problems at work for the dying patient—physical changes and emotional reactions.

Spirituality

The subject of spirituality and spiritual distress is an extremely complex problem faced by patient and caregivers. Some patients are very traditional in their religious practices and depend largely on, and receive much support from, religious objects and artifacts and their relationship with their clergyman. The nurse's actions of support center around allowing these patients to express these beliefs and needs. Often they will discuss freely the role they think their God has played in their illness.

For those patients who hold less-traditional beliefs and practices, it may be more difficult to anticipate and identify the actions that may offer solace to them. It is important here, as with all aspects of this kind of care, to establish communication and to listen. The patient and family will "tell" you in different ways what they need.

For those who have no allegiance with or ties to a religious institution or a belief in a Supreme Being, there are still ways in which the nurse can assist them to find spiritual comfort or at least to decrease spiritual distress. The nurse can help them explore their lives and identify those experiences that are noteworthy. Every person has worth—this is the message the nurse is helping to convey (Hospice-New Orleans 1984; Jackson 1979).

The choice of any of these approaches is, of course, determined by the patient.

Sexuality

The elderly dying patient may have already faced some alteration in sexual functioning. Sexual activity may decline and change in some characteristics, but it continues throughout life. Unexpected and drastic changes such as those that result from a terminal illness profoundly affect the core of a person's self-image. A person who has seen himself or herself as the initiator, and is now limited by the physical problems associated with a terminal illness, can be devastated by the fact that he or she is no longer able to participate in or perhaps has no interest in their usual sexual expression. Awareness of such a situation also can be devastating to their partner. Referral to a sexual counselor or psychologist may be necessary in some cases.

Patients and caregivers can express their sexuality by maintaining their established personal habits such as grooming and appearance. The role of the nurse is to assist them in this, by arranging for such items as a haircut and manicure, encouraging them to wear fresh, personally chosen clothing. These are simple interventions. The patient who is neglecting his or her appearance may indeed need affirmation of sexuality. Encouragements and praise can be used during conversation with the patient and spouse (Taylor 1983).

Individualized care

Physical condition in relation to therapy will constantly be questioned by the patient and caregivers. It is important to keep them as knowledgeable as they can be about the expected outcomes, the individualistic responses to therapies, and so forth, while assuring them that professional help will always be quickly available. The patient and family should receive visits and care from the health personnel or the hospice team at a level consistent with the progression of the disease process and consistent with the patient's and family's other needs, as expressed by them verbally and behaviorally. For example, frequent visits by the professional caregiver to see the hospitalized patient during a medical crisis, made in addition to those dictated by the medical regime, help provide reassurance that assistance is always near. For the patient at home, frequent home and phone visits by various team members will provide the same assurance. Answering telephone calls quickly also helps.

Family coping

Just as the patient is affected by the increased dependency that comes with illness that precedes death, so too is the whole family unit. The spouse may suddenly be faced with carrying the entire burden of responsibilities that always had been shared. Or, if there is no spouse, other family members will be faced with meeting these responsibilities. Normal routines and schedules are disrupted. And there is the burden of caring for the dying family member. In the home setting this means a physical and emotional effort that lasts 24 hours a day, 7 days a week; exhaustion, depression, and confusion can result. The support of a hospice home-care program to assist the spouse or family members can ease the physical burden by providing frequent team-member visits and assisting those involved to create a plan to minimize interruption of family-life activities (*e.g.*, making a schedule for rotating responsibility for certain tasks). Home care costs less than institutionalization and can reduce the pressure of financial burdens. Teaching simple care tasks and how to anticipate the patient's needs can help the spouse and family avoid the uncertainty and confusion that can result from caring for someone who is ill. Tasks that seem simple to the nurse (*e.g.*, how to change the sheets on a bed in which a person is lying) can be viewed as insurmountable hurdles by the inexperienced.

Legal and ethical issues

A problem that is not unique to the elderly, but which must be addressed is the right of the individual to refuse or discontinue curative medical treatment. This text will discuss only the right that is used when the medical treatment will not cure the patient.

This right is based on the constitutional right to privacy. It was first developed as a tort concept and evolves from the fourth amendment, which provides the right to "protect personal privacy and dignity against unwarranted intrusion by the "state" (California Western Law Review 1974). Several cases—Roe vs. Wade (1973), Doe vs. Bolton (1973), and Schmerber vs. California (1966)—have defined certain rights guaranteed by personal privacy. The right to privacy has also been described as a "fundamental personal right, emanating from the totality of the Constitutional scheme under which we live" (California Western Law Review 1974). The right to consent to treatment is central to this problem. A provider of care who renders that care without consent of the recipient is liable for suit based on the principles of tort liability between two or more private persons. This is true also if the recipient is treated beyond his or her wishes, which is more likely the case with terminal illness. The important concept to remember is that the patient makes the decision, not the provider. The consent, whether expressed or implied, must always be (Duquesne Law Review 1976): obtained, voluntary, given by a competent person, and informed (*i.e.*, the person affected must have enough information to make an intelligent decision).

Other legal topics that professionals who care for the dying elderly need to be familiar with are the "Living Will," and estate planning (discussed below) (Backer et al 1982). Is the Living Will endorsed in your state? Has this been discussed with the patient? Further reading on legal and ethical topics is suggested (Backer et al 1982; Ogg 1980). For further information contact the following agencies:

Concern for Dying
250 West 57th Street
Room 831
New York, New York 10107

Society for the Right to Die
250 West 57th Street
Room 929
New York, New York 10107

American Protestant Hospital Association
840 N. Lake Shore Drive
Room 607
Chicago, Illinois 60611

Catholic Hospital Association
1438 South Grand Boulevard
St. Louis, Missouri 63104

Estate planning

Estate planning is very complex and needs to be handled by the legal/financial counselor of the patient and family, but it must not be overlooked as a part of caring for the dying patient. Such issues as patient competency, instituting or revising a will, asset protection, and tax planning should be addressed.

Suggest to the family that they may want to consult their family lawyer "about unresolved matters concerning the will, insurance, or social security death benefits; and to call a social worker, if necessary, to assist with the many forms and bills the family must cope with at the time of death" (Taylor and Gideon 1981).

Financial crisis

Impending financial crisis related to fixed income, cost of illness treatment, insufficient insurance coverage, or lack of, or diminished, savings is a significant problem. Elements of the crisis must first be identified. The nurse may be the first to identify this need. Referral of the patient and family to Social Services is important. The patient's and family's financial situation should be evaluated to determine need and a concrete, step-by-step plan should be developed to resolve the crisis. The patient and caregiver should receive budget and financial counseling as appropriate to the situation. (For example, the patient and family could, as soon as possible, apply for disability and other resources, including job-related benefits, union benefits, Veterans Administration benefits, Aid and Attendance, Social Security, SSI, retirement funds, welfare benefits, food stamps, insurance, and so forth).

Grief

Engel (1964) and other researchers have described the grieving process, identifying its phases: shock and disbelief, developing awareness, restitution, and resolution. Knowledge of these phases has proved to be useful in anticipating the needs of the family or significant others during the bereavement period. It is also useful in anticipating the scope of survivors' needs during this very crucial period of successful re-integration into society (Clayton 1974; Earle et al 1976; Garfield 1978; Kuntz 1984; Pegels 1980; Raphael 1977). Studies of survivors also indicate that the incidences of illness and death increase during the bereavement period. The suicide rate is high among those who have lost a spouse, especially elderly white men (Clayton 1974; Kastenbaum and Aisenbug 1976; Pegels 1980).

While the patient is dying, he or she and the family experience grieving. They are grieving for the loss of life as they knew it, and are anticipating the separation that is inevitable. For some this occurs during periods of increased physical debilitation, whereas for others it is more evident during periods of lesser physical problems.

Grief is what the survivors experience during what has been labeled as bereavement. It is extremely painful emotionally; it is frightening. Its duration depends on many variables such as the underlying relationship with the deceased person, feelings of guilt, and the length of illness. The caregivers' grief is uniquely their own. They should never be made to feel that they should be expressing or experiencing something different. More and more is being learned about grief. Once it was thought that one to two years was a healthy grief period, now studies indicate that some people grieve for longer periods. At the same time, however, if a bereaved person is not progressing through his or her grief, professional guidance is indicated and should be encouraged. A nursing referral at this time would be indicated.

At times the bereaved wonder if they are sane, if they are grieving properly, or if their reactions are normal. A list of some of the common experiences of the bereaved are included in the boxed material below.

Common Experience of Bereaved

A feeling of tightness in the throat or heaviness in the chest

Difficulty with sleeping

Losing appetites yet having an empty feeling in the stomachs

Feeling restless and unable to concentrate

Feeling angry that the loved one has "left" them

Feeling guilty or angry over things that happened or didn't happen in the relationship

Frequent mood changes

Crying unexpectedly

Telling the story of the illness and death repeatedly

Sensing the presence of the loved one

(Data from Backer B, Hannon N, Russell N: Death and Dying: Individuals and Institutions. New York, John Wiley & Sons, 1982)

As Duch (1985) remarks, "There is marked variability in the intensity, duration, and fluctuation of these symptoms, some of which may be accounted for by cultural differences." Further, symptoms "may come and go cyclically, they may appear after a delay and they may last (but generally decrease) over 2 years or more" (Barrett and Schneweis 1980).

It is important to understand that the family who is in the crisis of dealing with the anticipated death of a beloved family member is still a normal family and the nursing diagnosis as presented in this chapter is not intended to be used in reference to an abnormal state. The same is true of their bereavement period. In either of these transition periods, if the members of the family unit exhibit abnormal responses to what is happening, the role of the nurse is to observe, assess, refer to, and consult with the appropriate professional resources. Conferring continues on an ongoing basis with a nurse specialist or person whose specialty is psychiatry, bereavement, or a related field. The nurse caring for the family unit would then have the added guidance and resources of this specialist.

Realistic hope

Through all of these needs, the nurse needs to assist the patient and family to maintain *realistic hope.* Earle et al (1976) states, "Realistic hope is not hope for cure or life forever but hope to achieve short-term to moderate-length goals, pleasures, or other meaningful activities." It is dependent on the attitudes and perceptions of what is happening by family, significant friends and influential members of the health-care team (Wallace 1961; Weisman 1972). It is "the ability to fulfill oneself as one is" (Earle et al 1976). Realistic hope may be exhibited in many ways. It arises "from a desirable self-image, healthy self-esteem and a belief in our ability to exert a degree of influence on the world surrounding us" (Weisman 1972).

Care for the professional caregiver

An individualized plan of care must always include the patient and family so that everyone can work toward the same goals. In this type of care, such a situation is a definite must. Many actions are dictated by the patient's physical condition and his or her responses to therapies, but beyond this area all actions will be dictated by the patient's and family's *expressed needs.* These needs may be expressed verbally or nonverbally and the nurse's observation and therapeutic interaction skills will determine how successful he or she is in identifying, clarifying, and validating those needs with the patient and family. Recognition of these needs will also aid the nurse in assisting the patient and family to find comfort and meaningfulness in a time of great stress and turmoil.

Care of the dying, whether elderly or young, is a unique interplay among a group of people comprising the professionals providing the physical care and emotional support and the patient and family. How does the professional caregiver protect himself or herself while giving so much?

Never allow feelings of isolation while providing this care. The patient and family will express needs on many levels, including financially, spiritually, ethically, and socially. These needs can be identified by the nurse, who should always use the resources of available experts. Call on social services, the clergy, occupational therapy, and other facilities to help round out and share the planned care.

Never forget that this kind of care is personally costly. The right answers cannot always be found and the correct responses cannot always be made, nor can every need be met. Failure to recognize this reality can lead to frustration, dissatisfaction, and other negative feelings. It is important for the professional caregiver to remember to talk with others who are trusted about what he or she is doing *and* his or her feelings. Other nurses are providing similar care and are experiencing similar feelings. Put aside time to discuss these matters. Caregivers need support.

Presented below are several situations that occur commonly when dealing with patients who are dying—and brief suggestions on how the situation can be handled constructively.

1. The family says the patient doesn't know he or she is going to die and they don't want you to tell him or her. You walk into the room and the patient asks you, "Am I going to die?" Here, your role is to use therapeutic communication techniques. Ask the patient what he or she believes. This question usually allows the patient to feel comfortable in sharing his or her greatest fears (Franks 1984). Your role as a nurse is to facilitate communication between the patient and family or to identify someone who can.

2. You feel like crying with the patient, but this conflicts with a nurse's role of remaining emotionally removed—to maintain professional distance. Give yourself the opportunity to share this special moment with your patient. It will not be appropriate with every patient in every situation, but it is a time of special sharing and part of a special relationship. Don't forget to use touch; it can eliminate barriers to communication.

3. You don't like the way the patient's care is being handled. Identify what bothers you. Does it bother the patient or family? Be diplomatic. Talk with your peers. You might consider talking with the doctor—you may be missing some information that could explain what is happening. Don't be afraid to ask questions.

4. The patient's situation closely resembles something in your own life. This explanation may appear to be simplistic—but this probably means that you're grieving again over a past loss. Accept that and share the recognition, if it seems appropriate.

5. The patient and family's values and needs are contrary to your own. This is where professionalism must take over. Identify for the patient and

family that this is what is happening, and allow them to express their feelings and beliefs. You don't have to agree. Help the patient to feel good about himself or herself. Get support for yourself from others.

6. You feel angry at the patient or family. Identify the reasons. Are they doing something you wouldn't do? Is it harmful? Can you share that with the family or another professional?

7. The family is abusive toward the nursing staff. Remember the real target of that anger is not you, but the terrible thing, *Death,* over which they have no control. Talk with your colleagues—share how you feel. Make assertive plans to intervene with the family before they make requests. Try to anticipate needs. Talk with them frequently, using a nonjudgmental attitude (Telesco 1984).

8. The patient dies. Remember it is normal to feel guilt, that in some way you've failed. You have been a witness to the impotence of medical and nursing knowledge and skills to remove this terrible burden from the patient and family. Deal with these feelings honestly.

9. Remember that not every nurse can tolerate being close with every dying patient. There will be those special patients who "get to you." Share that with your supporters. Explore it. Try to understand it. Above all—face and share it.

Hospice

In the past decade, a hospice system in England, the United States, and Canada has emerged to deal with many of the problems of dying patients in an integrated, coordinated way. The hospice movement is highly sophisticated, using scientific and creative approaches to problem solving, as well as application of theories of symptom-control to the care of the dying person and his or her family. The philosophy of this network is to provide homelike surroundings, physical care, and caring for those who are dying and their families, while preserving the individual's integrity and quality of life. They are designed to anticipate and cater to physical, psychosocial, spiritual, and financial needs. In the United States today there are around 1700 hospice programs, of which 275 are Medicare-certified (National Hospice Organization 1986). They provide predominantly home-care services. They also continue to oversee the care of the patient if hospitalization is required. Hospice programs also provide the professional caregiver with a support network and activities designed to reduce the stress of caring for dying patients.

An important focus of a hospice program is the building of a special relationship with both the elderly patient who is dying and the family. The care of someone who is dying is very special. The nurse will give a lot of himself or herself but also will be the witness to, and participator in, a very special and unique event.

Dr. Cicely Saunders, founder of St. Christopher's Hospice in England has said

There are important ways in which we heal our patients, and in which they heal us. Healing a person does not always mean curing a disease. Sometimes healing means learning to care for others, finding new wholeness in a family—being reconciled. Or it can mean easing the pain of dying or allowing someone to die when the time comes. . . . People nearing the end of their lives have so much to teach others, about the nature of relationships and about the meaning of life. They drop their masks and do not worry any more about inconsequentials (Ogg 1980).

Assessment

An *underlying principle* that must guide the actions of nurses who care for the dying elderly is to remember that health habits, how close the person's physical condition is to the accepted age-related norms, emotional maturity and adjustment, financial concerns, spiritual beliefs, and behaviors all play equally important roles in helping to determine and predict the responses that will occur. At the same time, the importance of existing interrelationships with the persons who are of significant importance to the dying person should not be diminished or negated. Studies indicate that group interaction provides many positive effects for elderly patients (Palmore 1979). It is important to remember that despite the good intentions of professional caregivers and loving family members, it is possible to unthinkingly separate the person who is facing death from these important aspects of his or her life. This must be avoided. Instead the existence of these relationships should help in the development of a plan of care.

Just as the nursing care of other patients requires use of the nursing process, so does care of elderly dying patients. The first phase, as always, is assessment and should include the pertinent areas discussed below.

Previous experience with death

Has someone close to the patient died (*e.g.,* spouse, other family member, friend, or acquaintance)? In the absence of tutored counseling, inexperience with death can precipitate individual and family crises. However, experience with death does not mean necessarily that this person will be able to "handle" this situation. It is important to explore with the patient what feelings and memories are present and how they are affecting him or her.

Established behaviors and response to death

Are beliefs ingrained or are they what the patient believes are most acceptable to society? First-hand experience with death will produce real emotions and reactions. Inexperience can lead to superficially accepting what is thought to be "correct." This superficial acceptance in turn can result in inadequate exploration of emotions and "correct" reactions.

Coping patterns throughout life will also indicate how a person deals with death. The nurse must bear in mind that one patient may accept new ideas or information whereas another may not. There are, of course, many degrees between these two extremes. If the dying person has, in the past, investigated and accepted some changes, then information provided at a rate that allows assimilation can assist him or her to do so in this situation also. On the other hand, previous refusal to explore or accept changes will mean this same behavior could impede successful counseling.

Facing the possibility of mortality

A person usually begins to explore this truth in later life. Life goals have been nearly met, children are grown with families of their own, and there is a need to understand one's place in the scheme of things. Questions and reactions begin to be considered, such as

Have I made a mark?

Will people remember me?

Will I be missed?

Has my life been worthwhile?

What have I accomplished?

I don't want to die—there are too many things I haven't done.

Other elderly persons, however, may not have allowed themselves to reflect on the subject. They have probably had these thoughts, but have not allowed themselves to fully explore them. When such a person faces death, it may be the first time that he or she faces these thoughts and feelings intensely. If this is the case, the absolute fear and panic that this person may experience can be better understood. Bear in mind that labeling a person as "elderly" does not guarantee that he or she will embrace death willingly.

Availability of support systems

Does the patient have a spouse? Are there family members? friends? church members? neighbors? What age group is this person in—young-old, mid-old, or old-old? The resources available in each of these groups may differ considerably. Financially, what are the patient's resources? Is he or she retired? on a fixed income? have savings? insurances? connections to government programs such as Medicare, Medicaid? other resources?

It is important to understand that not only is it necessary to know whether or not support people exist, but if they are willing to assist. The past events of these relationships may override the fact that one member is dying. Not everyone has a loving person on the sidelines who will put all else aside to help this person who is dying; this can be a hard lesson to learn. An example is the patient who wanted more than anything to live long enough to walk his daughter down the aisle at her wedding. Here, the hard thing to accept is that the daughter was embarrassed that her father would have to use a walker. She refused to allow him to do this. The wife and other children sided with the daughter. Not only did the father not attend the wedding, he died by himself in the hospital. The family relationships in this case were very complex. Essentially, the family felt that the father had not done much for them so there was no reason for them to do anything in return. Family dynamics are an important determinant in healthy dying.

Motivation to assist sometimes comes from a source other than concern for the dying person. An estranged or separated spouse may agree to assist the dying person if there is a trade-off. For example, it may be as direct as receiving part of the insurance money after the death occurs, or paying a personal "debt." This situation is important to recognize because motivation will dictate the limitations of the assistance provided.

Other frames of reference that will assist the nurse in understanding and anticipating needs and responses of the patient and family are developmental and growth tasks of that age group that influence an individual's capacity to deal with the added stress of dying (Miller 1981; Smith and Selye 1979; Sorenson and Luckman 1980). The technique of life review (deRamon 1983) can also be useful as a tool during this last phase of the patient's life, as is the therapeutic use of touch. Assisting the patient to find meaning in illness, worth in his or her life, and comfort or peace while dying are the goals (Kushner 1981; Travelbee 1966).

When trying to provide nursing care to the whole person and the family, the physical, psychosocial, emotional, financial, spiritual, and social dimensions must be considered. The care plans offered here deal mainly with the nonphysical needs of the patient, except where those needs have been determined to require some special considerations not covered in previous chapters. This selection of care plans is not all inclusive.

Nursing care plans

1. Nursing diagnosis: Anxiety related to
- *Patient's fear of death—loss of his world as he or she knows it*
- *Caregiver's fear of loss of the patient*
- *Patient's sense of abandonment by the caregiver(s), health-care providers, friends and others*

Goals

Patient and caregiver will verbalize fears of death and loss.
The ultimate goal is for the patient and caregiver to accept the impending death and loss while experiencing a sense of stability and assurance.

Nursing interventions

1. Allow and encourage patient and caregiver to verbalize fears; listen to them with non-judgmental attitude.
2. Increase frequency of home or inpatient visits as the patient's condition deteriorates and during periods of increased stress. Professional assistance should be available 24 hours a day, 7 days a week.
3. Schedule visits at different times, allowing maximum interaction for patient and families.
4. Plan for weekend and night needs of patient who is cared for at home. Example, a team member should be on call to respond directly by phone or visit.
5. Regulate the aide's visits according to physical needs of patient.
6. Arrange for volunteer visits if patient is cared for in a hospice program. This visit is one of a special friend, or a nonmedically oriented visitor who can provide a respite from the constant reminders of impending death. The volunteer also offers concrete services as needed: stays with the patient while the caregiver runs errands, grocery-shops for the family, etc.
7. Communication among all team members should be constant so that a realistic picture is maintained of the status of the patient and family and their needs.

2. Nursing diagnosis: Powerlessness related to feelings of dependency and associated with feelings of inability to effectively
* *Change the course of events*
* *Participate in family decision-making*
* *Participate in care decisions*

Goals

Patient will maintain a sense of independence by participating in: planning aspects of his or her care, family business, recreation, and by interacting with his family, friends, personnel, etc.

Patient will verbalize these feelings, identify the causes of these feelings, and make a practical plan to deal with them.

Nursing interventions

1. Help family and friends and caregiver understand ways to support independence:
   * Seek patient's opinion on issues of concern
   * Involve patient in plan of care, and other aspects
2. Encourage continued interaction of patient with family and friends
3. Assist patient, through appropriate counselling techniques, to develop realistic goals within the limitations of his or her illness (realistic hope). Don't always emphasize limitations.
   * Example: The patient may like gardening, but is confined to the home. Ramps could be built to allow access to the outside, but the nurse could also suggest bringing pots inside in which the patient could plant flowers.
4. Allow patient and family and friends to ventilate feelings about not being able to change the course of events.
5. Help patient to identify those things over which he or she does have power (*e.g.,* some of the above-mentioned issues: planning aspects of care, conferring on family business, etc.).
6. Assist family to follow the same procedures as the caregiver. The need here is to assist them to care for patient (with the assistance of professionals) and maintain their unique relationship with him or her.

3. Nursing diagnosis: Disturbance in self-concept: self-esteem, role performance, personal identity, and body image related to the physical effects of the disease process (e.g., increased weakness, loss of weight, odors) and a decrease of ability in the decision-making process.

Goal

Patient will maintain realistic hope and positive body image.

Nursing interventions

1. For the patient experiencing distress in areas of self-esteem, role performance, personal identity:
   • Assist the patient to continue to make decisions. This may be as simple as what to wear or as complex as helping the spouse decide how to deal with finances.
   • Explore this need with the family.
   • Allow and encourage patient to express feeling of change in his or her self-concept. Assist the patient with a realistic exploration of what this means. Listening is a powerful tool.
   • Encourage patient to communicate these emotions to family members and vice-versa. This lays a basis for realistic and practical accommodation. All parties will have a better picture of how the other(s) perceive what is happening.
   • Assist family and patient to achieve realistic hope.
2. For the patient experiencing distress related to body-image alteration:
   • Express acceptance of patient regardless of physical change.
   • Support caregiver and patient in coping with physical deterioration.
      a. Developing realistic plans for increased help, aids.
      b. Allow patient to continue to function as close to normally as possible.
   • Control odors by use of soaps, deodorizers, and so forth.
   • Encourage patient to express feelings about altered body image.

4. Nursing diagnosis: Compromised family coping related to patient or caregiver conflict in decision-making regarding
- *The place of patient's death (i.e., home vs. hospital vs. nursing home)*
- *Uncertainty concerning the approximate time of patient's death*
- *Protocol to follow if patient is to die at home**

Goals

Patient and caregiver will agree on the place for death.*

Caregiver will verbalize understanding of the inability to predict the time of death, and will be able to describe imminent death behaviors.

Nursing interventions

1. Family coping is compromised by conflict over where the death is to take place.
   - Discuss options openly.
   - Discuss psychological implications of the options. If agreement is not reached discuss feelings produced (*e.g.,* guilt).
2. Family coping compromised by uncertainty over approximate time death will occur.
   - Discuss truthfully and openly the inability to predict the exact time of death.
   - Review as often as necessary, over a period of time, the imminent death behaviors, why they occur, and what the caregiver can do about them.
     a. The arms and legs may become cool to the touch, and the underside of the patient's body may become darker in color. These signs result from the slowing of the blood circulation.
     b. The patient will spend an increasing amount of time asleep. This results from a change in the body metabolism (Hospice-New Orleans 1984).
     c. Review what caregiver can do about each of these signs (*e.g.,* keep warm blankets, preferably not electric, on patient to avoid chills and feelings of cold); plan to be with the patient when he or she is most alert (Hospice-New Orleans 1984). Reassure caregiver that if these behaviors are noted and staff is called in, time will be created for staff to stay with patient and caregiver.

* This conflict is sometimes an expression of uneasiness on the part of the caregiver about remaining in the same home while the memory of the death and pre-death experiences is still very vivid. It may also be an expression of the feeling of insufficient support by the caregiver. Reassurances that professional health-care workers will be available to assist as needed, may help the caregiver feel more secure.

continued

Goal

Nursing interventions

• Over a period of time before death becomes imminent, the family can be instructed (Taylor 1983)
    a. Not to call the emergency squad in the last minute of patient's life
    b. Make arrangements for the minister, priest, or rabbi to visit, if desired
    c. Make preliminary plans for the funeral and for notifying relatives and friends
3. Family coping is compromised by uncertainty over protocol to be followed for a death at home.

Caregiver will verbalize and then take the appropriate actions in case of death or emergency in the home.

• Give caregiver both verbal and written instructions to follow in case of death or emergency at home. (These can be obtained from the local police station for local guidelines. Also, request the patient's hospice program to make appropriate arrangements).

---

5. Nursing diagnosis: Spiritual distress related to decreased or absent hope, uncertainty of the meaning and purpose in life, and insufficient spiritual support.*

Goal

Patient and caregiver will verbalize satisfaction or dissatisfaction with their spirituality.

Nursing interventions

1. Discuss with the patient his or her perception of God in relation to his or her illness.
2. Offer (as the situation dictates) to read from the Bible, or other book chosen by patient.
3. Offer to pray with patient and caregiver.
4. By listening to patient's and caregiver's life philosophies and value systems offer acceptance and support.
5. Discuss contact with clergy, if appropriate.
6. Refer to clergy as appropriate.

continued

Nursing interventions

7. Allow the patient and caregiver to express spirituality individualistically. This may mean a departure from mainstream religious practices.

* More in-depth reading should be done in this area. The National Hospice Organization (1901 N. Fort Meyer Dr., Suite 402, Arlington, Virginia 22209) and its members are one source that provides this information to their patients and community (National Hospice Organization 1986).

---

6. Nursing diagnosis: Sexual dysfunction related to debilitating illness, changes in self-concept, changes in body image, altered body structure or function.

Goals

Patient and spouse will identify predictable or potential alterations in perception of sexuality or sexual function (*e.g.,* role reversal, role of body image, and weakness in sexual function). Patient and spouse will identify behaviors that can be developed as sexual gratification substitutes.
Patient and spouse will identify what helps each to be a sexual person.

Nursing interventions

1. Discuss with patient and spouse the role adjustments precipitated by illness.
2. Discuss with patient and spouse various sexual gratification alternatives (*e.g.,* lying down together, kissing, caressing, sharing feelings, being alone together).
3. Discuss with patient and spouse the physical and psychological traits that define male and female sexuality.
4. Discuss with patient and spouse the difference between sexual functioning and sexuality.

---

7. Nursing diagnosis: Knowledge deficit related to
- *Insufficient information on physical condition or medical regime*
- *Inability to anticipate medical crises*
- *Inexperience with personal threat of death*
- *Unfamiliarity with protocol to follow to obtain emergency care outside the hospital*

Goals

Patient or caregiver will verbalize an understanding of the illness and therapy plan.

Nursing interventions

1. Knowledge deficit of physical condition.
   - Discuss with the patient and caregiver the nature and extent of the disease process, using teaching/learning principles.
   - Allow time for active listening.
   - Share this responsibility with other professional team members.

continued

Goals	*Nursing interventions*
	• Encourage all team members to provide appropriate information on plans for therapy. • Offer explanations as conditions and plans change.
Patient/caregiver will verbalize the name, purpose, time for taking, side-effects, and adverse reactions of prescribed medicines.	2. Knowledge deficit of patient's medical regime. • Provide and review written schedule for administration. • Review medicines frequently. • Review procedures to follow to order drugs at home (*i.e.*, by phone and mail).
Patient will be medically stable at a level consistent with the disease process and treatment plan.	3. Knowledge deficit of how to anticipate medical crisis. • Provide periodic home or hospital visits as medical condition warrants to reassure patient he or she hasn't been abandoned by professional caregivers. • Perform appropriate lab or other tests to determine progress of disease process. • Provide appropriate medicine to make the patient comfortable. (see Chapter 14) • Re-hospitalize for care as patient's condition dictates or patient or patient's family desires.* • Consult other specialists as needed for palliative care.
Caregiver will verbalize and act on plan to follow if patient requires emergency care.	4. Knowledge deficit of how to handle a medical emergency that occurs at home. • Review steps for caregiver to follow if emergency care is needed. • Provide written instructions for caregiver to follow. These should include important phone numbers and persons to be contacted and the order in which they are to be contacted) • Intervene promptly if emergency care is requested by caregiver (Hospice-New Orleans 1984)

* The knowledge deficits mentioned here are common among dying patients. These deficits need to be addressed consistently and with planning. A dying person and his or her family face many dilemmas. *To not know* is one of the most serious.

8. Nursing diagnosis: Social isolation related to decreased energy to maintain social contacts, misunderstandings, misinformation, hesitancy by family and friends to continue a relationship with someone who has been labeled "dying."

Goals	*Nursing interventions*
Patient will express feelings of social isolation. Patient and caregiver will make and act on a plan to deal with their feelings.	1. Arrange to meet with patient's friends who visit and allow them to express their feelings and needs.
	2. Encourage friends to understand that behaving naturally, "being themselves," is very important.
	3. Provide an environment in which casual and upbeat conversations can occur.
	4. Encourage friends to continue to share social news and gossip with the dying person.
	5. Help friends to understand that a person who is dying doesn't concentrate on the process of dying 24 hr a day. They need the usual companionship that everyone needs.
	• Encourage friends to share their emotions. Explain that this can be frightening to do but also can help them to be more comfortable emotionally, while assisting with the comfort of the patient.

---

9. Nursing diagnosis: Alteration in family process related to increased dependency needs of the dying elderly patient and bereavement of the family after the death.

Goals	*Nursing interventions*
The family will identify the alteration(s) and begin to make a plan to deal with them. The bereaved will progress through the normal stages of grief.	1. Interventions for increased dependency needs
	• Assist family to make a plan for rotation of the responsibility for tasks.
	• Stress the need for frequent respite periods for primary caregiver and supplementary caregivers.
	• Provide frequent visits of health-care team members to reduce the stress of caregiver(s) during acute periods.
	• Teach caregiver(s) any necessary skills to make physical care of the patient easier (*e.g.,* how to give a bed bath or transfer a patient from a bed to a chair safely)

continued

Nursing interventions

2. Interventions for the bereavement period
   • Periodically assess any changes in the following
       a. Physical condition—appetite, sleep, weight
       b. Supportive contacts—number, type, who
       c. Financial status—housing, general finances, lifestyle
       d. Mood—general, feelings and activities on the anniversary date of the death, and longterm presence of: feelings of guilt, depression, and panic attacks.
   • Further assessment includes resumption of old activities, beginning new ones, visiting the grave, and a return to church if appropriate.
   • Allow the bereaved to share all these feelings and happenings. Ideally, as with hospice programs, contact with the bereaved family members should continue for one full year, with the intervention aimed at:
       a. Helping survivors deal with the reality of their loss.
       b. Helping them express emotions without fear of condemnation.
       c. Assisting them to adjust to living without the patient.
       d. Assisting them to slowly accept new relationships.

---

10. Nursing diagnosis: Dysfunctional grieving related to patient or caregiver having difficulty in identifying or expressing normal feelings associated with the grief process.

Goal

The bereaved will identify the need for further professional intervention.

Nursing interventions

1. Observe for signs of abnormal grief and assess.
2. Refer as needed to specialist for assistance in dealing with abnormal grief.

continued

Nursing interventions

3. Continue to give emotional support* to the bereaved, using the guidance of the specialist. Pathologic grief infers that the bereaved do not reach the recovery stage.

4. Assess for the following reactions, which are distortions of normal grief. They may be categorized as:
   • *Delayed:* The bereaved exhibits little emotion and continues with a busy life.
   • *Inhibited:* The bereaved exhibits various physical conditions and doesn't feel grief.
   • *Chronic:* The behaviors of the normal grief periods continue (Backer et al 1982).

* In a study of the elderly bereaved, Bornstein and coworkers found that only 13% of the poor-outcome group lived with their families, compared with 46% of the nondepressed group (Backer et al 1982). This finding makes clear the importance of social support during this period of vulnerability and loss.

References

Backer B, Hannon N, Russell N: Death and Dying: Individuals and Institutions. New York, John Wiley & Sons, 1982

Barrett CJ, Schneweis KM: An empirical search for the stages of widowhood. Omega 81:97–104, 1980

Bereavement Care Program Manual. New Orleans, Hospice-New Orleans, 1985

California Western Law Review: The right to die. California Western Law Review 10:613–627, 1974

Clayton PJ: Mortality and morbidity in the first year of widowhood. Arch Gen Psych 30:747–750, 1974

deRamon P: The final task: Life review for the dying patient. Nursing 83, February:44–49, 1983

Duch DM: Concepts and applications of bereavement programming. In Paradis LF (ed): Hospice Handbook: A Guide for Managers and Planners. Maryland, Aspen Systems Corporation, 1985

Dumont RG, Foss D: The American View of Death, Acceptance or Denial? Cambridge, Massachusetts, Schenkmann Publishing, 1972

Engel GL: Grief and grieving. Am J Nurs 64:93–98, 1964

Epstein C: Treating the patient dying in old age. In: Nursing the Dying Patient. Reston, Virginia, Reston Publishing, 1975

Franks LC: Does that mean I'm dying? RN Feb:25–26, 1984

Friedenberg E: Continuing education in aging and long-term care. In Earle AM, Argondizzio N, Kutscher A (eds): The Nurse As Caregiver for the Terminal Patient and His Family. New York, Columbia University Press, 1976

Garfield CA (ed): Psychosocial Care of the Dying Patient. New York, McGraw-Hill, 1978

Garner J: Palliative care: It's the quality of life remaining that matters. CMA J 115:179–180, 1976

Helsing KJ, Szklo M, Comstock G: Factors associated with mortality and widowhood. Am J Public Health 71:802, 1981

Hospice-New Orleans: Patient Care Manual. New Orleans, Hospice-New Orleans, 1984

Jackson EN: Wisely managing our grief: A pastoral viewpoint. Death Education 3:143–155, 1979

Joel LA: The economics of health care: trends and problems. (Keynote address, 12th Annual Meeting, American Academy of Nursing, Atlanta, Georgia, Dec 9, 1984)

Kaercher D: Hospice: A compassionate way of dealing with death. Better Homes and Gardens Nov:32–40, 1981

Kastenbaum R, Aisenberg R: The Psychology of Death. New York, Springer-Verlag, 1976

Kim MJ, McFarland G, McLane A: Nursing Diagnoses. St. Louis, Missouri, CV Mosby, 1984

Kron J: Designing a better place to die. New York Mar:43–49, 1976

Kuntz BB: I didn't think his death would hit me so hard. RN Feb:30, 1984

Kushner HS: When bad things happen to good people. Thorofare, New Jersey, Schocken Books, 1981

Lack S: The hospice concept—the adult with advanced cancer, pp 160–166 (reprint). Proceeding of the American Cancer Society 2nd National Conference on Human Values and Cancer, 1977

Lack S: Philosophy of a hospice program. New Haven, Connecticut, Hospice, Inc., 1977

McGill-Melzack R: The McGill pain questionnaire: Major properties and scoring methods. Pain 1:277, 1975

Markel WM, Simon VB: The hospice concept. CA-A Journal for Clinicians 28:225–237, 1978

Miller TW: Life events scaling: Clinical methodological issues. Nursing Res 30:317–321A, 1981

National Center for Health Statistics: Facts of Life and Death. Washington, DC, US Government Printing Office, 1978

National Hospice Organization. Personal communication. Virginia, September, 1986

Newsweek: Living with dying. May 1, 1978

Office of Cancer Communications: Eating Hints. NIH Publication #82-2079. Washington DC, US Department of Health and Human Services. National Cancer Institute, 1982

Office of Cancer Communications: Taking Time. NIH Publication #82-2059. Washington DC, US Department of Health and Human Services. National Cancer Institute, 1982

Ogg E: The right to die with dignity. Public Affairs Pamphlet No. 587. New York, 1980

Palmore E: Predictors of successful aging. The Gerontologist 19:427–36, 1979

Pegels CC: Health Care and the Elderly. Maryland, Aspen Systems, 1980

Raphael B: Preventive intervention with the recently bereaved. Arch Gen Psychiatry 34:1450–1454, 1977

Seidelson DE: Medical malpractice: Informal consent cases in full disclosure jurisdiction. Duquesne Law Review 14:309–347, 1976

Smith M, Selye H: Stress—reducing the negative effects of stress. Am J Nurs 79:1553–1555, 1979

Sorenson K, Luckman J: Modern unified theories of disease. In: A Psychophysiological Approach to Medical–Surgical Nursing. Philadelphia, WB Saunders, 1980

Stoddard S: The Hospice Movement: A Better Way of Caring for the Dying. New York, Random House, 1978

Taylor P: Understanding sexuality in the dying patient. Nurs 83, April:54–55, 1983

Taylor PB, Gideon M: Day in and day out you minister to others—but who will minister to you? Nurs 81, Oct:58–61, 1981

Telesco M: You killed my husband. RN Feb:27–28, 1984

Travelbee J: Interpersonal Aspects of Nursing. Philadelphia, FA Davis, 1966

Tucker S et al: Patient Care Standards, 2nd ed. St. Louis, Missouri, CV Mosby, 1980

U.S. Bureau of the Census. 1980

Vaughn N: The right to die. California Western Law Review 10:613–627, 1974

Weisman AD: On Dying and Denying. New York, Behavioral Publications, 1972

Zimmerman J: Hospice—Complete Care for the Terminally Ill. Urban and Schwarzenberg, 1981

Suggested reading

Connor S: The hospice movement. Family and Community Health: The Journal of Health Promotion & Maintenance. 5:39–53, 1982

Geltman R, Paige P: Symptom management in hospice care. Am J Nurs 83:78–55, 1983

International Work Group in Death, Dying and Bereavement, 1978: Assumptions and principles underlying standards for terminal care. Am J Nurs 79:296–297, 1979

Kubler-Ross E: On Death and Dying. New York, Macmillan, 1969

McNairn N: Helping the patient who wants to die at home. Nurs 81 Feb:66–68, 1981

Index

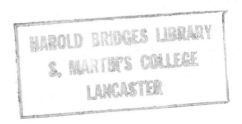